Edition

3

Updated

Basic Immunology

Functions and Disorders of the Immune System

Abul K. Abbas, MBBS
Professor and Chair
Department of Pathology
University of California San Francisco, School of Medicine
San Francisco, California

Andrew H. Lichtman, MD, PhD
Professor of Pathology
Harvard Medical School
Brigham and Women's Hospital
Boston, Massachusetts

Illustrated by David L. Baker, MA, and Alexandra Baker, MS, CMI

SAUNDERS

ELSEVIER

SAUNDERS
ELSEVIER

1600 John F. Kennedy Blvd. Ste 1800
Philadelphia, PA 19103-2899

BASIC IMMUNOLOGY: FUNCTIONS AND DISORDERS
OF THE IMMUNE SYSTEM

ISBN: 978-1-4160-5569-3

Copyright © 2011 by Saunders, an imprint of Elsevier Inc.

Previous editions copyrighted 2009, 2006, 2004, 2001

Library of Congress Cataloging-in-Publication Data
Abbas, Abul K.
  Basic immunology: functions and disorders of the immune system / Abul K. Abbas, Andrew H. Lichtman. – 3rd ed.
    p. ; cm.
Includes bibliographical references and index.
ISBN 978-1-4160-5569-3
1. Immunology. 2. Immunity. I. Lichtman, Andrew H. II. Title.
  [DNLM: 1. Immunity. 2. Hypersensitivity. 3. Immune System–physiology. 4. Immunologic Deficiency Syndromes. QW 504 A122b 2009]
QR181.A28 2009
616.07'9–dc22

2007030085

Acquisitions Editor: William Schmitt
Developmental Editor: Rebecca Gruliow
Editorial Assistant: Laura Stingelin
Design Direction: Gene Harris

Printed in China.

Last digit is the print number: 9 8 7 6 5

To Ann, Jonathan, Rehana,
Sheila, Eben, Ariella, Amos, Ezra

PREFACE

The third edition of *Basic Immunology* has been revised to incorporate recent advances in our understanding of the immune system and to improve upon how we present information to maximize its usefulness to students and teachers. We have been extremely gratified with how well the previous two editions of *Basic Immunology* have been received by students in the courses that we teach, and the guiding principles on which the book is based have not changed from the first edition. As teachers of immunology, we are becoming increasingly aware that assimilating detailed information and experimental approaches is difficult in many medical school and undergraduate courses. The problem of how much detail is appropriate has become a pressing one because of the continuous and rapid increase in the amount of information in all the biomedical sciences. This problem is compounded by the development of integrated curricula in many medical schools, with reduced time for didactic teaching and an increasing emphasis on social and behavioral sciences and primary health care. For all these reasons, we have realized the value for many medical students of presenting the principles of immunology in a concise and clear manner.

It is our view that several developments have come together to make the goal of a concise and modern consideration of immunology a realistic goal. Most importantly, immunology has matured as a discipline, so that it has now reached the stage when the essential components of the immune system, and how they interact in immune responses, are understood quite well. There are, of course, many details to be filled in, and the longstanding challenge of applying basic principles to human diseases remains a difficult task. Nevertheless, we can now teach our students, with reasonable confidence, how the immune system works. The second important development has been an increasing emphasis on the roots of immunology, which lie in its role in defense against infections. As a result, we are better able to relate experimental results, using simple models, to the more complex, but physi-ologically relevant, issue of host defense against infectious pathogens.

This book has been written to address the perceived needs of both medical school and undergraduate curricula and to take advantage of the new understanding of immunology. We have tried to achieve several goals. First, we have presented the most important principles governing the function of the immune system. Our principal objective has been to synthesize the key concepts from the vast amount of experimental data that emerge in the rapidly advancing field of immunology. The choice of what is most important is based largely on what is most clearly established by experimentation, what our students find puzzling, and what explains the wonderful efficiency and economy of the immune system. Inevitably, however, such a choice will have an element of bias, and our bias is toward emphasizing the cellular interactions in immune responses and limiting the description of many of the underlying biochemical and molecular mechanisms to the essential facts. We also have realized that in any concise discussion of complex phenomena, it is inevitable that exceptions and caveats will fall by the wayside. We have avoided such exceptions and caveats without hesitation, but we continue to modify conclusions as new information emerges. Second, we have focused on immune responses against infectious microbes, and most of our discussions of the immune system are in this context. Third, we have emphasized immune responses in humans (rather than experimental animals), drawing upon parallels with experimental situations whenever necessary. Fourth, we have made liberal use of illustrations to highlight important principles but have reduced factual details that may be found in more comprehensive textbooks. Fifth, we have discussed immunologic diseases also from the perspective of principles, emphasizing their relation to normal immune responses and avoiding details of clinical syndromes and treatments. We have added selected clinical cases in an Appendix, to illustrate how the principles of immunology may be applied to common human diseases. Finally, in order to make each chapter readable on its own, we have repeated key ideas in different places in the book. We feel such repetition will help students to grasp the most important concepts.

It is our hope that students will find this book clear, cogent, and manageable. Most importantly, we hope the book will convey our sense of wonder about the immune system and excitement about how the field has evolved and how it continues to be relevant to human health and disease. Finally, although we were spurred to tackle this project because of our associations with medical school courses, we hope the book will be valued more widely by students of allied health and biology as well. We will have succeeded if the book can answer many of the questions these students have about the immune system and, at the same time, encourage them to delve even more deeply into immunology.

Several individuals played key roles in the writing of this book. Our editor, Bill Schmitt, has been a constant source of encouragement and advice. We have been fortunate to again work with two wonderful illustrators, David and Alexandra Baker of DNA Illustrations, who have translated ideas into pictures that are informative and aesthetically pleasing. Ellen Sklar has shepherded the book through the production process with a calm efficiency and wonderful organization. Our development editor, Rebecca Gruliow, kept the project organized and on track despite pressures of time and logistics. To all of them we owe our many thanks.

Abul K. Abbas

Andrew H. Lichtman

CONTENTS

Chapter 1

INTRODUCTION TO THE IMMUNE SYSTEM

The Nomenclature, General Properties, and Components of the Immune System

Immunity is defined as resistance to disease, specifically infectious disease. The collection of cells, tissues, and molecules that mediate resistance to infections is called the **immune system**, and the coordinated reaction of these cells and molecules to infectious microbes is the **immune response**. Immunology is the study of the immune system and its responses to invading pathogens. **The physiologic function of the immune system is to prevent infections and to eradicate established infections**, and this is the principal context in which immune responses are discussed throughout this book.

The importance of the immune system for health is dramatically illustrated by the frequent observation that individuals with defective immune responses are susceptible to serious, often life-threatening infections (Fig. 1-1). Conversely, stimulating immune responses against microbes by the process of vaccination is the most effective method for protecting individuals against infections and is, for example, the approach that has led to the worldwide eradication of smallpox (Fig. 1-2). The emergence of the acquired immunodeficiency syndrome (AIDS) since the 1980s has tragically emphasized the importance of the immune system for defending individuals against infection. The impact of immunology, however, goes beyond infectious disease (see Fig. 1-1). The immune response is the major barrier to successful organ transplantation, an increasingly used therapy for organ failure. Attempts to treat cancers by stimulating immune responses against cancer cells are being tried for many

1

Role of the immune system	Implications
Defense against infections	Deficient immunity results in increased susceptibility to infections; exemplified by AIDS Vaccination boosts immune defenses and protects against infections
The immune system recognizes and responds to tissue grafts and newly introduced proteins	Immune responses are barriers to transplantation and gene therapy
Defense against tumors	Potential for immunotherapy of cancer

FIGURE 1-1 **The importance of the immune system in health and disease.** This table summarizes some of the physiologic functions of the immune system. Note that immune responses are also the causes of diseases. AIDS, acquired immunodeficiency syndrome.

human malignancies. Furthermore, abnormal immune responses are the causes of many inflammatory diseases with serious morbidity and mortality. Antibodies, one of the products of immune responses, are highly specific reagents for detecting a wide variety of molecules in the circulation and in cells and tissues and have therefore become invaluable reagents for laboratory testing in clinical medicine and research. Antibodies designed to block or eliminate potentially harmful molecules and cells are in widespread use for the treatment of immunologic diseases, cancers, and other types of disorders. For all of these reasons, the field of immunology has captured the attention of clinicians, scientists, and the lay public.

Disease	Maximum number of cases (year)	Number of cases in 2004	Percent change
Diphtheria	206,939 (1921)	0	-99.99
Measles	894,134 (1941)	37	-99.99
Mumps	152,209 (1968)	236	-99.90
Pertussis	265,269 (1934)	18,957	-96.84
Polio (paralytic)	21,269 (1952)	0	-100.0
Rubella	57,686 (1969)	12	-99.98
Tetanus	1,560 (1923)	26	-98.33
Haemophilus influenzae type b infection	~20,000 (1984)	16	-99.92
Hepatitis B	26,611 (1985)	6,632	-75.08

FIGURE 1-2 **The effectiveness of vaccination for some common infectious diseases.** This table illustrates the striking decrease in the incidence of selected infectious diseases for which effective vaccines have been developed. In some cases, such as with hepatitis B, a vaccine has become available recently, and the incidence of the disease is continuing to decrease. (Adapted from Orenstein WA, Hinman AR, Bart KJ, Hadler SC: Immunization. In Mandell GL, Bennett JE, Dolin R (eds): Principles and Practices of Infectious Diseases, 4th ed. New York, Churchill Livingstone, 1995; and Morbidity and Mortality Weekly Report 53:1213-1221, 2005.)

In this opening chapter of the book, we introduce the nomenclature of immunology, some of the important general properties of all immune responses, and the cells and tissues that are the principal components of the immune system. In particular, the following questions are addressed:

- What types of immune responses protect individuals from infections?
- What are the important characteristics of immunity, and what mechanisms are responsible for these characteristics?
- How are the cells and tissues of the immune system organized to find microbes and respond to them in ways that lead to their elimination?

We conclude the chapter with a brief overview of immune responses against microbes. The basic principles that are introduced in this chapter set the stage for more detailed discussions of immune responses in the remainder of the book. A glossary of the important terms used in the book is provided in Appendix I.

Innate and Adaptive Immunity

Host defense mechanisms consist of innate immunity, which mediates the initial protection against infections, and adaptive immunity, which develops more slowly and mediates the later, even more effective, defense against infections (Fig. 1-3). The term **innate immunity** (also called natural or native immunity) refers to the fact that this type of host defense is always present in healthy individuals, prepared to block the entry of microbes and to rapidly eliminate microbes that do succeed in entering host tissues. **Adaptive immunity** (also called specific or acquired immunity) is the type of host defense that is stimulated by microbes that invade tissues, that is, it adapts to the presence of microbial invaders.

The first line of defense in innate immunity is provided by epithelial barriers and by specialized cells and natural antibiotics present in epithelia, all of which function to block the entry of microbes. If microbes do breach epithelia and enter the tissues or

FIGURE 1-3 The principal mechanisms of innate and adaptive immunity. The mechanisms of innate immunity provide the initial defense against infections. Some of the mechanisms prevent infections (e.g., epithelial barriers) and others eliminate microbes (e.g., phagocytes, natural killer [NK] cells, the complement system). Adaptive immune responses develop later and are mediated by lymphocytes and their products. Antibodies block infections and eliminate microbes, and T lymphocytes eradicate intracellular microbes. The kinetics of the innate and adaptive immune responses are approximations and may vary in different infections.

circulation, they are attacked by phagocytes, specialized lymphocytes called natural killer cells, and several plasma proteins, including the proteins of the complement system. All of these agents of innate immunity specifically recognize and react against microbes but do not react against noninfectious foreign substances. Different components of innate immunity may be specific for molecules produced by different classes of microbes. In addition to providing early defense against infections, innate immune responses enhance adaptive immune responses against the infectious agents. The components and mechanisms of innate immunity are discussed in detail in Chapter 2.

Although innate immunity can effectively combat infections, many microbes that are pathogenic for humans (i.e., capable of causing disease) have evolved to resist innate immunity. Defense against these infectious agents is the task of the adaptive immune response, and this is why defects in the adaptive immune system result in increased susceptibility to infections. **The adaptive immune system consists of lymphocytes and their products, such as antibodies.** Whereas the mechanisms of innate immunity recognize structures shared by classes of microbes, the cells of adaptive immunity, namely, lymphocytes, express receptors that specifically recognize different substances produced by microbes as well as noninfectious molecules. These substances are called **antigens.** Adaptive immune responses are triggered only if microbes or their antigens pass through epithelial barriers and are delivered to lymphoid organs where they can be recognized by lymphocytes. Adaptive immune responses are specialized to combat different types of infections. For example, antibodies function to eliminate microbes in extracellular fluids, and activated T lymphocytes eliminate microbes living inside cells. These specialized mechanisms of adaptive immunity are described throughout the book. Adaptive immune responses often use the cells and molecules of the innate immune system to eliminate microbes, and adaptive immunity functions to greatly enhance these antimicrobial mechanisms of innate immunity. For instance, antibodies (a component of adaptive immunity) bind to microbes, and these coated microbes avidly bind to and activate phagocytes (a component of innate immunity), which ingest and destroy the microbes. Many similar examples of the cooperation

between innate and adaptive immunity are referred to in later chapters. By convention, the terms *immune system* and *immune response* refer to adaptive immunity, unless stated otherwise.

Types of Adaptive Immunity

The two types of adaptive immunity, *humoral immunity* and *cell-mediated immunity*, are mediated by different cells and molecules and are designed to provide defense against extracellular microbes and intracellular microbes, respectively (Fig. 1-4). Humoral immunity is mediated by proteins called **antibodies,** which are produced by cells called **B lymphocytes.** Antibodies are secreted into the circulation and mucosal fluids, and they neutralize and eliminate microbes and microbial toxins that are present outside of host cells, in the blood and in the lumens of mucosal organs, such as the gastrointestinal and respiratory tracts. One of the most important functions of antibodies is to stop microbes that are present at mucosal surfaces and in the blood from gaining access to and colonizing host cells and connective tissues. In this way, antibodies prevent infections from ever getting established. Antibodies cannot gain access to microbes that live and divide inside infected cells. Defense against such intracellular microbes is called cell-mediated immunity because it is mediated by cells called **T lymphocytes.** Some T lymphocytes activate phagocytes to destroy microbes that have been ingested by the phagocytes into intracellular vesicles. Other T lymphocytes kill any type of host cells that are harboring infectious microbes in the cytoplasm. Thus, the antibodies produced by B lymphocytes recognize extracellular microbial antigens, whereas T lymphocytes recognize antigens produced by intracellular microbes. Another important difference between B and T lymphocytes is that most T cells recognize only protein antigens, whereas antibodies are able to recognize many different types of molecules, including proteins, carbohydrates, and lipids.

Immunity may be induced in an individual by infection or vaccination (*active immunity*) or conferred on an individual by transfer of antibodies or lymphocytes from an actively immunized individual (*passive immunity*). An individual exposed to the antigens of a microbe mounts an active response to

FIGURE 1-4 Types of adaptive immunity. In humoral immunity, B lymphocytes secrete antibodies that eliminate extracellular microbes. In cell-mediated immunity, T lymphocytes either activate macrophages to destroy phagocytosed microbes or kill infected cells.

eradicate the infection and develops resistance to later infection by that microbe. Such an individual is said to be *immune* to that microbe, in contrast with a *naive* individual, not previously exposed to that microbe's antigens. We shall be concerned mainly with the mechanisms of active immunity. In passive immunity, a naive individual receives cells (e.g., lymphocytes, feasible only in genetically identical [inbred] animals) or molecules (e.g., antibodies) from another individual already immune to an infection; for the lifetime of the transferred antibodies or cells, the recipient is able to combat the infection. Passive immunity is therefore useful for rapidly conferring immunity even before the individual is able to mount an active response, but it

does not induce long-lived resistance to the infection. An excellent example of passive immunity is seen in newborns, whose immune systems are not mature enough to respond to many pathogens but who are protected against infections by acquiring antibodies from their mothers through the placenta and in milk.

Properties of Adaptive Immune Responses

Several properties of adaptive immune responses are crucial for the effectiveness of these responses in combating infections (Fig. 1-5).

Feature	Functional significance
Specificity	Ensures that distinct antigens elicit specific responses
Diversity	Enables immune system to respond to a large variety of antigens
Memory	Leads to enhanced responses to repeated exposures to the same antigens
Clonal expansion	Increases number of antigen-specific lymphocytes to keep pace with microbes
Specialization	Generates responses that are optimal for defense against different types of microbes
Contraction and homeostasis	Allows immune system to respond to newly encountered antigens
Nonreactivity to self	Prevents injury to the host during responses to foreign antigens

FIGURE 1-5 **Properties of adaptive immune responses.** The important properties of adaptive immune responses, and how each feature contributes to host defense against microbes, are summarized.

SPECIFICITY AND DIVERSITY

The adaptive immune system is capable of distinguishing among millions of different antigens or portions of antigens. Specificity for many different antigens implies that the total collection of lymphocyte specificities, sometimes called the lymphocyte repertoire, is extremely diverse. The basis of this remarkable specificity and diversity is that lymphocytes express clonally distributed receptors for antigens, meaning that the total population of lymphocytes consists of many different clones (each of which is made up of one cell and its progeny), and each clone expresses an antigen receptor that is different from the receptors of all other clones. The clonal selection hypothesis, formulated in the 1950s, correctly predicted that clones of lymphocytes specific for dif-

ferent antigens arise before encounter with these antigens, and each antigen elicits an immune response by selecting and activating the lymphocytes of a specific clone (Fig. 1-6). We now know how the specificity and diversity of lymphocytes are generated (see Chapter 4).

The diversity of lymphocyte means that very few cells, perhaps as few as one in 100,000 lymphocytes, are specific for any one antigen. In order to mount effective defense against microbes, these few cells have to proliferate to generate a large number of cells capable of combating the microbes. The remarkable effectiveness of immune responses is possible because of several features of adaptive immunity–marked expansion of the pool of lymphocytes specific for any antigen subsequent to exposure to that antigen, positive feedback loops that amplify immune responses, and selection mechanisms that preserve the most useful lymphocytes. We will describe these characteristics of the adaptive immune system in later chapters.

MEMORY

The immune system mounts larger and more effective responses to repeated exposures to the same antigen. The response to the first exposure to antigen, called the **primary immune response**, is mediated by lymphocytes, called **naive lymphocytes**, that are seeing antigen for the first time (Fig. 1-7). The term *naive* refers to the fact that these cells are "immunologically inexperienced," not having previously recognized and responded to antigens. Subsequent encounters with the same antigen lead to responses, called **secondary immune responses,** that usually are more rapid, larger, and better able to eliminate the antigen than are the primary responses (see Fig. 1-7). Secondary responses are the result of the activation of **memory lymphocytes,** which are long-lived cells that were induced during the primary immune response. Immunologic memory optimizes the ability of the immune system to combat persistent and recurrent infections, because each encounter with a microbe generates more memory cells and activates previously generated memory cells. Memory also is one of the reasons

Lymphocyte clones with diverse receptors arise in generative lymphoid organs

Clones of mature lymphocytes specific for many antigens enter lymphoid tissues

Antigen-specific clones are activated ("selected") by antigens

Antigen-specific immune responses occur

FIGURE 1-6 Clonal selection. Mature lymphocytes with receptors for many antigens develop before encounter with these antigens. A clone refers to a population of lymphocytes with identical antigen receptors and, therefore, specificities; all these cells are presumably derived from one precursor cell. Each antigen (e.g., the examples X and Y) selects a preexisting clone of specific lymphocytes and stimulates the proliferation and differentiation of that clone. The diagram shows only B lymphocytes giving rise to antibody-secreting effector cells, but the same principle applies to T lymphocytes. The antigens shown are surface molecules of microbes, but clonal selection also is true for soluble antigens.

why vaccines confer long-lasting protection against infections.

OTHER FEATURES OF ADAPTIVE IMMUNITY

Adaptive immune responses have other characteristics that are important for their functions (see Fig. 1-5). When lymphocytes are activated by antigens, they undergo proliferation, generating many thousands of clonal progeny cells, all with the same antigen specificity. This process, called **clonal expansion**, ensures that adaptive immunity keeps pace with rapidly proliferating microbes. Immune responses are specialized, and different responses are designed to best defend against different classes of microbes. All immune responses are self-limited and decline as the infection is eliminated, allowing the system to return to a resting state, prepared to respond to another infection. The immune system is able to react against an enormous number and variety of microbes and other foreign antigens, but it normally does not react against the host's own potentially antigenic substances—so-called self antigens.

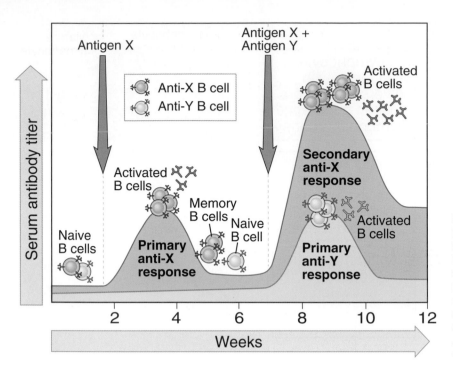

FIGURE 1-7   **Primary and secondary immune responses.** Antigens X and Y induce the production of different antibodies (a reflection of specificity). The secondary response to antigen X is more rapid and larger than the primary response (illustrating memory) and is different from the primary response to antigen Y (again reflecting specificity). Antibody levels decline with time after each immunization.

Cells of the Immune System

The cells of the immune system consist of lymphocytes, specialized cells that capture and display microbial antigens, and effector cells that eliminate microbes (Fig. 1-8). In the following section the important functional properties of the major cell populations are discussed; the details of the morphology of these cells may be found in histology textbooks.

LYMPHOCYTES

Lymphocytes are the only cells that produce specific receptors for antigens and are thus the key mediators of adaptive immunity. Although all lymphocytes are morphologically similar and rather unremarkable in appearance, they are extremely heterogeneous in lineage, function, and phenotype and are capable of complex biologic responses and activities (Fig. 1-9). These cells often are distinguishable by surface proteins that may be identified using panels of monoclonal antibodies. The standard nomenclature for these proteins is the *CD* (cluster of differentiation) numerical designation, which is used to delineate surface proteins that define a particular cell type or stage of cell differentiation and are recognized by a cluster or group of antibodies. (A list of CD molecules mentioned in the book is provided in Appendix II.)

As alluded to earlier, B lymphocytes are the only cells capable of producing antibodies; therefore, they are the cells that mediate humoral immunity. B cells express membrane forms of antibodies that serve as the receptors that recognize antigens and initiate the process of activation of the cells. Soluble antigens and antigens on the surface of microbes and other cells may bind to these B lymphocyte antigen receptors and elicit humoral immune responses. T lymphocytes are the cells of cell-mediated immunity. The antigen receptors of most T lymphocytes only recognize peptide fragments of protein antigens that are bound to specialized peptide display molecules

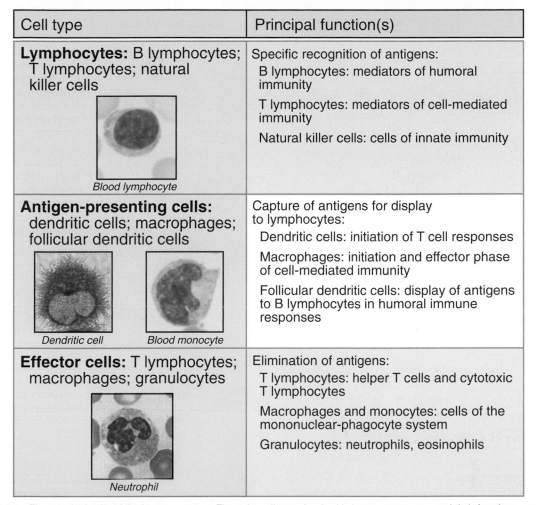

Cell type	Principal function(s)

Lymphocytes: B lymphocytes; T lymphocytes; natural killer cells
 	
Blood lymphocyte
	Specific recognition of antigens:
	  B lymphocytes: mediators of humoral immunity
	  T lymphocytes: mediators of cell-mediated immunity
	  Natural killer cells: cells of innate immunity

Antigen-presenting cells: dendritic cells; macrophages; follicular dendritic cells
 	
Dendritic cell   *Blood monocyte*
	Capture of antigens for display to lymphocytes:
	  Dendritic cells: initiation of T cell responses
	  Macrophages: initiation and effector phase of cell-mediated immunity
	  Follicular dendritic cells: display of antigens to B lymphocytes in humoral immune responses

Effector cells: T lymphocytes; macrophages; granulocytes
 	
Neutrophil
	Elimination of antigens:
	  T lymphocytes: helper T cells and cytotoxic T lymphocytes
	  Macrophages and monocytes: cells of the mononuclear-phagocyte system
	  Granulocytes: neutrophils, eosinophils

FIGURE 1-8 **The principal cells of the immune system.** The major cell types involved in immune responses, and their functions, are shown. Micrographs in the *left panels* illustrate the morphology of some of the cells of each type. Note that tissue macrophages are derived from blood monocytes.

called major histocompatibility complex (MHC) molecules, on the surface of specialized cells called antigen-presenting cells (APCs) (see Chapter 3). Among T lymphocytes, CD4+ T cells are called **helper T cells** because they help B lymphocytes to produce antibodies and help phagocytes to destroy ingested microbes. Some CD4+ T cells belong to a special subset that functions to prevent or limit immune responses; these are called **regulatory T lymphocytes.** CD8+ T lymphocytes are called **cytotoxic, or cytolytic, T lymphocytes (CTLs)** because they kill

("lyse") cells harboring intracellular microbes. A third class of lymphocytes is called **natural killer (NK) cells;** these cells also kill infected host cells, but they do not express the kinds of clonally distributed antigen receptors that B cells and T cells do and are components of innate immunity, capable of rapidly attacking infected cells.

All lymphocytes arise from stem cells in the bone marrow (Fig. 1-10). **B lymphocytes mature in the bone marrow, and T lymphocytes mature in an organ called the thymus;** these sites in which mature

| Antigen recognition | Effector functions |

FIGURE 1-9   Classes of lymphocytes. Different classes of lymphocytes recognize distinct types of antigens and differentiate into effector cells whose function is to eliminate the antigens. B lymphocytes recognize soluble or cell surface antigens and differentiate into antibody-secreting cells. Helper T lymphocytes recognize antigens on the surfaces of antigen-presenting cells and secrete cytokines, which stimulate different mechanisms of immunity and inflammation. Cytotoxic (cytolytic) T lymphocytes recognize antigens on infected cells and kill these cells. (Note that T lymphocytes recognize peptides that are displayed by major histocompatibility complex (MHC) molecules; this process is discussed in Chapter 3.) Natural killer cells recognize changes on the surface of infected cells and kill these cells. Regulatory T cells are not shown in the figure.

lymphocytes are produced are called the generative lymphoid organs. Mature lymphocytes leave the generative lymphoid organs and enter the circulation and the peripheral lymphoid organs, where they may encounter antigen for which they express specific receptors. A normal adult contains approximately 10^{12} lymphocytes in the circulation and lymphoid tissues.

When naive lymphocytes recognize microbial antigens and also receive additional signals

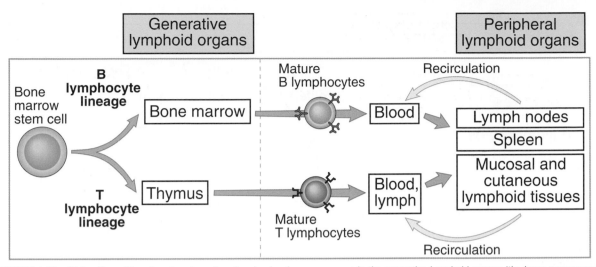

FIGURE 1-10 Maturation of lymphocytes. Lymphocytes develop from precursors in the generative lymphoid organs (the bone marrow and thymus). Mature lymphocytes enter the peripheral lymphoid organs, where they respond to foreign antigens and from where they recirculate in the blood and lymph.

induced by microbes, the antigen-specific lympho-cytes proliferate and differentiate into effector cells and memory cells (Fig. 1-11). **Naive lympho-cytes** express receptors for antigens but do not perform the functions that are required to eliminate antigens. These cells reside in and circulate between peripheral lymphoid organs and survive for several weeks or months, waiting to find and respond to antigen. If they are not activated by antigen, naive lymphocytes die by the process of apoptosis and are replaced by new cells that have arisen in the generative lymphoid organs. This cycle of cell loss and replacement maintains a stable number of lymphocytes, a phenom-enon called **homeostasis.** The differentiation of naive lymphocytes into effector cells and memory cells is initiated by antigen recognition, thus ensuring that the immune response that develops is specific for the antigen. **Effector cells** are the differentiated progeny of naive cells that have the ability to produce molecules that function to eliminate antigens. The effector cells in the B lymphocyte lineage are antibody-secreting cells, called **plasma cells.** Effector CD4+ T cells (helper T cells) produce proteins called cyto-kines that activate B cells and macrophages, thereby mediating the helper function of this lineage, and effector CD8+ T cells (CTLs) have the machinery

to kill infected host cells. The development and functions of these effector cells are discussed in later chapters. Most effector lymphocytes are short-lived and die as the antigen is eliminated, but some may migrate to special anatomic sites and live for long periods. This prolonged survival of effector cells is best documented for antibody-producing plasma cells, which develop in response to microbes in the peripheral lymphoid organs but may then migrate to the bone marrow and continue to produce small amounts of antibody long after the infection is eradi-cated. **Memory cells,** which also are generated from the progeny of antigen-stimulated lymphocytes, do survive for long periods of time in the absence of antigen. Therefore, the frequency of memory cells increases with age, presumably because of exposure to environmental microbes. In fact, memory cells make up less than 5% of peripheral blood T cells in a newborn, but 50% or more in an adult. Memory cells are functionally inactive—they do not perform effec-tor functions unless stimulated by antigen. When memory cells encounter the same antigen that induced their development, the cells rapidly respond to give rise to secondary immune responses. Very little is known about the signals that generate memory cells, the factors that determine whether the progeny of

A

Cell type	Stage		
	Naive cells	Effector cells	Memory cells
B lymphocytes	Antigen recognition	Proliferation — Differentiation	
Helper T lymphocytes	Antigen recognition	Proliferation — Differentiation	

B

Property	Stage		
	Naive cells	Effector cells	Memory cells
Antigen receptor	Yes	B cells: reduced T cells: Yes	Yes
Lifespan	Weeks or months	Usually short (days)	Long (years)

Effector function	None	Yes
		  B cells: antibody secretion
		  Helper T cells:
		    cytokine secretion
		  CTLs: cell killing
			None

Special characteristics B cells			
Affinity of Ig	Low	Variable	High (affinity maturation)
Isotype of Ig	Membrane-associated IgM, IgD	Membrane-associated and secreted IgM, IgG, IgA, IgE (class switching)	Various
T cells			
Migration	To lymph nodes	To peripheral tissues (sites of infection)	To lymph nodes and mucosal and other tissues

FIGURE 1-11 **Stages in the life history of lymphocytes. A,** Naive lymphocytes recognize foreign antigens to initiate adaptive immune responses. Some of the progeny of these lymphocytes differentiate into effector cells, whose function is to eliminate antigens. The effector cells of the B lymphocyte lineage are antibody-secreting plasma cells (some of which are long-lived). The effector cells of the CD4+ T lymphocyte lineage produce cytokines. (The effector cells of the CD8+ lineage are CTLs; these are not shown.) Other progeny of the antigen-stimulated lymphocytes differentiate into long-lived memory cells. **B,** The important characteristics of naive, effector, and memory cells in the B and T lymphocyte lineages are summarized. The processes of affinity maturation and class switching in B cells are described in Chapter 7. Ig, immunoglobulin.

antigen-stimulated lymphocytes will develop into effector or memory cells, or the mechanisms that keep memory cells alive in the absence of antigen or innate immunity.

ANTIGEN-PRESENTING CELLS

The common portals of entry for microbes— the skin, gastrointestinal tract, and respiratory tract—contain specialized antigen-presenting cells (APCs) located in the epithelium that capture antigens, transport them to peripheral lymphoid tissues, and display them to lymphocytes. This function of antigen capture and presentation is best understood for a cell type called **dendritic cells** because of their long processes. Dendritic cells capture protein antigens of microbes that enter through the epithelia and transport the antigens to regional lymph nodes. Here the antigen-bearing dendritic cells display portions of the antigens for recognition by T lymphocytes. If a microbe has invaded through the epithelium, it may be phagocytosed by macrophages that live in tissues and in various organs. Macrophages are also capable of presenting protein antigens to T cells. The process of antigen presentation to T cells is described in Chapter 3.

Cells that are specialized to display antigens to T lymphocytes have another important feature that gives them the ability to trigger T cell responses. These specialized cells respond to microbes by producing surface and secreted proteins that are required, together with antigen, to activate naive T lymphocytes to proliferate and differentiate into effector cells. Specialized cells that display antigens to T cells and provide additional activating signals sometimes are called "professional APCs." The prototypical professional APCs are dendritic cells, but macrophages and a few other cell types may serve the same function.

Less is known about cells that may capture antigens for display to B lymphocytes. B lymphocytes may directly recognize the antigens of microbes (either released or on the surface of the microbes), or macrophages lining lymphatic channels may capture antigens and display them to B cells. A type of dendritic cell called the follicular dendritic cell (FDC) resides in the germinal centers of lymphoid follicles in the peripheral lymphoid organs and displays antigens that stimulate the differentiation of B cells in the follicles. The role of FDCs is described in more detail in Chapter 7. FDCs do not present antigens to T cells and are quite different from the dendritic cells described earlier that function as APCs for T lymphocytes.

EFFECTOR CELLS

The cells that eliminate microbes are called effector cells and consist of lymphocytes and other leukocytes. The effector cells of the B and T lymphocyte lineages were mentioned earlier. The elimination of microbes often requires the participation of other, nonlymphoid leukocytes, such as granulocytes and macrophages. These leukocytes may function as effector cells in both innate immunity and adaptive immunity. In innate immunity, macrophages and some granulocytes directly recognize microbes and eliminate them (see Chapter 2). In adaptive immunity, the products of B and T lymphocytes call in other leukocytes and activate them to kill microbes.

Tissues of the Immune System

The tissues of the immune system consist of the generative (also called primary, or central) lymphoid organs, in which T and B lymphocytes mature and become competent to respond to antigens, and the peripheral (or secondary) lymphoid organs, in which adaptive immune responses to microbes are initiated (see Fig. 1-10). The generative lymphoid organs are described in Chapter 4, when we discuss the process of lymphocyte maturation. In the following section, we highlight some of the features of peripheral lymphoid organs that are important for the development of adaptive immunity.

PERIPHERAL LYMPHOID ORGANS

The peripheral lymphoid organs, which consist of the lymph nodes, the spleen, and the mucosal and cutaneous immune systems, are organized to optimize interactions of antigens, APCs, and lymphocytes in a way that promotes the development of adaptive immune responses. The immune system has to locate microbes that enter at any site in the body and then respond to these microbes and eliminate them. In addition, as we have mentioned earlier, in the normal immune system very few T and B lymphocytes are specific for any one antigen—perhaps as few as 1 in 100,000 cells. The anatomic organization of peripheral lymphoid organs enables APCs to concentrate antigens in these organs and lymphocytes to locate and respond to the antigens. This organization is complemented by a remarkable ability of lymphocytes to circulate throughout the body in such a way that naive lymphocytes preferentially go to the specialized organs in which antigen is concentrated and effector cells go to sites of infection, from where microbes have to be eliminated. Furthermore, different types of lymphocytes often need to communicate to generate effective immune responses. For instance, helper T cells specific for an antigen interact with and help B lymphocytes specific for the same antigen, resulting in antibody production. An important function of lymphoid organs is to bring these rare cells together in a way that will enable them to interact productively.

Lymph nodes are nodular aggregates of lymphoid tissues located along lymphatic channels throughout the body (Fig. 1-12). Fluid from all epithelia and connective tissues and most parenchymal organs is drained by lymphatics, which transport this fluid, called lymph, from the tissues to the lymph nodes. Therefore, the lymph contains a mixture of substances that are absorbed from epithelia and tissues. As the lymph passes through lymph nodes, APCs in the nodes are able to sample the antigens of microbes that may enter through epithelia into tissues. In addition, dendritic cells pick up antigens of microbes from epithelia and transport these antigens to the lymph nodes. The net result of these processes of antigen capture and trans-

FIGURE 1-12   The morphology of lymph nodes. A, This schematic diagram shows the structural organization and blood flow in a lymph node. **B,** This light micrograph shows a cross section of a lymph node with numerous follicles in the cortex, some of which contain lightly stained central areas (germinal centers), and the central medulla.

port is that the antigens of microbes that enter through epithelia or colonize tissues become concentrated in draining lymph nodes.

The **spleen** (Fig. 1-13) is an abdominal organ that serves the same role in immune responses to blood-borne antigens as that of lymph nodes in responses to

FIGURE 1-13 The morphology of the spleen. A, This schematic diagram shows a splenic arteriole surrounded by the periarteriolar lymphoid sheath (PALS) and attached follicle containing a prominent germinal center. The PALS and lymphoid follicles together constitute the white pulp. **B,** This light micrograph of a section of a spleen shows an arteriole with the PALS and a secondary follicle. These are surrounded by the red pulp, which is rich in vascular sinusoids.

lymph-borne antigens. Blood entering the spleen flows through a network of channels (sinusoids). Blood-borne antigens are trapped and concentrated by dendritic cells and macrophages in the spleen. The spleen contains abundant phagocytes, which ingest and destroy microbes in the blood.

The cutaneous and mucosal lymphoid systems are located under the epithelia of the skin and the gastro-intestinal and respiratory tracts, respectively. Pharyngeal tonsils and Peyer's patches of the intestine are two anatomically defined mucosal lymphoid tissues. At any time, more than half of the body's lymphocytes are in the mucosal tissues (reflecting the large size of these tissues), and many of these are memory cells. Cutaneous and mucosal lymphoid tissues are sites of immune responses to antigens that breach epithelia.

Within the peripheral lymphoid organs, T lymphocytes and B lymphocytes are segregated into different anatomic compartments (Fig. 1-14). In lymph nodes, the B cells are concentrated in discrete structures, called **follicles**, located around the periphery, or cortex, of each node. If the B cells in a follicle have recently responded to an antigen, this follicle may contain a central region called a **germinal center**. The role of germinal centers in the production of antibodies is described in Chapter 7. The T lymphocytes are concentrated outside, but adjacent to, the follicles, in the paracortex. The follicles contain the FDCs that are involved in the activation of B cells, and the paracortex contains the dendritic cells that present antigens to T lymphocytes. In the spleen, T lymphocytes are concentrated in periarteriolar lymphoid sheaths surrounding small arterioles, and B cells reside in the follicles.

The anatomic organization of peripheral lymphoid organs is tightly regulated to allow immune responses to develop. B lymphocytes are located in the follicles because FDCs secrete a protein that belongs to a class of cytokines called chemokines ("chemoattractant cytokines"), for which naive B cells express a receptor. (Chemokines and other cytokines are discussed in more detail in later chapters.) This chemokine is produced all the time, and it attracts B cells from the blood into the follicles of lymphoid organs. Similarly, T cells are segregated in the paracortex of lymph nodes and the periarteriolar lymphoid sheaths of the spleen, because naive T lymphocytes express a receptor, called

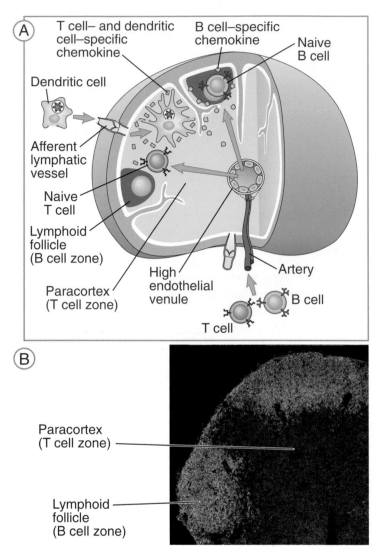

FIGURE 1-14 **Segregation of T and B lymphocytes in different regions of peripheral lymphoid organs.** **A,** This schematic diagram illustrates the path by which naive T and B lymphocytes migrate to different areas of a lymph node. The lymphocytes enter through a high endothelial venule (HEV), shown in cross section, and are drawn to different areas of the node by chemokines that are produced in these areas and bind selectively to either cell type. Also shown is the migration of dendritic cells, which pick up antigens from epithelia, enter through afferent lymphatic vessels, and migrate to the T cell–rich areas of the node. **B,** In this section of a lymph node, the B lymphocytes, located in the follicles, are stained green, and the T cells, in the parafollicular cortex, are red. The method used to stain these cells is called immunofluorescence. In this technique, a section of the tissue is stained with antibodies specific for T or B cells that are coupled to fluorochromes that emit different colors when excited at the appropriate wavelengths. The anatomic segregation of T and B cells also occurs in the spleen (not shown). (Courtesy of Drs. Kathryn Pape and Jennifer Walter, University of Minnesota Medical School, Minneapolis.)

CCR7, that recognizes chemokines that are produced in these regions of the lymph nodes and spleen. As a result, T lymphocytes are recruited from the blood into the parafollicular cortex region of the lymph node and the periarteriolar lymphoid sheaths of the spleen. When the lymphocytes are activated by microbial antigens, they alter their expression of the chemokine receptors. As a result, the B cells and T cells migrate toward each other and meet at the edge of follicles, where helper T cells interact with and help B cells to differentiate into antibody-producing cells (see Chapter 7). The activated lymphocytes ultimately exit the node through efferent lymphatic vessels and leave the spleen through veins. These activated lymphocytes end up in the circulation and can go to distant sites of infection.

LYMPHOCYTE RECIRCULATION AND MIGRATION INTO TISSUES

Naive lymphocytes constantly recirculate between the blood and peripheral lymphoid organs, where they may be activated by antigens to become effector cells, and the effector lymphocytes migrate to sites of infection, where microbes are eliminated

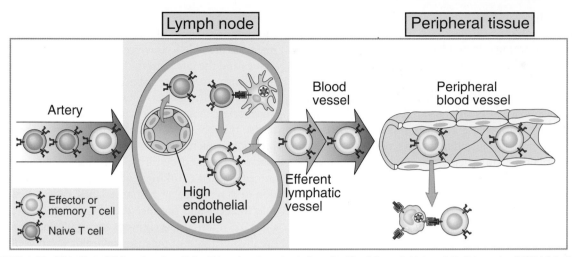

FIGURE 1-15 Migration of T lymphocytes. Naive T lymphocytes migrate from the blood through high endothelial venules (HEVs) into the T cell zones of lymph nodes, where the cells are activated by antigens. Activated T cells exit the nodes, enter the bloodstream, and migrate preferentially to peripheral tissues at sites of infection and inflammation. The adhesion molecules involved in the attachment of T cells to endothelial cells are described in Chapter 6.

(Fig. 1-15). Thus, lymphocytes at distinct stages of their lives migrate to the different sites where they are needed for their functions. This process of lymphocyte recirculation is best described for T lymphocytes. It also is most relevant for T cells, because effector T cells have to locate and eliminate microbes at any site of infection. By contrast, effector B lymphocytes remain in lymphoid organs and do not need to migrate to sites of infection. Instead, B cells secrete antibodies, and the antibodies enter the blood and find microbes and microbial toxins in the circulation or distant tissues. Therefore, we will largely limit our discussion of lymphocyte recirculation to T lymphocytes.

Naive T lymphocytes that have matured in the thymus and entered the circulation migrate to lymph nodes where they can find antigens that enter through lymphatic vessels that drain epithelia and parenchymal organs. These naive T cells enter lymph nodes through specialized postcapillary venules, called **high endothelial venules** (HEVs), that are present in lymph nodes. Naive T cells express a surface receptor called L-selectin that binds to carbohydrate ligands that are expressed only on the endothelial cells of HEVs. (Selectins are a family of proteins involved in cell-cell adhesion that contain conserved structural features, including a lectin, or carbohydrate-binding, domain. More information about these proteins is in Chapter 6.) Because of the interaction of L-selectin with its ligand, naive T cells bind loosely to HEVs. In response to chemokines

produced in the T cell zones of the lymph nodes, the naive T cells bind strongly to HEVs and then migrate through the HEVs into this region, where antigens are displayed by dendritic cells.

In the lymph node, naive T cells move around rapidly, scanning the surfaces of dendritic cells searching for antigens. If a T cell specifically recognizes an antigen, that T cell is transiently arrested on the antigen-presenting dendritic cell, forms stable conjugates with the APCs, and is activated. Such an encounter between an antigen and a specific lymphocyte is likely to be a random event, but most T cells in the body circulate through some lymph nodes at least once a day. As a result, some of the cells in the total population of T lymphocytes have an excellent chance of encountering antigens for which these cells express specific receptors. As we mentioned earlier and will describe in more detail in Chapter 3, the likelihood of the correct T cell finding its antigen is increased in peripheral lymphoid organs, particularly lymph nodes, because microbial antigens are concentrated in the same regions of these organs through which naive T cells circulate. In response to the microbial antigen, the naive T cells are activated to proliferate and differentiate. During this process, the cells reduce expression of adhesion molecules and chemokine receptors that keep naive cells in the lymph nodes. At the same time, T cells increase their expression of receptors for a phospholipid called sphingosine

1-phosphate, and since the concentration of this phospholipid is higher in the blood than in lymph nodes, activated cells are drawn out of the nodes into the circulation. The net result of these changes is that differentiated effector T cells leave the lymph nodes and enter the circulation. These effector cells preferentially migrate into the tissues that are colonized by infectious microbes, where the T lymphocytes perform their function of eradicating the infection. This process is described in more detail in Chapter 6, where cell-mediated immune reactions are discussed.

Memory T cell populations appear to consist of some cells that recirculate through lymph nodes, where they can mount secondary responses to captured antigens, and other cells that migrate to sites of infection, where they can respond rapidly to eliminate the infection.

We do not know much about lymphocyte circulation through the spleen or other lymphoid tissues or about the circulation pathways of naive and activated B lymphocytes. The spleen does not contain HEVs, but the general pattern of lymphocyte migration through this organ probably is similar to migration through lymph nodes. B lymphocytes appear to enter lymph nodes through HEVs, but after they respond to antigen, their differentiated progeny either remain in the lymph nodes or migrate mainly to the bone marrow.

Overview of Immune Responses to Microbes

Now that we have described the major components of the immune system, it is useful to summarize the key features of immune responses to microbes. The focus here is on the physiologic function of the immune system—defense against infections. In subsequent chapters, each of these features is discussed in more detail.

THE EARLY INNATE IMMUNE RESPONSE TO MICROBES

The principal barriers between the host and the environment are the epithelia of the skin and the gastrointestinal and respiratory tracts. Infectious microbes usually enter through these routes and attempt to colonize the host. Epithelia serve as physical and functional barriers to infections, simultaneously impeding

the entry of microbes and interfering with their growth through production of natural antimicrobial agents. If microbes are able to traverse these epithelia and enter tissues and the circulation, they encounter the defense mechanisms of innate immunity, which are designed to react rapidly against microbes and their products. Phagocytes, including neutrophils and macrophages, ingest microbes into vesicles and destroy them by producing microbicidal substances in these vesicles; macrophages and dendritic cells also secrete soluble proteins called **cytokines,** which stimulate inflammation and lymphocyte responses. NK cells kill virus-infected cells and produce the macrophage-activating cytokine interferon-γ (IFN-γ). Many plasma proteins are involved in host defense, including the proteins of the complement system, which are activated by microbes, and whose products kill microbes and coat (opsonize) them for phagocytosis by macrophages and neutrophils. In addition to combating infections, innate immune responses stimulate subsequent adaptive immunity, providing signals that are essential for initiating the responses of antigen-specific T and B lymphocytes. The combined actions of the mechanisms of innate immunity can eradicate some infections and keep other pathogens in check until the more powerful adaptive immune response kicks in.

THE ADAPTIVE IMMUNE RESPONSE

The adaptive immune system uses three main strategies to combat most microbes.

- Secreted antibodies bind to extracellular microbes, block their ability to infect host cells, and promote their ingestion and subsequent destruction by phagocytes.
- Phagocytes ingest microbes and kill them, and helper T cells enhance the microbicidal abilities of the phagocytes.
- Cytotoxic T lymphocytes destroy cells infected by microbes that are inaccessible to antibodies.

The goal of the adaptive response is to activate these defense mechanisms against microbes that are in different anatomic locations, such as intestinal lumens, the circulation, or inside cells. All adaptive immune responses develop in steps, each of which corresponds to particular reactions of lymphocytes (Fig. 1-16). We start this overview of adaptive immunity with the first step, which is the recognition of antigens.

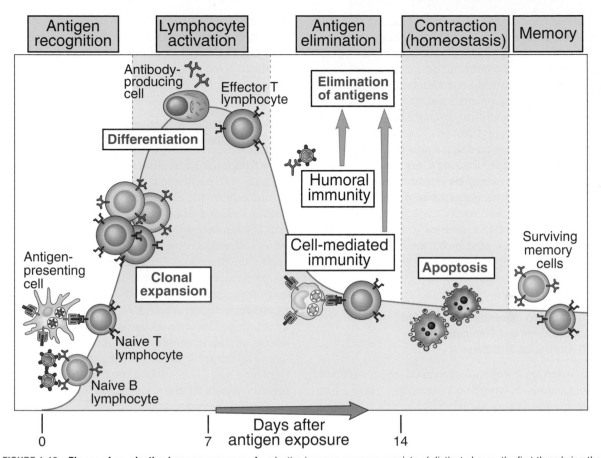

FIGURE 1-16 **Phases of an adaptive immune response.** An adaptive immune response consists of distinct phases, the first three being the recognition of antigen, the activation of lymphocytes, and elimination of antigen (the effector phase). The response declines as antigen-stimulated lymphocytes die by apoptosis, restoring homeostasis, and the antigen-specific cells that survive are responsible for memory. The duration of each phase may vary in different immune responses. The *y*-axis represents an arbitrary measure of the magnitude of the response. These principles apply to both humoral immunity (mediated by B lymphocytes) and cell-mediated immunity (mediated by T lymphocytes).

The Capture and Display of Microbial Antigens

Microbes that enter through epithelia, and their protein antigens, are captured by dendritic cells that are resident in these epithelia, and the cell-bound antigens are transported to draining lymph nodes. Protein antigens are processed in the dendritic cells to generate peptides that are displayed on the surface of the APCs bound to MHC molecules. Naive T cells recognize these peptide-MHC complexes—this is how T cell responses are initiated. Protein antigens also are

recognized by B lymphocytes in the lymphoid follicles of the peripheral lymphoid organs. Polysaccharides and other nonprotein antigens are captured in the lymphoid organs and are recognized by B lymphocytes but not by T cells.

As part of the innate immune response, the dendritic cells that present the antigen to naive T cells are activated to express molecules called costimulators and to secrete cytokines, both of which are needed, in addition to the antigen, to stimulate the proliferation and differentiation of T lymphocytes. The innate immune response to some microbes and polysaccharide antigens also results in the activation of complement, generating cleavage products of complement proteins that enhance the proliferation and differentiation of B lymphocytes. Thus, antigen (often referred to as "signal 1") and molecules produced during innate immune responses ("signal 2") function cooperatively to activate antigen-specific lymphocytes. The requirement for microbe-triggered signal 2 ensures that the adaptive immune response is induced by microbes and not by harmless substances. Signals generated in lymphocytes by the engagement of antigen receptors and receptors for costimulators lead to the transcription of various genes, which encode cytokines, cytokine receptors, effector molecules, and proteins that control cell cycling. All of these molecules are involved in the responses of the lymphocytes.

Cell-Mediated Immunity: Activation of T Lymphocytes and Elimination of Cell-Associated Microbes

When naive T cells are activated by antigen and costimulators in lymphoid organs, they secrete cytokine growth factors and respond to other cytokines secreted by APCs. The combination of signals (antigen, costimulation and cytokines) stimulates the proliferation of the T cells and their differentiation into effector T cells. Different subsets of T cells differentiate into effector cells with distinct functional properties. Naive CD4+ T cells become helper T cells, and naive CD8+ T cells become CTLs. The helper T cells and CTLs that are generated in the lymphoid organ may migrate back into the blood and then into any site where the antigen (microbe) is present. The effector T cells are reactivated by antigen at sites of infection and perform the functions that are responsible for elimination of the microbes. Helper T cells produce cytokines and express cell surface molecules that bind to receptors on B cells and macrophages and thereby promote antibody production or macrophage killing of ingested microbes. Some helper T cells function to recruit and activate neutrophils, which then phagocytose and destroy microbes. CTLs directly kill cells harboring microbes in the cytoplasm. These microbes may be viruses that infect many cell types or bacteria that are ingested by macrophages but have learned to escape from phagocytic vesicles into the cytoplasm (where they are inaccessible to the killing machinery of phagocytes, which is largely confined to vesicles). By destroying the infected cells, CTLs eliminate the reservoirs of infection.

Humoral Immunity: Activation of B Lymphocytes and Elimination of Extracellular Microbes

On activation, B lymphocytes proliferate and then differentiate into plasma cells that secrete different classes of antibodies with distinct functions. Many polysaccharide and lipid antigens have multiple identical antigenic determinants (epitopes) that are able to engage many antigen receptor molecules on each B cell and initiate the process of B cell activation. Typical globular protein antigens are not able to bind to many antigen receptors, and the full response of B cells to protein antigens requires help from CD4+ T cells. B cells ingest protein antigens, degrade them, and display peptides bound to MHC molecules for recognition by helper T cells. The helper T cells express cytokines and cell surface proteins, which work together to activate the B cells.

Some of the progeny of the expanded B cell clones differentiate into antibody-secreting cells. Each B cell secretes antibodies that have the same antigen binding site as the cell surface antibodies (B cell receptors) that first recognized the antigen. Polysaccharides and lipids stimulate secretion mainly of a class of antibody called immunoglobulin M (IgM). Protein antigens stimulate helper T cells, which induce the production of antibodies of different classes (IgG, IgA, and IgE). This production of different antibodies, all with the same specificity, is called **heavy chain class (isotype) switching**; it provides plasticity in the antibody response, enabling antibodies to serve many functions. Helper T cells also stimulate the production of antibodies with higher and higher affinity for the antigen. This process, called **affinity maturation**, improves the quality of the humoral immune response.

The humoral immune response combats microbes in many ways. Antibodies bind to microbes and prevent them from infecting cells, thereby neutralizing the microbes. Antibodies coat (opsonize) microbes and target them for phagocytosis, because phagocytes (neutrophils and macrophages) express receptors for the antibodies. Additionally, antibodies activate a system of serum proteases called complement, and complement products promote phagocytosis and destruction of microbes. Specialized types of antibodies and specialized transport mechanisms for antibodies serve distinct roles at particular anatomic sites, including the lumens of the respiratory and gastrointestinal tracts or the placenta and fetus.

DECLINE OF IMMUNE RESPONSES AND IMMUNOLOGICAL MEMORY

A majority of effector lymphocytes induced by an infectious pathogen die by apoptosis after the microbe is eliminated, thus returning the immune system to its basal resting state. This return to a stable or steady state is called homeostasis. It occurs because microbes provide essential stimuli for lymphocyte survival and activation and effector cells are short-lived. Therefore, as the stimuli are eliminated, the activated lymphocytes are no longer kept alive.

The initial activation of lymphocytes generates long-lived memory cells, which may survive for years after the infection. Memory cells are an expanded pool of antigen-specific lymphocytes (more numerous than the naive cells specific for any antigen that are present before encounter with that antigen), and memory cells respond faster and more effectively against the antigen than do naive cells. This is why the generation of memory cells is an important goal of vaccination.

SUMMARY

■ The physiologic function of the immune system is to protect individuals against infections.

■ Innate immunity is the early line of defense, mediated by cells and molecules that are always present and ready to eliminate infectious microbes. Adaptive immunity is the form of immunity that is stimulated by microbes, has a fine specificity for foreign substances, and responds more effectively against each successive exposure to a microbe.

■ Lymphocytes are the cells of adaptive immunity and are the only cells with clonally distributed receptors for antigens.

■ Adaptive immunity consists of humoral immunity, in which antibodies neutralize and eradicate extracellular microbes and toxins, and cell-mediated immunity, in which T lymphocytes eradicate intracellular microbes.

■ Adaptive immune responses consist of sequential phases: antigen recognition by lymphocytes, activation of the lymphocytes to proliferate and to differentiate into effector and memory cells, elimination of the microbes, decline of the immune response, and long-lived memory.

■ Different populations of lymphocytes serve distinct functions and may be distinguished by the expression of particular membrane molecules.

■ B lymphocytes are the only cells that produce antibodies. B lymphocytes express membrane antibodies that recognize antigens, and effector B cells secrete the antibodies that neutralize and eliminate the antigen.

■ T lymphocytes recognize peptide fragments of protein antigens displayed on other cells. Helper T lymphocytes activate phagocytes to destroy ingested microbes and activate B lymphocytes to produce antibodies. CTLs are cytotoxic: They kill infected cells harboring microbes in the cytoplasm.

■ APCs capture antigens of microbes that enter through epithelia, concentrate these antigens in lymphoid organs, and display the antigens for recognition by T cells.

■ Lymphocytes and APCs are organized in peripheral lymphoid organs, where immune responses are initiated and develop.

■ Naive lymphocytes circulate through the peripheral lymphoid organs searching for foreign antigens. Effector T lymphocytes migrate to peripheral sites of infection, where they function to eliminate infectious microbes. Effector B lymphocytes remain in lymphoid organs and the bone marrow, from where they secrete antibodies that enter the circulation and find and eliminate microbes.

REVIEW QUESTIONS

1 *What are the two types of adaptive immunity, and what types of microbes do these adaptive immune responses combat?*

2 *What are the principal classes of lymphocytes, how do they differ in function, and how may they be identified and distinguished?*

3 *What are the important differences among naive, effector, and memory T and B lymphocytes?*

4 *Where are T and B lymphocytes located in lymph nodes, and how is their anatomic separation maintained?*

5 *How do naive and effector T lymphocytes differ in their patterns of migration?*

Chapter 2

INNATE IMMUNITY

The Early Defense Against Infections

All multicellular organisms, including plants, invertebrates, and vertebrates, possess intrinsic mechanisms for defending themselves against microbial infections. Because these defense mechanisms are always present, ready to recognize and eliminate microbes, they are said to constitute **innate immunity** (also called natural, or native, immunity). The components of innate immunity make up the innate immune system. The shared characteristic of the mechanisms of innate immunity is that they recognize and respond to microbes but do not react against nonmicrobial substances. Innate immunity may also be triggered by host cells that are damaged by microbes. Innate immunity contrasts to adaptive immunity, which must be stimulated by and adapts to encounters with microbes before it can be effective. Furthermore, adaptive immune responses may be directed against microbial as well as nonmicrobial antigens.

For many years it was believed that innate immunity is nonspecific and weak and is not effective in combating most infections. We now know that, in fact, innate immunity specifically targets microbes and is a powerful early defense mechanism capable of controlling and even eradicating infections before adaptive immunity becomes active. Innate immunity not only provides the early defense against infections but also instructs the adaptive immune system to respond to different microbes in ways that are effective for combating these microbes. Conversely, the adaptive immune response often uses mechanisms of innate immunity to eradicate infections. Thus, a constant bidirectional cross-talk occurs between innate immunity and adaptive immunity. For these reasons, great interest exists in defining the mechanisms of innate immunity and learning how to harness these mechanisms for optimizing defense against infections.

Before we consider adaptive immunity—the topic that most of this book is devoted to—we discuss the early defense reactions of innate immunity in this chapter. The discussion focuses on three main questions:

- How does the innate immune system recognize microbes?
- How do the different components of innate immunity function to combat different kinds of microbes?
- How do innate immune reactions stimulate adaptive immune responses?

We start by describing how the cells of innate immunity detect the presence of microbes.

Recognition of Microbes by the Innate Immune System

The specificity of innate immunity is different in several respects from the specificity of lymphocytes, the recognition systems of adaptive immunity (Fig. 2-1).

The components of innate immunity recognize structures that are shared by various classes of microbes and are not present on host cells. Each component of innate immunity may recognize many bacteria, or viruses, or fungi. For instance, phagocytes express receptors for bacterial lipopolysaccharide (LPS), also called endotoxin, which is present in the cell wall of many bacterial species but is not produced by mammalian cells. Other receptors of phagocytes recognize terminal mannose residues, which are typical of bacterial but not mammalian glycoproteins. Phagocytes recognize and respond to double-stranded RNA, which is found in many viruses but not in mammalian cells, and to unmethylated CpG oligonucleotides, which are common in microbial DNA but are not abundant in mammalian DNA. The microbial molecules that are the targets of innate immunity are sometimes called *pathogen-associated molecular patterns*, to indicate that they are shared by microbes of the same type. The receptors of innate immunity that recognize these shared structures are called *pattern*

recognition receptors. Some components of innate immunity are capable of binding to host cells but are prevented from being activated by these cells. For instance, if the plasma proteins of the complement system are deposited on host cells, the activation of these complement proteins is blocked by regulatory molecules that are present on the host cells but are not present on microbes.

The components of innate immunity have evolved to recognize structures of microbes that are often essential for the survival and infectivity of these microbes. This characteristic of innate immunity makes it a highly effective defense mechanism because a microbe cannot evade innate immunity simply by mutating or not expressing the targets of innate immune recognition: Microbes that do not express functional forms of these structures lose their ability to infect and colonize the host. In contrast, microbes frequently evade adaptive immunity by mutating the antigens that are recognized by lymphocytes, because these antigens are usually not required for the life of the microbes.

The innate immune system can also recognize molecules that are released from stressed or necrotic cells. The subsequent response serves to eliminate these cells. Such molecules have been grouped under *damage-associated molecular patterns.*

The receptors of the innate immune system are encoded in the germline and are not produced by somatic recombination of genes. These germline-encoded pattern recognition receptors have evolved as a protective adaptation against potentially harmful microbes. In contrast, the antigen receptors of lymphocytes, namely, antibodies and T cell receptors, are produced by random recombination of receptor genes during the maturation of these cells (see Chapter 4). Gene recombination can generate many more structurally different receptors than can be produced from inherited germline genes, but these different receptors cannot have a predetermined specificity for microbes. Therefore, the specificity of adaptive immunity is much more diverse than that of innate immunity, and the adaptive immune system is capable of recognizing many more chemically distinct structures. It is estimated that the total population of lymphocytes can recognize more than a billion different antigens; by contrast, all of the receptors of innate immunity

	Innate immunity	Adaptive immunity
Specificity	For structures shared by classes of microbes ("molecular patterns") Different microbes Identical mannose receptors	For structural detail of microbial molecules (antigens); may recognize nonmicrobial antigens Different microbes Distinct antibody molecules
Receptors	Encoded in germline; limited diversity Toll-like receptor *N*-formyl methionyl receptor Mannose receptor	Encoded by genes produced by somatic recombination of gene segments; greater diversity Ig TCR
Distribution of receptors	Nonclonal: identical receptors on all cells of the same lineage	Clonal: clones of lymphocytes with distinct specificities express different receptors
Discrimination of self and nonself	Yes; host cells are not recognized or they may express molecules that prevent innate immune reactions	Yes; based on selection against self-reactive lymphocytes; may be imperfect (giving rise to autoimmunity)

FIGURE 2-1 **The specificity of innate immunity and adaptive immunity.** The important features of the specificity and receptors of innate and adaptive immunity are summarized, with selected examples, some of which are illustrated in the *boxed panels.* Ig, Immunoglobulin (antibody); TCR, T cell receptor.

probably recognize less than a thousand microbial patterns. Furthermore, the receptors of the adaptive immune system are clonally distributed, meaning that each clone of lymphocytes (B cells and T cells) has a different receptor specific for a particular antigen. In contrast, in the innate immune system the receptors are nonclonally distributed; that is, identical receptors are expressed on all the cells of a particular type,

such as macrophages. Therefore, many cells of innate immunity may recognize and respond to the same microbe.

The innate immune system does not react against the host. This inability of the innate immune system to react against an individual's own, or "self," cells and molecules is due partly to the inherent specificity of innate immunity for microbial structures and partly to the fact that mammalian cells express regulatory molecules that prevent innate immune reactions. The adaptive immune system also discriminates between self and nonself; in the adaptive immune system, lymphocytes capable of recognizing self antigens are produced, but they die or are inactivated on encounter with self antigens.

The innate immune system usually responds in the same way to repeat encounters with a microbe, whereas the adaptive immune system responds more efficiently to each successive encounter with a microbe. In other words, the adaptive immune system remembers, and adapts to, its encounters with a microbe. This is the phenomenon of immunologic memory. It ensures that host defense reactions are highly effective against repeated or persistent infections. Memory is a defining characteristic of adaptive immunity and is not seen in innate immunity.

The two principal types of reactions of the innate immune system are inflammation and antiviral defense. Inflammation consists of the recruitment and activation of leukocytes. Defense against intracellular viruses is mediated mainly by natural killer (NK) cells and the cytokines, interferons, which are described later.

CELLULAR RECEPTORS FOR MICROBES

The receptors that the innate immune system uses to react against microbes are expressed on phagocytes, dendritic cells, and many other cell types, including lymphocytes and epithelial and endothelial cells, all of which participate in defense against various classes of microbes. These receptors are expressed in different cellular compartments where microbes may be located. Some are present on the cell surface; others are present in the endoplasmic reticulum and are rapidly recruited to vesicles (endosomes) into which microbial products are ingested; and still others are in the cytoplasm, where they function as sensors of cytoplasmic microbes (Fig. 2-2). Several classes of these receptors have been identified that are specific for different types of microbial products ("molecular patterns").

Toll-like receptors (TLRs) are homologous to a *Drosophila* protein called Toll, which was discovered for its role in dorsal-ventral patterning and later shown to be essential for protecting the flies against infections. TLRs are specific for different components of microbes (Fig. 2-3). For instance, TLR-2 is essential for responses to several bacterial lipoglycans, TLR-3, -7, and -8 for viral nucleic acids (such as double-

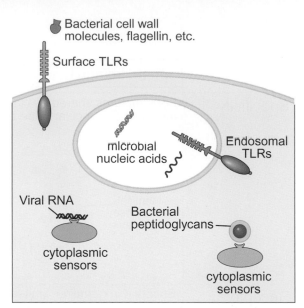

FIGURE 2-2 Cellular locations of receptors of the innate immune system. Some receptors, such as Toll-like receptors (TLRs), are located on cell surfaces; other TLRs are in endosomes (they may be resident in the endoplasmic reticulum and may be rapidly translocated to endosomes in response to microbe entry); and some receptors for viral RNA and for bacterial peptides are in the cytoplasm.

stranded RNA), TLR-4 for bacterial LPS (endotoxin), TLR-5 for a component of bacterial flagella called flagellin, and TLR-9 for unmethylated CG-rich (CpG) oligonucleotides, which are more abundant in bacteria than in mammalian cells. Some of these TLRs are present on the cell surface, where they recognize products of extracellular microbes, and other TLRs are in endosomes, into which microbes are ingested. Signals generated by engagement of TLRs activate transcription factors that stimulate expression of genes encoding cytokines, enzymes, and other proteins involved in the antimicrobial functions of activated phagocytes and dendritic cells (discussed later). Two of the most important transcription factors activated by TLR signals are NF-κB (nuclear factor κB), which promotes expression of various cytokines and endothelial adhesion molecules, and IRF-3 (interferon response factor-3), which stimulates production of type I interferons, cytokines that block viral replication.

Many other receptor types are involved in innate immune responses to microbes. A cell surface receptor recognizes peptides that begin with N-formyl methionine, which is peculiar to bacterial proteins. A receptor for terminal mannose residues is involved in the phagocytosis of bacteria. Several cytoplasmic receptors recognize viral nucleic acids or bacterial

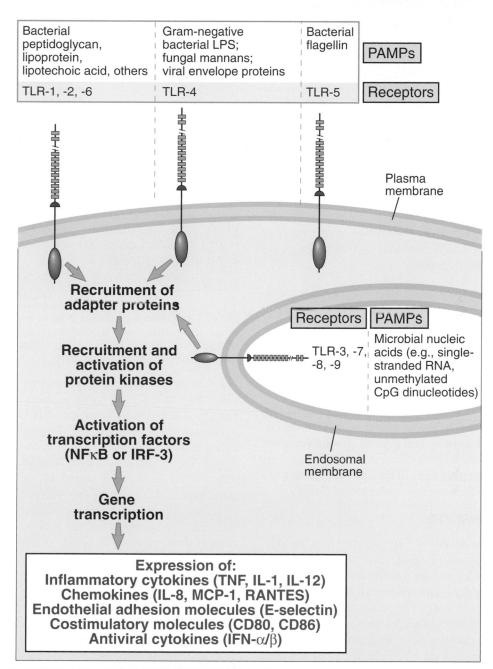

Bacterial peptidoglycan, lipoprotein, lipotechoic acid, others	Gram-negative bacterial LPS; fungal mannans; viral envelope proteins	Bacterial flagellin	PAMPs
TLR-1, -2, -6	TLR-4	TLR-5	Receptors

Plasma membrane

Recruitment of adapter proteins

Recruitment and activation of protein kinases

Activation of transcription factors (NFκB or IRF-3)

Gene transcription

Receptors	PAMPs
TLR-3, -7, -8, -9	Microbial nucleic acids (e.g., single-stranded RNA, unmethylated CpG dinucleotides)

Endosomal membrane

Expression of:
Inflammatory cytokines (TNF, IL-1, IL-12)
Chemokines (IL-8, MCP-1, RANTES)
Endothelial adhesion molecules (E-selectin)
Costimulatory molecules (CD80, CD86)
Antiviral cytokines (IFN-α/β)

FIGURE 2-3   Specificities and functions of Toll-like receptors (TLRs). Different TLRs respond to different products of microbes. All of the TLRs activate similar signaling mechanisms, resulting in cellular responses that are central to innate immunity. IFN, interferon; IL, interleukin; IRF-3, interferon response factor-3; LPS, lipopolysaccharide; MCP-1 and RANTES are two chemokines; NFκB, nuclear factor κB; PAMPs, pathogen-associated molecular patterns; TNF, tumor necrosis factor.

peptides (see Fig. 2-2). Other cytoplasmic receptors that participate in innate immune reactions recognize microbes as well as components of dead cells, including uric acid and DNA itself. Some of these receptors associate with a multi-protein complex called the *inflammasome*, which transmits signals that activate an enzyme that cleaves a precursor of the cytokine interleukin-1 (IL-1) to generate its biologically active form. IL-1 is a powerful inducer of the inflammatory reaction to microbes and damaged tissues. Gain-of-function mutations affecting components of the inflammasome are the cause of rare human diseases that are called autoinflammatory syndromes. In these diseases, the clinical manifestations are the result of excessive IL-1 production, and IL-1 antagonsists are highly effective therapies.

With this introduction to some of the characteristics of innate immunity, we proceed to a description of the individual components of the innate immune system and how these components function in host defense against infections.

Components of Innate Immunity

The innate immune system consists of epithelia, which provide barriers to infection, cells in the circulation and tissues, and several plasma proteins. These components play different but complementary roles in blocking the entry of microbes and in eliminating microbes that enter the tissues of the host.

EPITHELIAL BARRIERS

The common portals of entry of microbes, namely, the skin, gastrointestinal tract, and respiratory tract, are protected by continuous epithelia that provide physical and chemical barriers against infection (Fig. 2-4). The three major interfaces between the body and the external environment are the skin, the gastrointestinal tract, and the respiratory tract. Microbes may enter hosts from the external environment through these interfaces by physical contact, ingestion, and breathing. All three portals of entry are lined by continuous epithelia that physically interfere with the entry of microbes. Epithelial cells also produce peptide antibiotics that kill bacteria. In addition, epithelia contain a type of lymphocyte, called intraepithelial lymphocytes, that belongs to the T cell lineage but expresses antigen receptors of limited diversity.

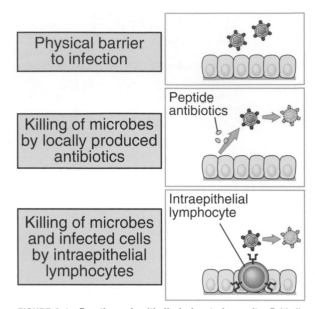

FIGURE 2-4 Functions of epithelia in innate immunity. Epithelia present at the portals of entry of microbes provide physical barriers, produce antimicrobial substances, and harbor lymphocytes that are believed to kill microbes and infected cells.

Some of these T cells express receptors composed of two chains, called γ and δ chains, that are similar, but not identical, to the highly diverse $\alpha\beta$ T cell receptors expressed on a majority of T lymphocytes (see Chapters 4 and 5). Intraepithelial lymphocytes, including $\gamma\delta$ T cells, often recognize microbial lipids and other structures that are shared by microbes of the same type. Intraepithelial lymphocytes presumably serve as sentinels against infectious agents that attempt to breach the epithelia, but the specificity and functions of these cells remain poorly understood.

PHAGOCYTES: NEUTROPHILS AND MONOCYTES/MACROPHAGES

The two types of circulating phagocytes, neutrophils and monocytes, are blood cells that are recruited to sites of infection, where they recognize and ingest microbes for intracellular killing. Neutrophils (also called polymorphonuclear leukocytes [PMNs]) are the most abundant leukocytes in the blood, numbering 4000 to 10,000 per μL (Fig. 2-5). In response to infections, the production of neutrophils from the bone marrow increases rapidly, and their number may rise to 20,000 per μL of blood. The production of neutrophils is stimulated by cytokines, known as colony-stimulating factors, that

FIGURE 2-5 Morphology of neutrophils. This light micrograph of a blood neutrophil shows the multilobed nucleus, because of which these cells also are called polymorphonuclear leukocytes, and the faint cytoplasmic granules (mostly lysosomes).

are secreted by many cell types in response to infections and act on bone marrow stem cells to stimulate proliferation and maturation of neutrophil precursors. Neutrophils are the first cell type to respond to most infections, particularly bacterial and fungal infections.

They ingest microbes in the circulation, and they rapidly enter extravascular tissues at sites of infection, where they also ingest microbes and die after a few hours.

Monocytes are less abundant than neutrophils, numbering 500 to 1000 per μL of blood (Fig. 2-6). They, too, ingest microbes in the blood and in tissues. Unlike neutrophils, monocytes that enter extravascular tissues survive in these sites for long periods; in the tissues, these monocytes differentiate into cells called **macrophages** (see Fig. 2-6). Blood monocytes and tissue macrophages are two stages of the same cell lineage, which often is called the mononuclear phagocyte system. Resident macrophages are found in connective tissues and in every organ in the body, where they serve the same function as that of mononuclear phagocytes newly recruited from the circulation.

Neutrophils and monocytes migrate to extravascular sites of infection by binding to endothelial

FIGURE 2-6 Stages in the maturation of mononuclear phagocytes. Mononuclear phagocytes arise from precursors in the bone marrow. The circulating blood stage is the monocyte; a light micrograph and an electron micrograph of a blood monocyte are shown, illustrating the phagocytic vacuoles and lysosomes. In the tissues, these cells become macrophages; they may be activated by microbes, and they may differentiate into specialized forms that are resident in different tissues. The electron micrograph of a portion of an activated macrophage shows numerous phagocytic vacuoles and cytoplasmic organelles. CNS, central nervous system. (From Fawcett DW: Bloom & Fawcett Textbook of Histology, 12th ed. Philadelphia, WB Saunders, 1994.)

FIGURE 2-7   The sequence of events in the migration of blood leukocytes to sites of infection. At sites of infection, macrophages and dendritic cells that have encountered microbes produce cytokines (e.g., tumor necrosis factor [TNF] and interleukin-1 [IL-1]) that activate the endothelial cells of nearby venules to produce selectins, ligands for integrins, and chemokines. Selectins mediate weak tethering and rolling of blood neutrophils on the endothelium, integrins mediate firm adhesion of neutrophils, and chemokines activate the neutrophils and stimulate their migration through the endothelium to the site of infection. Blood monocytes and activated T lymphocytes use the same mechanisms to migrate to sites of infection. PECAM-1, platelet-endothelial cell adhesion molecule-1.

adhesion molecules and in response to chemoattractants that are produced on encounter with microbes. Leukocyte migration from the blood into tissues is a multistep process that consists of initial loose attachment of the leukocytes to endothelial cells, followed by firm adhesion and transmigration through the endothelium (Fig. 2-7). If an infectious microbe breaches an epithelium and enters the subepithelial tissue, resident macrophages recognize the microbe and respond by producing cytokines (described in more detail later). Two of these cytokines, called tumor necrosis factor (TNF) and interleukin-1 (IL-1), act on the endothelium of small vessels at the site of infection. These cytokines stimulate the endothelial cells to rapidly express two adhesion molecules called E-selectin and P-selectin (the name **selectin** referring to the carbohydrate-binding,

or lectin, property of these molecules). Circulating neutrophils and monocytes express surface carbohydrates that bind weakly to the selectins. The neutrophils become tethered to the endothelium, flowing blood disrupts this binding, the bonds re-form downstream, and so on, resulting in the "rolling" of the leukocytes on the endothelial surface. Leukocytes express another set of adhesion molecules that are called **integrins** because they "integrate" extrinsic signals into cytoskeletal alterations. Integrins are present in a low-affinity state on unactivated leukocytes. As these cells are rolling on the endothelium, tissue macrophages that encountered the microbe, and the endothelial cells responding to the macrophage-derived TNF and IL-1, produce cytokines called **chemokines** (chemoattractant cytokines). Chemokines bind to glycoproteins on the luminal surface of endothelial cells and are thus displayed at a high concentration to the leukocytes that are rolling on the endothelium. These chemokines stimulate a rapid increase in the affinity of the leukocyte integrins for their ligands on the endothelium. Concurrently, TNF and IL-1 act on the endothelium to stimulate expression of ligands for integrins. The firm binding of integrins to their ligands arrests the rolling leukocytes on the endothelium. The cytoskeleton of the leukocytes is reorganized, and the cells spread out on the endothelial surface. Chemokines also stimulate the motility of leukocytes. As a result, the leukocytes begin to migrate between endothelial cells, through the vessel wall, and along the chemokine concentration gradient to the site of infection. The sequence of selectin-mediated rolling, integrin-mediated firm adhesion, and chemokine-mediated motility leads to the migration of blood leukocytes to an extravascular site of infection within minutes after the infection. (As we shall see in Chapter 6, the same sequence of events is responsible for the migration of activated T lymphocytes into infected tissues.) The accumulation of leukocytes at sites of infection, with concomitant vascular dilation and increased leakage of fluid and proteins in the tissue, is called **inflammation.** Inherited deficiencies in integrins and selectin ligands lead to defective leukocyte recruitment to sites of infection and increased susceptibility to infections. These disorders are called leukocyte adhesion deficiencies.

Neutrophils and macrophages use several types of receptors to recognize microbes in the blood and extravascular tissues and to initiate responses that function to destroy the microbes (Fig. 2-8). These receptors are the TLRs and other pattern recognition receptors, discussed earlier. Some of these receptors are involved mainly in activating the phagocytes; these include TLRs, receptors for formyl methionine peptides, and receptors for cytokines, mainly IFN-γ and chemokines. Other receptors are involved in phagocytosis of microbes as well as activation of the phagocytes (described next); these include mannose receptors and scavenger receptors. Receptors for products of complement activation and for antibodies avidly bind microbes that are coated with complement proteins or antibodies (the latter only in adaptive immunity) and function in ingestion of microbes and in the activation of the phagocytes. The process of coating microbes for efficient recognition by phagocytes is called **opsonization.**

Neutrophils and macrophages ingest (phagocytose) microbes and destroy the ingested microbes in intracellular vesicles (Fig. 2-9). Phagocytosis is a process that begins with membrane receptors binding to the microbe, followed by extension of the phagocyte plasma membrane around the microbe. The membrane then closes up and pinches off, and the microbe is internalized in a membrane-bound vesicle, called a phagosome. The phagosomes fuse with lysosomes to form phagolysosomes. At the same time as the microbe is being bound by the phagocyte's receptors and ingested, the receptors deliver signals that activate several enzymes in the phagolysosomes. One of these enzymes, called phagocyte oxidase, converts molecular oxygen into superoxide anion and free radicals. These substances are called reactive oxygen species (ROS), and they are toxic to the ingested microbes. A second enzyme, called inducible nitric oxide synthase, catalyzes the conversion of arginine to nitric oxide (NO), also a microbicidal substance. The third set of enzymes are lysosomal proteases, which break down microbial proteins. All of these microbicidal substances are produced mainly within lysosomes and phagolysosomes, where they act on the ingested microbes but do not damage the phagocytes. In some instances, the same enzymes and ROS may be liberated into the extracellular space and may injure host tissues. This is the reason why inflammation, normally a protective host response to infections, may cause tissue injury as well. Inherited deficiency of the phagocyte oxidase enzyme is the cause of an immunodeficiency disease called chronic granulomatous disease. In this disorder, phagocytes are unable to eradicate intracellular microbes, and the host tries to contain the infection by calling in more macrophages and lymphocytes, resulting in collections of cells around the microbes that are called granulomas.

In addition to killing phagocytosed microbes, macrophages perform several functions that play important roles in defense against infections (see Fig. 2-8). Macrophages produce cytokines that recruit and activate leukocytes. Macrophages secrete growth factors and enzymes that function to repair injured tissue and replace it with connective tissue. Macrophages stimulate T lymphocytes and enhance adaptive immunity.

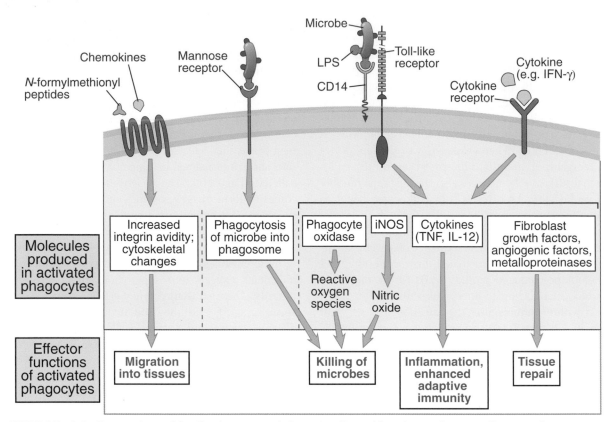

FIGURE 2-8 **Activating receptors and functional responses of phagocytes.** Neutrophils and macrophages use diverse membrane receptors to recognize microbes, microbial products, and substances produced by the host in infections. These receptors activate cellular responses that function to stimulate inflammation and eradicate microbes. Toll-like receptors (TLRs) and the receptor for IFN-γ work synergistically in some but not all the responses shown, and activate the microbicidal functions of the macrophages. Note that only selected examples of receptors of different classes are shown, and other phagocytic receptors are shown in Figure 2-9. Cytokines other than IFN-γ may activate macrophages to produce growth factors that are involved in tissue remodeling and repair; these distinct functional responses are sometimes grouped under "alternative macrophage activation" (implying other than activation by the best-defined signals, TLRs and IFN-γ). The biochemical signaling pathways used by these receptors are complex; their common feature is that they stimulate the production of transcription factors, which result in the production of various proteins. IFN-γ, interferon-γ; iNOS, inducible nitric oxide synthase; LPS, lipopolysaccharide.

Finally, macrophages respond to products of T cells and function as effector cells of cell-mediated immunity (Chapter 6).

DENDRITIC CELLS

Dendritic cells respond to microbes by producing cytokines that recruit leukocytes and initiate adaptive immune responses. Dendritic cells constitute an important bridge between innate and adaptive immu-

nity. We will return to a discussion of the properties and functions of these cells in Chapter 3, in the context of antigen display, which is a major function of dendritic cells.

NATURAL KILLER CELLS

Natural killer (NK) cells are a class of lymphocytes that recognize infected and stressed cells and respond by killing these cells and by secreting the

FIGURE 2-9 Phagocytosis and intra-cellular killing of microbes. Macrophages and neutrophils express many surface receptors that may bind microbes for subsequent phagocytosis; selected examples of such receptors are shown. Microbes are ingested into phagosomes, which fuse with lysosomes, and the microbes are killed by enzymes and several toxic substances produced in the phagolysosomes. The same substances may be released from the phagocytes and may kill extracellular microbes (*not shown*). iNOS, inducible nitric oxide synthase; Mac-1 is an integrin; NO, nitric oxide; ROS, reactive oxygen species.

FIGURE 2-10 **Functions of natural killer (NK) cells. A,** NK cells
kill host cells infected by intracellular microbes, thus eliminating
reservoirs of infection. **B,** NK cells respond to interleukin-12 (IL-12)
produced by macrophages and secrete interferon-γ (IFN-γ), which
activates the macrophages to kill phagocytosed microbes.

macrophage-activating cytokine IFN-γ (Fig. 2-10).
NK cells make up approximately 10% of the lymphocytes in the blood and peripheral lymphoid organs.
These cells contain abundant cytoplasmic granules and
express characteristic surface markers, but they do not
express immunoglobulins and T cell receptors, the
antigen receptors of B and T lymphocytes, respectively.

Activation of NK cells triggers the discharge of proteins contained in the NK cells' cytoplasmic granules
toward the infected cells. These NK cell granule proteins include molecules that enter the infected cells
and activate enzymes that induce apoptotic death. The
cytotoxic mechanisms of NK cells are the same as the
mechanisms used by CTLs to kill infected cells (see
Chapter 6). The net result of these reactions is that
NK cells kill infected host cells. By killing infected host
cells, NK cells, like CTLs, function to eliminate cellular reservoirs of infection and thus eradicate infections
by obligate intracellular microbes, such as viruses.

Activated NK cells also synthesize and secrete the
cytokine IFN-γ. IFN-γ activates macrophages to
become more effective at killing phagocytosed
microbes. Thus, NK cells and macrophages function
cooperatively to eliminate intracellular microbes: Macrophages ingest microbes and produce IL-12, IL-12
activates NK cells to secrete IFN-γ, and IFN-γ in turn
activates the macrophages to kill the ingested microbes.
As discussed in Chapter 6, essentially the same
sequence of reactions involving macrophages and T
lymphocytes is central to the cell-mediated arm of
adaptive immunity.

**The activation of NK cells is determined by a
balance between engagement of activating and
inhibitory receptors** (Fig. 2-11). The activating
receptors recognize cell surface molecules that commonly are expressed on stressed cells, including those
infected with viruses and intracellular bacteria. Other
types of stress that lead to the expression of ligands
for activating receptors are DNA damage and malignant transformation; thus, NK cells function to eliminate irreparably injured and tumor cells. One of the
well-defined activating receptors of NK cells is called
NKG2D; it recognizes molecules that resemble class I
major histocompatibility complex (MHC) proteins
and is expressed in response to many types of cellular
stress. Another activating receptor is specific for IgG
antibodies bound to cells. The recognition of antibody-coated cells results in killing of these cells, a
phenomenon called **antibody-dependent cellular
cytotoxicity (ADCC).** NK cells are the principal
mediators of ADCC. The role of this reaction in antibody-mediated immunity is described in Chapter 8.
Activating receptors on NK cells have signaling subunits that contain **immunoreceptor tyrosine-based
activation motifs (ITAMs)** in their cytoplasmic tails.
ITAMs, which also are present in subunits of lymphocyte antigen receptors, become phosphorylated on
tyrosine residues when the receptors bind their ligands.
The phosphorylated ITAMs bind and promote the
activation of cytoplasmic protein tyrosine kinases, and
these enzymes phosphorylate, and thereby activate,
other substrates in several different downstream signal
transduction pathways, eventually leading to cytotoxic
granule exocytosis and production of IFN-γ.

**The inhibitory receptors of NK cells are specific
for self class I MHC molecules, which are expressed**

FIGURE 2-11 Activating and inhibitory receptors of natural killer (NK) cells. A, Healthy host cells express self class I major histocompatibility complex (MHC) molecules, which are recognized by inhibitory receptors, thus ensuring that NK cells do not attack normal host cells. Note that healthy cells may express ligands for activating receptors (as shown) or may not express such ligands, but they are not attacked by NK cells because they engage the inhibitory receptors. **B,** NK cells are activated by infected cells in which ligands for activating receptors are expressed (often at high levels) and class I MHC expression is reduced so that the inhibitory receptors are not engaged. The result is that the infected cells are killed.

*Figure panel labels:*

(A) Inhibitory receptor engaged

Activating receptor
NK cell
Activating ligand for NK cell
Inhibitory receptor
Self class I MHC–self peptide complex
Normal cell

NK cell not activated; no cell killing

(B) Inhibitory receptor not engaged

NK cell

Virus inhibits class I MHC expression

Virus-infected cell (class I MHC negative)

NK cell activated; killing of infected cell

on all healthy nucleated cells and function to block signaling by activating receptors. (In Chapter 3 we will describe the important function of MHC molecules in displaying peptide antigens to T lymphocytes.) Two major families of NK cell inhibitory receptors are the killer cell immunoglobulin-like receptors (KIRs), so called because they share structural homology with immunoglobulin molecules (described in Chapter 4), and receptors consisting of a protein called CD94 and a lectin subunit called NKG2. Both families of inhibitory receptors contain in their cytoplasmic domains structural motifs called **immunoreceptor tyrosine-based inhibitory motifs (ITIMs),** which become phosphorylated on tyrosine residues when the receptors bind class I MHC molecules. The phosphorylated ITIMs bind and promote the activation of cytoplasmic protein tyrosine phosphatases. These phosphatases remove phosphate groups from the tyrosine residues of various signaling molecules, thereby blocking the activation of NK cells through activating receptors. Therefore, when the inhibitory receptors of NK cells encounter self MHC molecules, the NK cells are shut off (see Fig. 2-11). Many viruses have mechanisms to block expression of

class I molecules in infected cells, which allows them to evade killing by virus-specific CD8+ cytotoxic T lymphocytes (CTLs) (see Chapter 6). When this happens, the NK cell inhibitory receptors are not engaged, and if the virus induces expression of activating ligands at the same time, the NK cells become activated and eliminate the virus-infected cells. The ability of NK cells to protect against infections is enhanced by cytokines secreted by macrophages and dendritic cells that have encountered microbes. Three of these NK-activating cytokines are interleukin-15 (IL-15), type I interferons (IFNs), and IL-12. IL-15 is important for the development and maturation of NK cells, and IFNs and IL-12 enhance the killing functions of NK cells.

The role of NK cells and CTLs in defense illustrates how hosts and microbes are engaged in a constant evolutionary struggle: The host uses CTLs to recognize MHC-displayed viral antigens, viruses shut off MHC expression, and NK cells have evolved to respond to the absence of MHC molecules. Whether the host or the microbe wins this kind of evolutionary struggle will, of course, determine the outcome of the infections. The same principles may apply to the functions of NK cells in eradication of tumors, many of which also attempt to evade CTL-mediated killing by reducing expression of class I MHC molecules.

OTHER CLASSES OF LYMPHOCYTES

Several types of lymphocytes that have some features of T and B lymphocytes also function in the early defense against microbes and may be considered as part of the innate immune system. A unifying characteristic of these lymphocytes is that they express somatically rearranged antigen receptors (like classical T and B cells), but they have limited diversity. As mentioned earlier, **γδ T cells** are present in epithelia. **NK-T cells,** some of which express surface molecules typically found on NK cells, are present in epithelia and lymphoid organs. They recognize microbial lipids bound to a class I MHC–related molecule called CD1. **B-1 cells** are a population of B lymphocytes that are found mostly in the peritoneal cavity and mucosal tissues, where they produce antibodies in response to microbes and microbial toxins that pass through the walls of the intestine. Most of the circulating IgM antibodies found in the blood of normal individuals, called natural antibodies, are the products of B-1 cells, and many of these antibodies are specific for carbohydrates that are present in the cell walls of many bacteria. Another type of B lymphocyte, called **marginal zone B cells,** is present at the edges of lymphoid follicles in the spleen and other organs and also is involved in rapid antibody responses to blood-borne polysaccharide-rich microbes. Thus, these populations of lymphocytes make responses that are characteristic of adaptive immunity (e.g., antibody production) but have features of innate immunity (i.e., rapid responses and limited diversity of antigen recognition).

THE COMPLEMENT SYSTEM

The complement system is a collection of circulating and membrane-associated proteins that are important in defense against microbes. Many complement proteins are proteolytic enzymes, and complement activation involves the sequential activation of these enzymes, sometimes called an enzymatic cascade. The complement cascade may be activated by any of three pathways (Fig. 2-12). The **alternative pathway** is triggered when some complement proteins are activated on

microbial surfaces and cannot be controlled, because complement regulatory proteins are not present on microbes (but are present on host cells). This pathway is a component of innate immunity. The **classical pathway** is triggered after antibodies bind to microbes or other antigens and is thus a component of the humoral arm of adaptive immunity. The **lectin pathway** is activated when a plasma protein, mannose-binding lectin, binds to terminal mannose residues on the surface glycoproteins of microbes. This lectin activates proteins of the classical pathway, but because it is initiated by a microbial product, in the absence of antibody, it is a component of innate immunity. Activated complement proteins function as proteolytic enzymes to cleave other complement proteins, in an enzymatic cascade that can be rapidly amplified. The central component of complement is a plasma protein called C3, which is cleaved by enzymes generated in the early steps. The major proteolytic fragment of C3, called C3b, becomes covalently attached to microbes and is able to activate downstream complement proteins on the microbial surface. The three pathways of complement activation differ in how they are initiated, but they share the late steps and perform the same effector functions.

The complement system serves three functions in host defense. First, C3b coats microbes and promotes the binding of these microbes to phagocytes, by virtue of receptors for C3b that are expressed on the phagocytes. Thus, microbes that are opsonized with complement proteins are rapidly ingested and destroyed by phagocytes. Second, some proteolytic fragments of complement proteins, especially C5a and C3a, are chemoattractants for phagocytes, and they promote leukocyte recruitment (inflammation) at the site of complement activation. Third, complement activation culminates in the formation of a polymeric protein complex that inserts into the microbial cell membrane, disturbing the permeability barrier and causing either osmotic lysis or apoptotic death of the microbe. A more detailed discussion of the activation and functions of complement is presented in Chapter 8, where we consider the effector mechanisms of humoral immunity.

CYTOKINES OF INNATE IMMUNITY

In response to microbes, dendritic cells, macrophages, and other cells secrete cytokines that

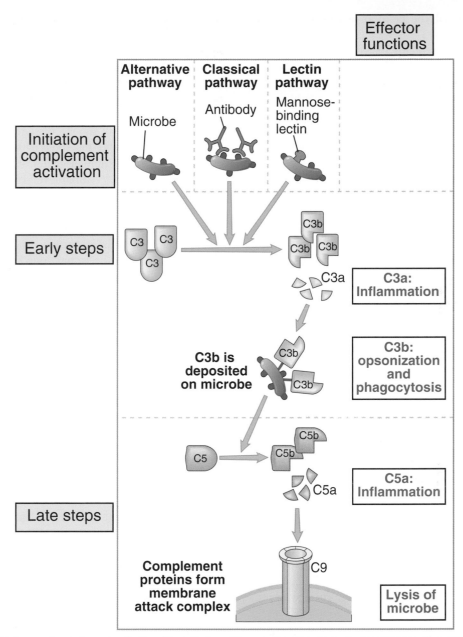

FIGURE 2-12 **Pathways of complement activation.** The activation of the complement system may be initiated by three distinct pathways, all of which lead to the production of C3b (the early steps). C3b initiates the late steps of complement activation, culminating in the production of numerous peptides and polymerized C9 (which forms the membrane attack complex, so called because it creates holes in plasma membranes). The principal functions of proteins produced at different steps are shown. The activation, functions, and regulation of the complement system are discussed in much more detail in Chapter 8.

mediate many of the cellular reactions of innate immunity (Fig. 2-13). As we mentioned earlier, cytokines are soluble proteins that mediate immune and inflammatory reactions and are responsible for communications between leukocytes and between leukocytes and other cells. Most of the molecularly defined cytokines are called **interleukins**, by convention, implying that these molecules are produced by leukocytes and act on leukocytes. (In reality, this is too limited a definition, because many cytokines are produced by or act on cells other than leukocytes, and many cytokines that fulfill these criteria are given other names for historical reasons.) In innate immunity, the principal sources of cytokines are dendritic cells and macrophages activated by recognition of microbes. Binding of bacterial components such as LPS or of viral molecules such as double-stranded RNA to TLRs of dendritic cells and macrophages is a powerful stimulus for cytokine secretion by the cells. Cytokines also are produced in cell-mediated immunity. In this type of adaptive immunity, the major sources of cytokines are helper T lymphocytes (see Chapter 5).

Cytokines are secreted in small amounts in response to an external stimulus and bind to high-affinity receptors on target cells. Most cytokines act on the cells that produce them (autocrine actions) or on adjacent cells (paracrine actions). In innate immune reactions against infections, enough dendritic cells and macrophages may be activated that large amounts of cytokines are produced, and they may be active distant from their site of secretion (endocrine actions).

The cytokines of innate immunity serve various functions in host defense. As discussed earlier in this chapter, TNF, IL-1, and chemokines are the principal cytokines involved in recruiting blood neutrophils and monocytes to sites of infection. At high concentra-tions, TNF promotes thrombus formation on the endothelium and reduces blood pressure by a combination of reduced myocardial contractility and vascular dilatation and leakiness. Severe, disseminated gram-negative bacterial infections sometimes lead to a potentially lethal clinical syndrome called **septic shock,** which is characterized by low blood pressure (the defining feature of shock), disseminated intravascular coagulation, and metabolic disturbances. The early clinical and pathologic manifestations of septic shock are caused by very high levels of TNF, which is produced in response to the bacteria. Dendritic cells and macrophages also produce IL-12 in response to LPS and other microbial molecules. The role of IL-12 in activating NK cells, ultimately leading to macrophage activation, has been mentioned previously. NK cells produce IFN-γ, whose function as a macrophage-activating cytokine also has been described earlier. Because IFN-γ is produced by T cells as well, it is considered a cytokine of both innate immunity and adaptive immunity. In viral infections, dendritic cells, macrophages, and other infected cells produce cytokines called type I interferons, which inhibit viral replication and prevent spread of the infection to uninfected cells. A type I IFN called IFN-α is used clinically to treat chronic viral hepatitis.

OTHER PLASMA PROTEINS OF INNATE IMMUNITY

Several circulating proteins in addition to complement proteins are involved in defense against infections. Plasma mannose-binding lectin (MBL) is a protein that recognizes microbial carbohydrates and can coat microbes for phagocytosis or activate the complement cascade by the lectin pathway. MBL belongs to the collectin family of proteins, which share homology to

---

FIGURE 2-13 Cytokines of innate immunity. A, Dendritic cells and macrophages responding to microbes produce cytokines that stimulate inflammation (leukocyte recruitment) and activate natural killer (NK) cells to produce the macrophage-activating cytokine IFN-γ. **B,** Some important characteristics of the major cytokines of innate immunity are listed. Note that IFN-γ and TGF-β are cytokines of both innate and adaptive immunity and are referred to again in Chapter 5. The name *tumor necrosis factor* (TNF) arose from an experiment showing that a cytokine induced by LPS killed tumors in mice. We now know that this effect is the result of TNF-induced thrombosis of tumor blood vessels, which is an exaggerated form of a reaction seen in inflammation. The name *interferon* arose from the ability of these cytokines to "interfere" with viral infection. IFN-γ is a weak antiviral cytokine compared with the type I IFNs. IFN, interferon; LPS, lipopolysaccharide; MHC, major histocompatibility complex; NK, natural killer; TGF-β, transforming growth factor-β.

(A) **Activation of dendritic cells, macrophages and NK cells**

Microbes

IL-12

IFN-γ

Natural killer cell

Macrophage

TNF, IL-1, chemokines

Inflammation

Neutrophil

Blood vessel

(B)

Cytokine	Principal cell source(s)	Principal cellular targets and biologic effects
Tumor necrosis factor (TNF)	Macrophages, T cells	Endothelial cells: activation (inflammation, coagulation) Neutrophils: activation Hypothalamus: fever Liver: synthesis of acute phase proteins Muscle, fat: catabolism (cachexia) Many cell types: apoptosis
Interleukin (IL-1)	Macrophages, endothelial cells, some epithelial cells	Endothelial cells: activation (inflammation, coagulation) Hypothalamus: fever Liver: synthesis of acute phase proteins T cells: T_H17 differentiation
Chemokines	Macrophages, dendritic cells, endothelial cells, T lymphocytes, fibroblasts, platelets	Leukocytes: Increased integrin affinity, chemotaxis, activation
Interleukin-12 (IL-12)	Dendritic cells, macrophages,	NK cells and T cells: IFN-γ production, increased cytotoxic activity T cells: T_H1 differentiation
Interferon-γ (IFN-γ)	NK cells, T lymphocytes	Activation of macrophages Stimulation of some antibody responses
Type I IFNs (IFN-α, IFN-β)	IFN-α: dendritic cells, macrophages IFN-β: fibroblasts	All cells: anti-viral state, increased class I MHC expression NK cells: activation
Interleukin-10 (IL-10)	Macrophages, dendritic cells, T cells	Macrophages, dendritic cells: inhibition of IL-12 production, reduced expression of costimulators and class II MHC molecules
Interleukin-6 (IL-6)	Macrophages, endothelial cells, T cells	Liver: synthesis of acute phase proteins B cells: proliferation of antibody-producing cells T cells: T_H17 differentiation
Interleukin-15 (IL-15)	Macrophages, others	NK cells: proliferation T cells: proliferation
Interleukin-18 (IL-18)	Macrophages	NK cells and T cells: IFN-γ production
TGF-β	Many cell types	Inhibition of inflammation T cells: differentiation of T_H17, regulatory T cells

collagen and contain a carbohydrate-binding (lectin) domain. Surfactant proteins in the lung also belong to the collectin family and protect the airways from infection. C-reactive protein (CRP) binds to phosphorylcholine on microbes and coats the microbes for phagocytosis by macrophages, which express a receptor for CRP. The circulating levels of many of these plasma proteins increase rapidly after infection. This protective response is called the **acute phase response** to infection.

Innate immune responses to different types of microbes may vary and are designed to best eliminate these microbes. Extracellular bacteria and fungi are combated by phagocytes and the complement system and by acute phase proteins. Defense against intracellular bacteria and viruses is mediated by phagocytes, dendritic cells, and NK cells, with cytokines providing the communications between the leukocytes.

Evasion of Innate Immunity by Microbes

Pathogenic microbes have evolved to resist the mechanisms of innate immunity and are thus able to enter and colonize their hosts (Fig. 2-14). Some intracellular bacteria resist destruction inside phagocytes. *Listeria monocytogenes* produces a protein that enables it to escape from phagocytic vesicles and enter the cytoplasm of infected cells, where it is no longer susceptible to reactive oxygen species and nitric oxide (which are produced mainly in phagolysosomes). The cell walls of mycobacteria contain a lipid that inhibits fusion of vesicles containing ingested bacteria with lysosomes. Other microbes have cell walls that are resistant to the actions of complement proteins. As discussed in Chapters 6 and 8, the same mechanisms enable microbes to resist the effector mechanisms of cell-mediated and humoral immunity, the two arms of adaptive immunity.

Role of Innate Immunity in Stimulating Adaptive Immune Responses

So far we have focused on how the innate immune system recognizes microbes and functions to combat infections. We mentioned at the beginning of this chapter that, in addition to its defense functions, the innate immune response to microbes serves an important warning function by alerting the adaptive immune system that an effective immune response is needed.

Mechanism of immune evasion	Organism (example)	Mechanism
Resistance to phagocytosis	Pneumococci	Capsular polysaccharide inhibits phagocytosis
Resistance to reactive oxygen species in phagocytes	Staphylococci	Production of catalase, which breaks down reactive oxygen intermediates
Resistance to complement activation (alternative pathway)	*Neisseria meningitidis*	Sialic acid expression inhibits C3 and C5 convertases
	Streptococci	M protein blocks C3 binding to organism, and C3b binding to complement receptors
Resistance to antimicrobial peptide antibiotics	*Pseudomonas*	Synthesis of modified LPS that resists action of peptide antibiotics

FIGURE 2-14 **Evasion of innate immunity by microbes.** Selected examples by which microbes may evade or resist innate immunity are shown.

In this final section of the chapter, we summarize some of the mechanisms by which innate immune responses stimulate adaptive immune responses.

Innate immune responses generate molecules that function as "second signals," together with antigens, to activate T and B lymphocytes. In Chapter 1 we introduced the concept that full activation of antigen-specific lymphocytes requires two signals: Antigen itself is "signal 1," and microbes, innate immune responses to microbes, and host cells damaged by microbes all may provide "signal 2" (Fig. 2-15). This requirement for microbe-dependent second signals ensures that lymphocytes respond to infectious agents and not to harmless, noninfectious substances. In experimental situations or for vaccination, adaptive immune responses may be induced by antigens without microbes. In all such instances, the

antigens have to be administered with substances, called **adjuvants,** that elicit the same innate immune reactions as microbes do. In fact, many potent adjuvants are the products of microbes. The nature and mechanisms of action of second signals are described in detail in the discussion of the activation of T and B lymphocytes (see Chapters 5 and 7, respectively). Here it is useful to describe two illustrative examples of second signals that are generated during innate immune reactions.

Microbes (or IFN-γ produced by NK cells in response to microbes) stimulate dendritic cells and macrophages to produce two types of second signals that can activate T lymphocytes (Fig. 2-16A). First, the dendritic cells and macrophages express surface molecules called **costimulators,** which bind to receptors on naive T cells and function together with antigen recognition to activate the T cells. Second, the dendritic cells and macrophages secrete the cytokine IL-12, which stimulates the differentiation of naive T cells into the effector cells of cell-mediated adaptive immunity.

Blood-borne microbes activate the complement system by the alternative pathway (see Fig. 2-16B). One of the proteins produced during complement activation, called C3d, becomes covalently attached to the microbe. When B lymphocytes recognize microbial antigens by their antigen receptors, at the same time the B cells recognize the C3d bound to the microbe by a receptor for C3d. The combination of antigen recognition and C3d recognition initiates the process of B cell differentiation into antibody-secreting cells. Thus, a complement product serves as the second signal for humoral immune responses.

These examples illustrate an important feature of second signals—namely, that these signals not only stimulate adaptive immunity but also guide the nature of the adaptive immune response. Intracellular and phagocytosed microbes need to be eliminated by cell-mediated immunity, the adaptive response mediated by T lymphocytes. Microbes that are encountered and ingested by dendritic cells or macrophages induce the second signals—that is, costimulators and IL-12—that stimulate T cell responses. By contrast, blood-borne microbes need to be combated by antibodies, which are produced by B lymphocytes during humoral immune responses. Blood-borne microbes activate the plasma complement system, which in turn stimulates

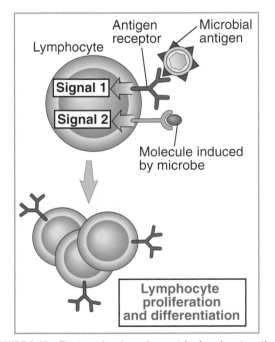

FIGURE 2-15 The two-signal requirement for lymphocyte activation. Antigen recognition by lymphocytes provides signal 1 for the activation of the lymphocytes, and components of microbes or substances produced during innate immune responses to microbes provide signal 2. In this illustration, the lymphocytes could be T cells or B cells. By convention, the major second signals for T cells are called *costimulators* because they function together with antigens to stimulate the cells. The nature of second signals for T and B lymphocytes is described in later chapters.

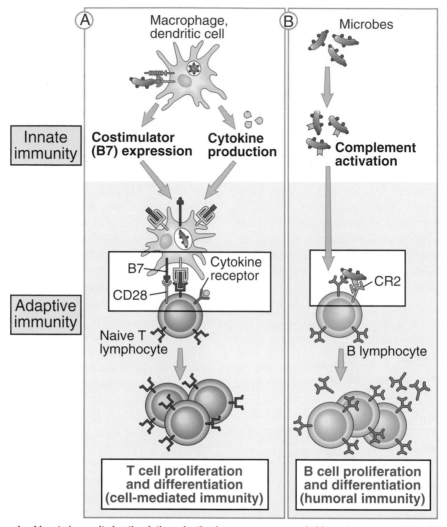

FIGURE 2-16 **The role of innate immunity in stimulating adaptive immune responses. A,** Macrophages respond to phagocytosed microbes by expressing costimulators (e.g., B7 proteins, which are recognized by the CD28 receptor of T cells) and by secreting cytokines (e.g., interleukin-12 [IL-12]). Costimulators and IL-12 function, together with antigen recognition, to activate the T cells. **B,** The complement system is activated by microbes and generates proteins, such as C3d, which become attached to the microbes. B lymphocytes recognize microbial antigens by their antigen receptors and recognize C3d by a receptor called the type 2 complement receptor (CR2). Signals from the antigen receptor and CR2 function cooperatively to activate the B cells. Note that in both examples, the second signals act on lymphocytes that also specifically recognize antigens of microbes, this recognition providing signal 1.

B cell activation and antibody production. Thus, different types of microbes induce different innate immune responses, which then stimulate the types of adaptive immunity that are best able to combat different infectious pathogens.

SUMMARY

■ All multicellular organisms contain intrinsic mechanisms of defense against infections, which constitute innate immunity.

■ The mechanisms of innate immunity respond to microbes and not to nonmicrobial substances, are specific for structures present on various classes of microbes, are mediated by receptors encoded in the germline, and are not enhanced by repeat exposures to microbes.

■ TLRs, which are expressed on plasma membranes and in endosomes of many cell types, are a major class of innate immune system receptors that recognize different microbial products, including bacterial cell wall constituents and viral nucleic acids.

■ The principal components of innate immunity are epithelia, phagocytes, dendritic cells, NK cells, cytokines, and plasma proteins, including the proteins of the complement system.

■ Epithelia provide physical barriers against microbes, produce antibiotics, and contain lymphocytes that may prevent infections.

■ The principal phagocytes, neutrophils and monocytes/macrophages, are blood cells that are recruited to sites of infection, a process mediated by binding to endothelial adhesion molecules that are induced by the cytokines TNF and IL-1, and by responding to soluble chemoattractants, including chemokines, complement fragments, and bacterial peptides.

■ Once at the site of infection, neutrophils and macrophages recognize microbes by several receptors, ingest the microbes for intracellular destruction, secrete cytokines, and respond in other ways that contribute to elimination of microbes and repair of infected tissues.

■ NK cells kill host cells infected by intracellular microbes and produce the cytokine IFN-γ, which activates macrophages to kill phagocytosed microbes.

■ The complement system is a family of proteins that are activated sequentially on encounter with some microbes and by antibodies (in the humoral arm of adaptive immunity). Complement proteins coat (opsonize) microbes for phagocytosis, stimulate inflammation, and lyse microbes.

■ Cytokines of innate immunity function to stimulate inflammation (TNF, IL-1, chemokines), activate NK cells (IL-12), activate macrophages (IFN-γ), and prevent viral infections (type I IFNs).

■ In addition to providing the early defense against infections, innate immune responses provide second signals for the activation of B and T lymphocytes. The requirement for these second signals ensures that adaptive immunity is elicited by microbes (the natural inducers of innate immune reactions) and not by nonmicrobial substances.

REVIEW QUESTIONS

1 *How does the specificity of innate immunity differ from that of adaptive immunity?*

2 *What are examples of microbial substances recognized by the innate immune system, and what are the receptors for these substances?*

3 *What are the mechanisms by which the epithelium of the skin prevents the entry of microbes?*

4 *How do phagocytes ingest and kill microbes?*

5 *What is the role of MHC molecules in the recognition of infected cells by NK cells, and what is the physiologic significance of this recognition?*

6 *What are the roles of the following cytokines in defense against infections: (a) TNF, (b) IL-12, and (c) type I interferon?*

7 *How do innate immune responses enhance adaptive immunity?*

Chapter 3

ANTIGEN CAPTURE AND PRESENTATION TO LYMPHOCYTES

What Lymphocytes See

Adaptive immune responses are initiated when the antigen receptors of lymphocytes recognize antigens. B and T lymphocytes differ in the types of antigens they recognize. The antigen receptors of B lymphocytes—namely, membrane-bound antibodies—can recognize a wide variety of macromolecules (proteins, polysaccharides, lipids, and nucleic acids), as well as small chemicals in soluble or cell surface–associated form. Therefore, B cell–mediated humoral immune responses may be generated against many types of microbial cell wall and soluble antigens. Most T lymphocytes, on the other hand, can see only peptide fragments of protein antigens, and can do so only when these peptides are presented by specialized peptide display molecules on host cells. Therefore, T cell–mediated immune responses may be generated only against the protein antigens of microbes that are associated with host cells. This chapter focuses on the nature of the antigens that are recognized by lymphocytes. Chapter 4 describes the receptors that lymphocytes use to detect these antigens.

The induction of immune responses by antigens is a remarkable process that has to overcome many seemingly insurmountable barriers. The first of these barriers is the low frequency of naive lymphocytes specific for any one antigen, which may be less than 1 in 10^5 lymphocytes. This small fraction of the body's lymphocytes has to locate and react rapidly to the antigen, wherever it is introduced. Second, different kinds of microbes need to be combated by different types of adaptive immune responses. In fact, the immune system has to react in different ways even to the same microbe at different stages of its life. For instance, if a microbe, such as a virus, has entered the circulation and is free in the blood, the immune system needs to produce antibodies that bind the microbe, prevent it from infecting host cells, and help to eliminate it. But after the microbe has infected host cells, it is safe from antibodies, which cannot get inside the cells, so activation of cytotoxic T lymphocytes (CTLs) may be necessary to kill the infected cells and eliminate the reservoir of infection. Thus, we are faced with two important questions:

- How do the rare lymphocytes specific for any microbial antigen find that microbe, especially considering that microbes may enter anywhere in the body?
- How does the immune system produce the effector cells and molecules best able to eradicate a particular type of infection, such as antibodies against extracellular microbes and CTLs to kill infected cells harboring microbes in their cytoplasm?

The answer to both questions is that the immune system has developed a highly specialized system for capturing and displaying antigens to lymphocytes. A large amount of research by immunologists, cell biologists, and biochemists has led to a sophisticated understanding of how protein antigens are captured, broken down, and displayed for recognition by T lymphocytes. This is the major topic of discussion in this chapter. We know less about how antigens are captured for recognition by B lymphocytes. B cells are capable of recognizing many more different types of molecules than are T cells, without the need for specialized processing and often not on the surface of host cells. At the end of the chapter we summarize our limited understanding of how protein and nonprotein antigens are presented to B cells.

Antigens Recognized by T Lymphocytes

The majority of T lymphocytes recognize peptide antigens that are bound to and displayed by major histocompatibility complex (MHC) molecules of antigen-presenting cells (APCs). The MHC is a

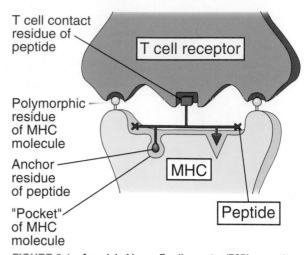

FIGURE 3-1   A model of how a T cell receptor (TCR) recognizes a complex of a peptide antigen displayed by a major histocompatibility complex (MHC) molecule. MHC molecules are expressed on antigen-presenting cells and function to display peptides derived from protein antigens. Peptides bind to the MHC molecules by anchor residues, which attach the peptides to pockets in the MHC molecules. The TCR of every T cell recognizes some residues of the peptide and some (polymorphic) residues of the MHC molecule.

genetic locus whose principal products function as the peptide display molecules of the immune system. In every individual, different clones of T cells can see peptides only when these peptides are displayed by that individual's MHC molecules. This property of T cells is called **MHC restriction.** Thus, each T cell has a dual specificity: The T cell receptor (TCR) recognizes some residues of peptide antigen and also recognizes residues of the MHC molecule that is displaying that peptide (Fig. 3-1). The properties of MHC molecules and the significance of MHC restriction are described later in this chapter. How T cells learn to recognize peptides presented only by self MHC molecules is described in Chapter 4. It should be noted that there are relatively small subpopulations of T cells that recognize lipid and other nonpeptide antigens displayed by nonpolymorphic class I MHC–like molecules.

The specialized cells that capture microbial antigens and display them for recognition by T lymphocytes are called **antigen-presenting cells.** Naive T lymphocytes need to see protein antigens presented by dendritic cells, the most effective "professional" APCs, to initiate clonal expansion and effector cell differentiation. Differentiated effector T cells again need to see antigens, presented by various APCs, to activate the effector functions of the T cells in humoral and cell-mediated immune responses. We first describe the way in which APCs present antigens to trigger immune responses and then examine the role of MHC molecules in these processes.

Capture of Protein Antigens by Antigen-Presenting Cells

Protein antigens of microbes that enter the body are captured mainly by dendritic cells and concen- trated in the peripheral lymphoid organs, where immune responses are initiated (Fig. 3-2). Microbes usually enter the body through the skin (by contact), the gastrointestinal tract (by ingestion), and the respiratory tract (by inhalation). (Some insect-borne microbes may be injected into the bloodstream as a result of insect bites.) All of the interfaces between the body and the external environment are lined by continuous epithelia, whose principal function is to provide a physical barrier to infection. The epithelia and subepithelial tissues contain a network of dendritic cells; the same cells are present in the T cell–rich areas of peripheral lymphoid organs and, in smaller numbers, in most other organs (Fig. 3-3). In the skin, the epidermal dendritic cells are called Langerhans

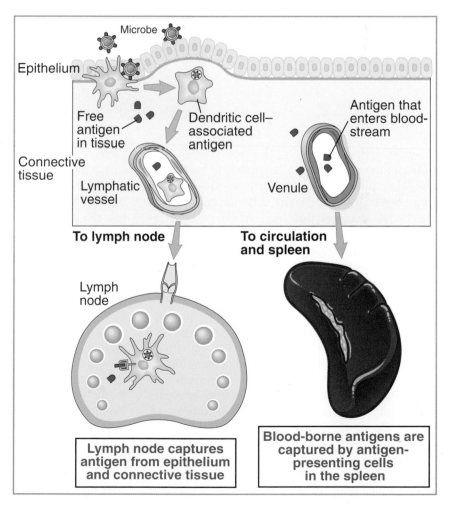

FIGURE 3-2 **The capture and display of microbial antigens.** Microbes enter through an epithelium and are captured by antigen-presenting cells resident in the epithelium, or they enter lymphatic vessels or blood vessels. The microbes and their antigens are transported to peripheral lymphoid organs, the lymph nodes, and the spleen, where protein antigens are displayed for recognition by T lymphocytes.

Ⓐ Dendritic cell (Langerhans cell) in epidermis

Ⓑ Follicle   Dendritic cell in lymph node

FIGURE 3-3 Dendritic cells. A, Immature dendritic cells reside in epithelia, such as the skin, and form a network of cells with interdigitating processes, seen as blue cells on the section of skin immunohistochemically stained with an antibody that recognizes dendritic cells. (The micrograph of the skin is courtesy of Dr. Y-J. Liu, M. D. Anderson Cancer Center, Houston, Texas.) **B,** Mature dendritic cells reside in the T cell–rich areas of lymph nodes (and spleen, not shown) and are seen in the section of a lymph node stained with fluorochrome-conjugated antibodies against dendritic cells (*red*) and B cells in follicles (*green*). (Courtesy of Drs. Kathryn Pape and Jennifer Walter, University of Minnesota Medical School, Minneapolis.)

cells. Epithelial dendritic cells are said to be "immature," because they are inefficient at stimulating T lymphocytes. These immature dendritic cells express membrane receptors that bind microbes, such as receptors for terminal mannose residues on glycoproteins, a typical feature of microbial but not mammalian glycoproteins. Dendritic cells use these receptors to capture and endocytose microbial antigens. Some soluble microbial antigens may enter dendritic cells by pinocytosis. At the same time, microbes stimulate innate immune reactions by binding to Toll-like receptors (TLRs) and other sensors of microbes in the dendritic cells, as well as in epithelial cells and resident macrophages in the tissue (see Chapter 2). This results in production of inflammatory cytokines such as tumor necrosis factor (TNF) and interleukin-1 (IL-1). The combination of the TLR signaling and cytokines activates the dendritic cells, resulting in several changes in phenotype and function.

Activated dendritic cells lose their adhesiveness for epithelia and begin to express the surface receptor

CCR7 that is specific for chemoattracting cytokines (chemokines) produced in the T cell zones of lymph nodes. These chemokines direct the dendritic cells to exit the epithelium and migrate through lymphatic vessels to the lymph nodes draining that epithelium (Fig. 3-4). During the process of migration, the dendritic cells mature from cells designed to capture antigens into APCs capable of stimulating T lymphocytes. This maturation is reflected in increased synthesis and stable expression of MHC molecules, which display antigen to T cells, and of other molecules, called costimulators, that are required for full T cell responses (discussed later in the chapter). Soluble antigens in the lymph are picked up by dendritic cells that reside in the lymph nodes, and blood-borne antigens are handled in essentially the same way by dendritic cells in the spleen.

The net result of this sequence of events is that the protein antigens of microbes that enter the body are transported to and concentrated in the regions of lymph nodes where the antigens are most likely to

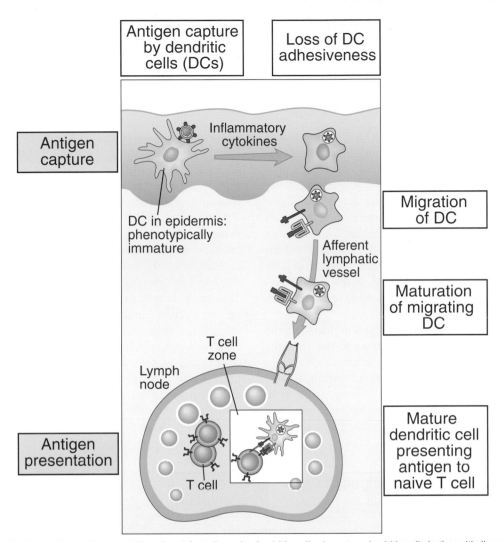

FIGURE 3-4 **The capture and presentation of protein antigens by dendritic cells.** Immature dendritic cells in the epithelium (skin, in the example shown, where the dendritic cells are called Langerhans cells) capture microbial antigens and leave the epithelium. The dendritic cells migrate to draining lymph nodes, being attracted there by chemokines produced in the nodes. During their migration, and probably in response to the microbe, the dendritic cells mature; and in the lymph nodes, the dendritic cells present antigens to naive T lymphocytes. Dendritic cells at different stages of their maturation may express different membrane proteins. Immature dendritic cells express surface receptors that capture microbial antigens, whereas mature dendritic cells express high levels of major histocompatibility complex (MHC) molecules and costimulators, which function to stimulate T cells.

encounter T lymphocytes. Recall that naive T lymphocytes continuously recirculate through lymph nodes and also express CCR7, which promotes their entry into the T cell zones of lymph nodes. Therefore, dendritic cells bearing captured antigen and naive T cells poised to recognize antigens come together in lymph nodes. This process is remarkably efficient; it is esti-

mated that if microbial antigens are introduced at any site in the body, a T cell response to these antigens begins in the lymph nodes draining that site within 12 to 18 hours.

Different types of APCs serve distinct functions in T cell–dependent immune responses. Dendritic cells are the principal inducers of such responses, because these cells are the most potent APCs for activating naive T lymphocytes. Dendritic cells not only initiate T cell responses but may also influence the nature of the response. For instance, various subsets of dendritic cells can direct the differentiation of naive CD4+ T cells into distinct populations that function in defense against different types of microbes (see Chapter 5). Another important type of APC is the macrophage, which is abundant in all tissues. In cell-mediated immune reactions, macrophages phagocytose microbes and display the antigens of these microbes to effector T cells, which activate the macrophages to kill the microbes (see Chapter 6). B lymphocytes ingest protein antigens and display them to helper T cells within lymphoid tissues; this process is important for the development of humoral immune responses (see Chapter 7). As is discussed later in this chapter, all nucleated cells can present antigens derived from microbes in the cytoplasm to CTLs.

Dendritic cells also are involved in initiating the responses of CD8+ T lymphocytes to the antigens of intracellular microbes. The sequence of antigen capture and transport to lymphoid organs is best understood for the presentation of antigens of extracellular microbes to CD4+ T lymphocytes. But some microbes, such as viruses, rapidly infect host cells and can be eradicated only by CTLs destroying the infected cells. The immune system, and especially CD8+ T lymphocytes, must be able to recognize and respond to the antigens of these intracellular microbes. However, viruses may infect any type of host cells, not only dendritic cells, and these infected cells may not produce all of the signals that are needed to initiate T cell activation. How, then, are naive CD8+ T lymphocytes able to respond to the intracellular antigens of infected cells? A likely mechanism is that dendritic cells ingest infected cells and display the antigens present in the infected cells for recognition by CD8+ T lymphocytes (Fig. 3-5). This process is called **cross-presentation** (or cross-priming), to indicate that one cell type, the dendritic cells, can present the antigens of other cells, the infected cells, and prime (or activate) naive T lymphocytes specific for these antigens. The dendritic cells that ingest infected cells may also present microbial antigens to CD4+ helper T lymphocytes. Thus, both classes of T lymphocytes, CD4+ and CD8+ cells, specific for the same microbe are activated close to one another. As we shall see in Chapter 6, this process may be important for the antigen-stimulated differentiation of naive CD8+ T cells to effector CTLs, which often requires help from CD4+ cells. Once the CD8+ T cells have differentiated into CTLs, they kill

FIGURE 3-5   **Cross-presentation of microbial antigens from infected cells by professional antigen-presenting cells (APCs).** Cells infected with intracellular microbes, such as viruses, are ingested (captured) by professional APCs, and the antigens of the infectious microbes are broken down and presented in association with the major histocompatibility complex (MHC) molecules of the APCs. T cells recognize the microbial antigens and co-stimulators expressed on the APCs, and the T cells are activated. In most cases, the term *cross-presentation* (or cross-priming) is applied to CD8+ T cells—cytotoxic T lymphocytes (CTLs)—recognizing class I MHC–associated antigens (as shown); the same cross-presenting APC may display class II MHC–associated antigens from the microbe for recognition by CD4+ helper T cells.

infected host cells without any need for dendritic cells or signals other than recognition of antigen (see Chapter 6).

Now that we know how protein antigens are captured, transported to, and concentrated in peripheral lymphoid organs, the next question is how are these antigens displayed to T lymphocytes? To answer this question, we first need to understand what MHC molecules are and how they function in immune responses.

The Structure and Function of Major Histocompatibility Complex Molecules

MHC molecules are membrane proteins on APCs that display peptide antigens for recognition by T lymphocytes. The MHC was discovered as the genetic locus that is the principal determinant of acceptance or rejection of tissue grafts exchanged between individuals. In other words, individuals that are identical at their MHC locus (inbred animals and identical twins) will accept grafts from one another, and individuals that differ at their MHC loci will reject such grafts. Graft rejection is, of course, not a natural biologic phenomenon, and therefore MHC genes, and the molecules they encode, could not have evolved only

to mediate graft rejection. We now know that the physiologic function of MHC molecules is to display peptides derived from protein antigens to antigen-specific T lymphocytes. This function of MHC molecules is the explanation for the phenomenon of MHC restriction of T cells, which was mentioned earlier.

The collection of genes that make up the MHC locus is found in all mammals (Fig. 3-6) and includes genes that encode MHC and other proteins. Human MHC proteins are called **human leukocyte antigens (HLAs)** because these proteins were discovered as antigens of leukocytes that could be identified with specific antibodies. In all species, the MHC locus contains two sets of highly polymorphic genes, called the class I and class II MHC genes. These genes encode the class I and class II MHC molecules that display peptides to T cells. In addition to the polymorphic genes, the MHC locus contains many nonpolymorphic genes. Some of these nonpolymorphic genes code for proteins involved in antigen presentation, and others code for proteins whose function is not known.

Class I and class II MHC molecules are membrane proteins that each contains a peptide-binding cleft at the amino-terminal end. Although the two classes of molecules differ in subunit composition, they are very similar in overall structure (Fig. 3-7).

FIGURE 3-6 The genes of the major histocompatibility complex (MHC) locus. Schematic maps of the human MHC (called the HLA complex) and the mouse MHC (called the H-2 complex) are shown, illustrating the major genes that code for molecules involved in immune responses. Sizes of genes and intervening DNA segments are not shown to scale. Class II loci are shown as single blocks but each consists of at least two genes. Class III MHC locus refers to genes that encode molecules other than peptide display molecules; this term is not used commonly. There are also multiple class I–like genes and pseudogenes (not shown). HLA, human leukocyte antigen; LT, lymphotoxin; TAP, transporter associated with antigen processing; TNF, tumor necrosis factor.

FIGURE 3-7   The structure of class I and class II major histocompatibility complex (MHC) molecules. The schematic diagrams (at *left*) and models (at *right*) of the crystal structures of class I MHC and class II MHC molecules illustrate the domains of the molecules and the fundamental similarities between them. Both types of MHC molecules contain peptide-binding clefts and invariant portions that bind CD8 (the α3 domain of class I) or CD4 (the β2 domain of class II). β2m, β2-microglobulin; Ig, immunoglobulin. (Crystal structures courtesy of Dr. P. Bjorkman, California Institute of Technology, Pasadena, California.)

Each class I molecule consists of an α chain noncovalently attached to a protein called β_2-microglobulin that is encoded by a gene outside the MHC. The amino-terminal α1 and α2 domains of the class I MHC molecule form a peptide-binding cleft, or groove, that is large enough to accommodate peptides of 8 to 11 amino acids. The floor of the peptide-binding cleft is the region that binds peptides for display to T lymphocytes, and the sides and tops of the cleft are the regions that are contacted by the T cell receptor (which, of course, contacts part of the displayed peptide as well) (see Fig. 3-1). The polymorphic residues of class I molecules, that is, the amino acids that differ among different individuals' MHC molecules, are located in the α1 and α2 domains of the α chain. Some of these polymorphic residues contribute to variations in the floor of the peptide-binding cleft and thus in the ability of different MHC molecules to bind peptides. Other polymorphic residues contribute to variations in the tops of the clefts and thus influence recognition by T cells. The α3 domain is invariant and contains the binding site for the T cell co-receptor CD8. As we shall see in Chapter 5, T cell activation requires recognition of MHC-associated peptide antigen by the TCR and simultaneous recognition of the MHC molecule by the co-receptor. Therefore, CD8+ T cells can only respond to peptides displayed by class I MHC molecules, the MHC molecules to which the CD8 co-receptor binds.

Each class II MHC molecule consists of two chains, called α and β. The amino-terminal regions of both chains, called the α1 and β1 domains, contain polymorphic residues and form a cleft that is large enough to accommodate peptides of 10 to 30 residues. The nonpolymorphic β2 domain contains the binding site for the T cell co-receptor CD4. Because CD4 binds to class II MHC molecules, CD4+ T cells can only respond to peptides presented by class II MHC molecules.

Several features of MHC genes and molecules are important for the normal function of these molecules (Fig. 3-8):

MHC genes are codominantly expressed, meaning that the alleles inherited from both parents are expressed equally. Because there are three polymorphic class I genes, called HLA-A, HLA-B, and HLA-C in humans, and each person inherits one set of these genes from each parent, any cell can express six different class I molecules. In the class II locus, every individual inherits one pair of HLA-DP genes (called DPA1 and DPB1, encoding the α and β chains), one pair of HLA-DQ genes (DQA1 and DQB1, encoding the α and β chains), one HLA-DRα gene (DRA1), and one or two HLA-DRβ genes (DRB1 and DRB3, -4 or -5). Thus, a heterozygous individual can inherit six or eight class II MHC alleles, three or four from each parent (one set each of DP and DQ, and one or two of DR). Because of the extra DRβ genes, and because some DQα molecules encoded on one chromosome can associate with DQβ molecules encoded from the other chromosome, the total number of expressed class II molecules may be considerably more than 6.

The set of MHC alleles present on each chromosome is called an **MHC haplotype.** In humans, each HLA allele is given a numerical designation. For instance, an HLA haplotype of an individual could be HLA-A2, HLA-B5, HLA-DR3, and so on. All heterozygous individuals, of course, have two HLA haplotypes, one from each chromosome.

MHC genes are highly polymorphic, meaning that many different alleles are present among the different individuals in the population. The polymorphism is so great that any two individuals in an outbred population are unlikely to have exactly the same MHC genes and molecules. Because the polymorphic residues determine which peptides are presented by which MHC molecules, the existence of multiple alleles ensures that there are always some members of the population that will be able to present any particular microbial protein antigen. The evolution of MHC polymorphism ensures that a population will be able to deal with the diversity of microbes and will not succumb to a newly encountered or mutated microbe, because at least some individuals will be able to mount effective immune responses to the peptide antigens of these microbes. The variations in MHC molecules (accounting for the polymorphism) result from inheritance of distinct DNA sequences and are not induced by gene recombination (as they are in antigen receptors; see Chapter 4).

Class I molecules are expressed on all nucleated cells, but class II molecules are expressed mainly on dendritic cells, macrophages and B lymphocytes. The physiologic significance of this strikingly different expression pattern is described later in the chapter.

Feature	Significance
Codominant expression: Both parental alleles of each MHC gene are expressed	Increases number of different MHC molecules that can present peptides to T cells
Polymorphic genes: Many different alleles are present in the population	Ensures that different individuals are able to present and respond to different microbial peptides
MHC-expressing cell types: **Class II:** Dendritic cells, macrophages, B cells	CD4+ helper T lymphocytes interact with dendritic cells, macrophages, B lymphocytes
Class I: All nucleated cells	CD8+ CTLs can kill any virus-infected cell

FIGURE 3-8 Properties of major histocompatibility complex (MHC) molecules and genes. Some of the important features of MHC molecules are listed, with their significance for immune responses. CTLs, cytotoxic T lymphocytes.

Class II molecules also are expressed on thymic epithelial cells and endothelial cells and can be induced on other cell types by the cytokine interferon-γ.

The peptide-binding clefts of MHC molecules bind peptides derived from protein antigens and display these peptides for recognition by T cells (Fig. 3-9). There are pockets in the floors of the peptide-binding clefts of most MHC molecules. The side chains of amino acids in the peptide antigens fit into these MHC pockets and anchor the peptides in the cleft of the MHC molecule. Peptides that are anchored in the cleft by these side chains (also called

FIGURE 3-9 Binding of peptides to major histocompatibility complex (MHC) molecules. A, These top views of the crystal structures of MHC molecules show how peptides (in *yellow*) lie on the floors of the peptide-binding clefts and are available for recognition by T cells. (Courtesy of Dr. P. Bjorkman, California Institute of Technology, Pasadena, California.) **B,** The side view of a cut-out of a peptide bound to a class II MHC molecule shows how anchor residues of the peptide hold it in the pockets in the cleft of the MHC molecule. (From Scott CA, Peterson PA, Teyton L, Wilson IA: Crystal structures of two I-Ad-peptide complexes reveal that high affinity can be achieved without large anchor residues. Immunity 8:319-329, 1998. © Cell Press; with permission.) These structures are the basis for the schematic view of peptide recognition by T cells shown in Figure 3-1.

anchor residues) contain some residues that bow upward and are recognized by the antigen receptors of T cells.

Several features of the interaction of peptide antigens with MHC molecules are important for under-

standing the peptide display function of MHC molecules (Fig. 3-10).

Each MHC molecule can present only one peptide at a time, because there is only one cleft, but each MHC molecule is capable of presenting many different peptides. So long as the pockets of the MHC molecule can accommodate the anchor residues of the peptide, that peptide can be displayed by the MHC molecule. Therefore, only one or two residues in a peptide have to fit into an MHC molecule's cleft. Thus, MHC molecules are said to have a "broad" specificity for peptide binding: Each molecule can bind many but not all possible peptides. This feature is essential for the antigen display function of MHC molecules, because each individual has only a few different MHC molecules that must be able to present a vast number and variety of antigens.

MHC molecules bind only peptides and not other types of antigens. This is why MHC-restricted CD4+ T cells and CD8+ T cells can recognize and respond to only protein antigens, the natural source of peptides.

MHC molecules acquire their peptide cargo during their biosynthesis and assembly inside cells. Therefore, MHC molecules display peptides derived from microbes that are inside host cells, and this is why MHC-restricted T cells recognize cell-associated microbes and are the mediators of immunity to intracellular microbes. Of importance, class I MHC molecules acquire peptides from cytosolic proteins and class II molecules from proteins in intracellular vesicles. The mechanisms and significance of these processes are discussed later in the chapter. Only peptide-loaded MHC molecules are stably expressed on cell surfaces. The reason for this is that MHC molecules must assemble both their chains and bound peptides to achieve a stable structure, and "empty" molecules are degraded inside cells. This requirement for peptide binding ensures that only "useful" MHC molecules, that is, those that are displaying peptides, are expressed on cell surfaces for recognition by T cells. Once peptides bind to MHC molecules and are displayed on the cell surface, they stay bound for a long time, even up to days. The slow off-rate ensures that after an MHC molecule has acquired a peptide, it will display the peptide long enough

Feature	Significance	
Broad specificity	Many different peptides can bind to the same MHC molecule	
Each MHC molecule displays one peptide at a time	Each T cell responds to a single peptide bound to an MHC molecule	
MHC molecules bind only peptides	MHC-restricted T cells respond only to protein antigens, and not to other chemicals	Lipids / Carbohydrate sugars / Nucleic acids / Proteins / Peptides
Peptides are acquired during intracellular assembly	Class I and class II MHC molecules display peptides from different cellular compartments	Peptide in endocytic vesicle / $\alpha + \beta +$ Ii / Class II MHC / β_2-microglobulin / α / Cytosolic peptide, transported into ER / Class I MHC
Stable surface expression of MHC molecule requires bound peptide	Only MHC molecules that are displaying peptides are expressed for recognition by T cells	MHC molecule with bound peptide / "Empty" MHC molecule
Very slow off-rate	MHC molecule displays bound peptide for long enough to be located by T cell	β_2-microglobulin / α / Peptide / Days

FIGURE 3-10 Features of peptide binding to major histocompatibility complex (MHC) molecules. Some of the important features of peptide binding to MHC molecules are listed, with their significance for immune responses. ER, endoplasmic reticulum.

to maximize the chance that a particular T cell will find the peptide it can recognize and initiate a response.

In each individual, the MHC molecules can display peptides derived from foreign, that is, microbial, proteins as well as peptides from that individual's own proteins. This inability of MHC molecules to discriminate between foreign antigens and self antigens raises two questions. First, at any time, the quantity of self proteins is certain to be much greater than that of any microbial antigens. Why, then, are the available MHC molecules not constantly occupied by self peptides and unable to present foreign antigens? The likely answer is that new MHC molecules are constantly being synthesized, ready to accept peptides, and they are adept at capturing any peptides that are present in cells. Also, a single T cell may need to see a peptide displayed by only as few as 0.1% to 1% of the approximately 10^5 MHC molecules on the surface of an APC, so that even rare MHC molecules displaying a peptide are enough to initiate an immune response. The second problem is that if MHC molecules are constantly displaying self peptides, why do we not develop immune responses to self antigens, so-called autoimmune responses? The answer to this question is that T cells specific for self antigens are either killed or inactivated; this process is discussed in Chapter 9. Although it seems puzzling that MHC molecules present self peptides, this is actually the key to the normal surveillance function of T cells. Thus, T cells are constantly patrolling the body looking at MHC-associated peptides, not reacting to peptides derived from self proteins but able to respond to rare microbial peptides.

MHC molecules are capable of displaying peptides but not intact microbial protein antigens. It follows that there must be mechanisms for converting naturally occurring proteins into peptides able to bind to MHC molecules. This conversion, called **antigen processing,** is described next.

Processing and Presentation of Protein Antigens

Extracellular proteins that are internalized by specialized APCs (dendritic cells, macrophages, and B cells) are processed in vesicles and displayed by class II MHC molecules, whereas proteins in the cytosol of any nucleated cell are processed in the cytoplasm and displayed by class I MHC molecules (Fig. 3-11). These two pathways of antigen processing involve different cellular organelles and proteins (Fig. 3-12). They are designed to sample all of the proteins present in the extracellular and intracellular environments. The segregation of antigen-processing pathways also ensures that different classes of T lymphocytes recognize antigens from different compartments, as is discussed later.

PROCESSING OF INTERNALIZED ANTIGENS FOR DISPLAY BY CLASS II MAJOR HISTOCOMPATIBILITY COMPLEX MOLECULES

APCs may internalize extracellular microbes or microbial proteins by several mechanisms (Fig. 3-13). Microbes may bind to surface receptors specific for microbial products or to receptors that recognize antibodies or products of complement activation that are attached to the microbes. B lymphocytes internalize proteins that specifically bind to the cells' antigen receptors (see Chapter 7). Some APCs may phagocytose microbes or pinocytose proteins without any specific recognition event. After internalization into APCs by any of these pathways, the microbial proteins enter acidic intracellular vesicles, called endosomes or phagosomes, which may fuse with lysosomes. In these vesicles the proteins are broken down by proteolytic enzymes, generating many peptides of varying lengths and sequences.

APCs constantly synthesize class II MHC molecules in the endoplasmic reticulum (ER). Each newly synthesized class II molecule carries with it an attached protein called the invariant chain, which contains a sequence (called the class II invariant chain peptide [CLIP]) that binds tightly to the peptide-binding cleft of the class II molecule. Thus, the cleft of the newly synthesized class II molecule is occupied. This "inaccessible" class II molecule begins its transport to the cell surface in an exocytic vesicle, which then fuses with the endosomal vesicle containing peptides derived from ingested extracellular proteins. The same endosomal vesicle contains a class II–like protein called DM, whose function is to remove CLIP from the class II MHC molecule. After removal of CLIP, the cleft of the class II molecule becomes

FIGURE 3-11 **Pathways of intracellular processing of protein antigens.** The class II MHC pathway converts protein antigens that are endocytosed into vesicles of antigen-presenting cells into peptides that bind to class II MHC molecules for recognition by CD4+ T cells. The class I MHC pathway converts proteins in the cytoplasm into peptides that bind to class I MHC molecules for recognition by CD8+ T cells. CTL, cytotoxic T lymphocyte; ER, endoplasmic reticulum; MHC, major histocompatibility complex.

available to accept peptides. If the class II MHC molecule is able to bind one of the peptides generated from the ingested proteins, the complex becomes stable and is delivered to the cell surface. If the MHC molecule does not find a peptide it can bind, the empty molecule is unstable and is degraded by proteases in the endosomes. One protein antigen may give rise to many peptides, only a few of which (perhaps only one or two) may bind to the MHC molecules present in the individual. Therefore, only these peptides derived from the intact antigen stimulate immune responses in that individual; such peptides are said to be the **immunodominant epitopes** of the antigen.

PROCESSING OF CYTOSOLIC ANTIGENS FOR DISPLAY BY CLASS I MAJOR HISTOCOMPATIBILITY COMPLEX MOLECULES

Antigenic proteins may be produced in the cytoplasm from viruses that are living inside infected cells, from some phagocytosed microbes that may leak from, or be transported out of, the vesicles into the cytoplasm, and from mutated or altered host genes, as in tumors. All of these proteins, as well as the cell's own nonfunctional cytoplasmic proteins, are targeted for destruction by proteolysis. These proteins are unfolded, covalently tagged with multiple copies of a small peptide called ubiquitin, and "threaded" through a

Feature	Class II MHC Pathway	Class I MHC pathway
Composition of stable peptide-MHC complex	Polymorphic α and β chains, peptide	Polymorphic α chain, β_2-microglobulin, peptide
Types of APCs	Dendritic cells, mononuclear phagocytes, B lymphocytes; some endothelial cells, thymic epithelium	All nucleated cells
Responsive T cells	CD4+ T cells (helper T cells)	CD8+ T cells (CTLs)
Source of protein antigens	Endosomal/lysosomal proteins (mostly internalized from extracellular environment)	Cytosolic proteins (mostly synthesized in the cell; may enter cytosol from phagosomes)
Enzymes responsible for peptide generation	Endosomal and lysosomal proteases (e.g., cathepsins)	Cytosolic proteasome
Site of peptide loading of MHC	Specialized vesicular compartment	Endoplasmic reticulum
Molecules involved in transport of peptides and loading of MHC molecules	Invariant chain, DM	TAP

FIGURE 3-12 Features of the pathways of antigen processing. APCs, antigen-presenting cells; CTL, cytotoxic T lymphocyte; MHC, major histocompatibility complex; TAP, transporter associated with antigen processing.

proteolytic organelle called the proteasome, where the unfolded proteins are degraded by enzymes (Fig. 3-14). Some classes of proteasomes efficiently cleave cytosolic proteins into peptides with the size and sequence properties typical of class I MHC–binding peptides. But the cell faces another challenge: The peptides are in the cytoplasm, while the MHC molecules are being synthesized in the ER, and the two have to come together. This problem is overcome by a specialized transport molecule, called transporter associated with antigen processing (TAP), which is located in the ER membrane. TAP binds peptides

from the cytoplasm and actively pumps them across the ER membrane into the interior of the ER. (This, of course, is the reverse of the normal direction of protein traffic, which is from the site of synthesis in the ER out into the cytoplasm or to the plasma membrane.) Newly synthesized class I MHC molecules are loosely attached to the interior face of the TAP molecule. Thus, as peptides enter the ER, they can be captured by the class I molecules. (Recall that in the ER, the class II MHC molecules are not able to bind peptides because of the invariant chain.) If a class I molecule finds a peptide with the right fit, the complex is

Uptake of extracellular proteins into vesicular compartments of APC

Processing of internalized proteins in endosomal/lysosomal vesicles

Biosynthesis and transport of class II MHC molecules to endosomes

Association of processed peptides with class II MHC molecules in vesicles

Expression of peptide-MHC complexes on cell surface

FIGURE 3-13 The class II major histocompatibility complex (MHC) pathway of processing of internalized vesicular antigens. Protein antigens are ingested by antigen-presenting cells (APCs) into vesicles, where they are degraded into peptides. Class II MHC molecules enter the same vesicles and lose the CLIP peptide that occupies the cleft of newly synthesized class II molecules. These class II molecules are able to bind peptides derived from the endocytosed protein. The DM molecule facilitates the removal of CLIP and subsequent binding of the antigenic peptide. The peptide–class II MHC complexes are transported to the cell surface and are recognized by CD4+ T cells. ER, endoplasmic reticulum.

Production of proteins in the cytosol

Proteolytic degradation of cytosolic proteins

Transport of peptides from cytosol to ER

Assembly of peptide–class I complexes in ER

Surface expression of peptide–class I complexes

Virus

Phagosome

Viral protein synthesis in cytoplasm

Protein antigen of ingested microbe transported to cytosol

Ubiquitinated unfolded protein

Proteasome

Peptides

TAP

Class I MHC α chain

ER

β_2m

Golgi

Exocytic vesicle

CD8

CD8+ T lymphocyte

FIGURE 3-14 **The class I major histocompatibility complex (MHC) pathway of processing of cytosolic antigens.** Proteins enter the cytoplasm of cells either from phagocytosed microbes or from endogenous synthesis by microbes, such as viruses, that reside in the cytoplasm of infected cells. Cytoplasmic proteins are unfolded, ubiquitinated, and degraded in proteasomes. The peptides that are produced are transported by the transporter associated with antigen processing (TAP) into the endoplasmic reticulum (ER), where the peptides may be further trimmed by an ER-resident aminopeptidase and then bind to newly synthesized class I MHC molecules. The peptide–class I MHC complexes are transported to the cell surface and are recognized by CD8+ T cells.

stabilized and transported to the cell surface. During this transport, the class I MHC–peptide complex may intersect endosomes, but now the class I molecule is not available to bind peptides, and, being stable, it is able to resist proteolysis by endosomal proteases. If a class I MHC molecule does not find a peptide in the ER, the molecule becomes unstable and is degraded by proteases.

The co-evolution of microbes and their hosts is well illustrated by the numerous strategies that viruses have developed to block the class I MHC pathway of antigen presentation. These strategies include removing newly synthesized MHC molecules from the ER, inhibiting the transcription of MHC genes, and blocking peptide transport by TAP. By inhibiting the class I MHC pathway, viruses reduce presentation of their own antigens to CD8[+] T cells and are thus able to evade the adaptive immune system. These viral evasion strategies are partly counterbalanced by the ability of natural killer cells of the innate immune system to recognize and kill virally infected cells that have lost class I MHC expression (see Chapter 2). We will discuss the mechanisms of immune evasion by viruses in more detail in Chapter 6.

THE PHYSIOLOGIC SIGNIFICANCE OF MAJOR HISTOCOMPATIBILITY COMPLEX-ASSOCIATED ANTIGEN PRESENTATION

It is expected that such a precisely regulated system for protein antigen processing and presentation plays an important role in stimulating immune responses. In fact, many fundamental features of T cell–mediated immunity are closely linked to the peptide display function of MHC molecules.

The restriction of T cell recognition to MHC-associated peptides ensures that T cells see and respond only to cell-associated antigens. This is partly because MHC molecules are cell membrane proteins and partly because peptide loading and subsequent expression of MHC molecules are dependent on intracellular biosynthetic and assembly steps. In other words, MHC molecules can be loaded with peptides only inside cells, where the antigens of phagocytosed and intracellular pathogens are present. Therefore, T lymphocytes can recognize the antigens of only phagocytosed and intracellular microbes, which are the types of microbes that have to be combated by T cell–mediated immunity.

By segregating the class I and class II pathways of antigen processing, the immune system is able to respond to extracellular and intracellular microbes in different ways that are best able to combat these microbes (Fig 3-15). Extracellular microbes are captured by APCs, including B lymphocytes and macrophages, and are presented by class II molecules, which, of course, are expressed mainly on these APCs (and on dendritic cells). Because of the specificity of CD4 for class II, class II–associated peptides are recognized by CD4[+] T lymphocytes, which function as helper cells. These helper T cells help B lymphocytes to produce antibodies, and they help phagocytes to destroy ingested microbes, thereby activating the two effector mechanisms best able to eliminate extracellular and ingested microbes. Neither of these mechanisms is effective against viruses and other pathogens that survive and replicate in the cytoplasm of host cells. Cytosolic antigens are processed and displayed by class I MHC molecules, which are expressed on all nucleated cells—again, as expected, because all nucleated cells can be infected with some viruses. Class I–associated peptides are recognized by CD8[+] T lymphocytes, which differentiate into CTLs. The CTLs kill the infected cells and eradicate the infection, this being the most effective mechanism for eliminating cytoplasmic microbes. Thus, the nature of the protective immune response to different microbes is optimized by linking several features of antigen presentation and T cell recognition: the pathways of processing of vesicular and cytosolic antigens, the cellular expression of class II and class I MHC molecules, the specificity of CD4 and CD8 co-receptors for class II and class I molecules, and the functions of CD4[+] cells as helper cells and of CD8[+] cells as CTLs. This function of MHC-associated antigen processing pathways is important because T cells themselves cannot distinguish between extracellular and intracellular microbes. In fact, as mentioned at the beginning of this chapter, the same virus can be extracellular early after infection and becomes intracellular once the infection is established. During its extracellular life, it is combated by antibodies and phagocytes activated by helper T cells, but once the virus has found a haven

FIGURE 3-15 **The role of major histocompatibility complex (MHC)-associated antigen presentation in the recognition of microbes by CD4+ and CD8+ T cells. A,** Protein antigens of microbes that are endocytosed from the extracellular environment by macrophages and B lymphocytes enter the class II MHC pathway of antigen processing. As a result, these proteins are recognized by CD4+ helper T lymphocytes, whose functions are to activate macrophages to destroy phagocytosed microbes and activate B cells to produce antibodies against extracellular microbes and toxins. **B,** Protein antigens of microbes that live in the cytoplasm of infected cells enter the class I MHC pathway of antigen processing. As a result, these proteins are recognized by CD8+ cytotoxic T lymphocytes, whose function is to kill infected cells.

in the cytoplasm of cells, it can be eradicated only by CTL-mediated killing of the infected cells. The segregation of class I and class II antigen presentation pathways ensures the correct, specialized immune response against microbes in different locations.

This chapter began with two questions: How do rare antigen-specific lymphocytes find antigens, and how are the appropriate immune responses generated against extracellular and intracellular microbes? Understanding the biology of APCs and the role of MHC molecules in displaying the peptides of protein antigens has provided satisfying answers to both questions, specifically for T cell–mediated immune responses.

FUNCTIONS OF ANTIGEN-PRESENTING CELLS IN ADDITION TO ANTIGEN DISPLAY

APCs not only display peptides for recognition by T cells but, in response to microbes, also express "second signals" for T cell activation. The "two-signal" concept of lymphocyte activation was introduced in Chapters 1 and 2 (see Fig. 2-16), and we will return to this concept when we discuss the responses of T and B cells (see Chapters 5 and 7). Recall that antigen is the necessary signal 1, and signal 2 is provided by microbes or APCs reacting to microbes. Different types of microbial products and innate immune responses may activate APCs to express molecules that are the second signals for lymphocyte activation. For instance, many bacteria produce a substance called lipopolysaccharide (LPS), also called endotoxin. When the bacteria are captured by APCs for presentation of their protein antigens, LPS acts on the same APCs, via a TLR, and stimulates the expression of costimulators and the secretion of cytokines. The costimulators and cytokines act in concert with antigen recognition by the T cell to stimulate the proliferation and differentiation of the T cells.

Antigens Recognized by B Cells and Other Lymphocytes

B lymphocytes use membrane-bound antibodies to recognize a wide variety of antigens, including proteins, polysaccharides, lipids, and small chemicals. These antigens may be expressed on microbial surfaces (e.g., capsular or envelope antigens) or they may be in soluble form (e.g., secreted toxins). B cells differentiate in response to antigen and other signals into cells that secrete antibodies (see Chapter 7). The secreted antibodies enter the circulation and mucosal fluids and bind to the antigens, leading to their neutralization and elimination. The antigen receptors of B cells and the antibodies that are secreted usually recognize antigens in the native conformation, without any requirement for antigen processing or display by a specialized system. Macrophages in lymphatic sinuses may capture antigens that enter lymph nodes and present the antigens, in intact (unprocessed) form, to B lymphocytes in the follicles. However, it is not known if there is a requirement for a specialized population of APCs to present antigens to naive B cells in order to initiate humoral immune responses.

The B cell–rich lymphoid follicles of the lymph nodes and spleen contain a population of cells called follicular dendritic cells (FDCs), whose function is to display antigens to activated B cells. The antigens that FDCs display are coated with antibodies or by complement byproducts such as C3b and C3d. FDCs

use receptors for one end of antibody molecules, called Fc receptors, to bind the antigen-antibody complexes, and receptors for complement proteins, to bind antigens with these proteins attached. These antigens are seen by specific B lymphocytes during humoral immune responses, and they function to select B cells that bind the antigens with high affinity. This process is discussed in Chapter 7.

Although our focus in this chapter has been on peptide recognition by MHC-restricted CD4+ and CD8+ T cells, there are other, smaller populations of T cells that recognize different types of antigens. Natural killer T cells (NK-T cells) are specific for lipids displayed by class I–like CD1 molecules, and γδ T cells recognize a wide variety of molecules, some displayed by class I–like molecules and others apparently requiring no specific processing or display. The functions of these cells and the significance of their unusual specificities are poorly understood.

SUMMARY

■ The induction of immune responses to the protein antigens of microbes is dependent on a specialized system for capturing and displaying these antigens for recognition by the rare naive T cells specific for any antigen. Microbes and microbial antigens that enter the body through epithelia are captured by professional APCs, mainly dendritic cells, located in the epithelia and transported to regional lymph nodes, or are captured by APCs resident in lymph nodes and spleen. The protein antigens of the microbes are displayed by the APCs to naive T lymphocytes that recirculate through the lymphoid organs.

■ Molecules encoded in the MHC perform the function of displaying peptides derived from protein antigens.

■ Proteins that are ingested by APCs from the extracellular environment are proteolytically degraded within the vesicles of the APCs, and the peptides that are generated bind to the clefts of newly synthesized class II MHC molecules. Class II MHC molecules are recognized by CD4, because of which CD4+ helper T cells are specific for class II MHC–associated peptides that are derived mainly from extracellular proteins.

■ Proteins that are produced by microbes living in the cytoplasm of infected cells, or enter the cytoplasm from phagosomes, are degraded by proteasomes, transported into the ER by TAP, and bind to the clefts of newly synthesized class I MHC molecules. Class I MHC molecules are recognized by CD8, because of which CD8[+] cytotoxic T lymphocytes are specific for class I MHC–associated peptides derived from cytosolic proteins.

■ The role of MHC molecules in antigen display ensures that T cells only see cell-associated protein antigens, and the correct type of T cell (helper or cytotoxic cell) responds to the type of microbe that T cell is best able to combat.

■ Microbes activate APCs to express membrane proteins (called costimulators) and to secrete cytokines that provide signals that function in concert with antigens to stimulate specific T cells. The requirement for these second signals ensures that T cells respond to microbial antigens and not to harmless, nonmicrobial substances.

■ B lymphocytes recognize proteins as well as nonprotein antigens, even in their native conformations. It is not known if a specialized system of antigen display is essential for the induction of B cell responses. FDCs display antigens to germinal center B cells and select the high-affinity B cells during humoral immune responses.

REVIEW QUESTIONS

1 When antigens enter through the skin, in what organs are they concentrated? What cell type(s) play important roles in this process of antigen capture?

2 What are MHC molecules? What are human MHC molecules called? How were they discovered, and what is their function?

3 What are the differences between the antigens that are displayed by class I and class II MHC molecules?

4 Describe the sequence of events by which class I and class II MHC molecules acquire antigens for display.

5 Which functional subsets of T cells recognize antigens presented by class I and class II MHC molecules? What molecules on T cells contribute to their specificity for either class I or class II MHC–associated peptide antigens?

Chapter 4

ANTIGEN RECOGNITION IN THE ADAPTIVE IMMUNE SYSTEM

Structure of Lymphocyte Antigen Receptors and the Development of Immune Repertoires

The recognition of antigen is the initiating event in lymphocyte responses. **Specific antigen recognition is the task of two structurally similar types of cell surface receptors of lymphocytes: membrane-bound antibodies on B cells and T cell receptors (TCRs) on T lymphocytes.**

The principal function of cellular receptors in the immune system, as in other biologic systems, is to detect external stimuli (antigens, for the adaptive immune system) and trigger responses of the cells on which the receptors are expressed. To recognize a large number and variety of antigens, the antigen receptors of lymphocytes must be able to bind to and distinguish between many, often closely related, chemical structures. Antigen receptors are clonally distributed, meaning that each clone of lymphocytes having a particular specificity has a unique receptor, different from the receptors of all other clones. (Recall that a clone consists of a parent cell and its progeny.) The total number, or repertoire, of lymphocyte specificities is very large, because the immune system consists of many clones with distinct specificities. Although each clone of B lymphocytes or T lymphocytes recognizes a different antigen, the antigen receptors transmit biochemical signals that are fundamentally the same in all lymphocytes and are unrelated to specificity. These features of lymphocyte recognition and antigen receptors raise two important questions:

67

- How do the antigen receptors of lymphocytes recognize extremely diverse antigens and transmit quite conserved activating signals to the cells?

- How is the vast diversity of receptor structures generated in lymphocytes? The diversity of antigen recognition implies the existence of many structurally different antigen receptor proteins, more than can reasonably be encoded in the inherited genome (germline). Therefore, there must be special mechanisms for generating this diversity.

In this chapter, we describe the structures of the antigen receptors of B and T lymphocytes and how these receptors recognize antigens. We also discuss how the diversity of antigen receptors is generated during the process of lymphocyte maturation, thus giving rise to the repertoire of mature lymphocytes. The process of antigen-induced lymphocyte activation is described in later chapters.

Antigen Receptors of Lymphocytes

The antigen receptors of B and T lymphocytes have several features that are important for the functions of these receptors in adaptive immunity (Fig. 4-1).

The antigen receptors of B and T lymphocytes recognize chemically different structures. B lymphocyte antigen receptors (membrane-bound antibodies) and the antibodies that B cells secrete are able to recognize the shapes, or conformations, of native macromolecules, including proteins, lipids, carbohydrates, and nucleic acids, as well as simple small chemical groups and parts of macromolecules. This broad specificity of B cells for structurally different types of molecules enables antibodies to recognize diverse microbes and toxins in their native form. In striking contrast, most T cells see only peptides, and only when these peptides are displayed on antigen-presenting cells (APCs) bound to membrane proteins encoded in the major histocompatibility complex (MHC) genetic locus. Thus, T cells are able to detect cell-associated microbes (see Chapter 3).

Antigen receptor molecules consist of regions, or domains, that are involved in antigen recognition and, therefore, vary between clones of lymphocytes, and other regions that are required for structural integrity and for effector functions and are relatively conserved among all clones. The antigen-recognizing portions of the receptors are called the **variable (V) regions,** and the conserved portions are the **constant (C) regions.** Even within the V regions, much of the sequence variability is concentrated within short stretches, which are called hypervariable regions, or complementarity-determining regions (CDRs), because they form the parts of the receptor that bind antigens (i.e., they are complementary to the shapes of antigens). By concentrating sequence variation in small regions of the receptor, it is possible to maximize the variability while retaining the basic structures of the receptors. Furthermore, as we will see later in this chapter, there are special genetic mechanisms for introducing variations in the antigen-recognizing regions of these receptors while using a limited set of genes to code for most of the receptor polypeptides.

Antigen receptors are noncovalently attached to other invariant molecules whose function is to deliver to the inside of the cell the activation signals that are triggered by antigen recognition (see Fig. 4-1). Thus, the two functions of lymphocyte receptors for antigen—specific antigen recognition and signal transduction—are mediated by different polypeptides. This again allows variability to be segregated in one set of molecules (the receptors themselves) while leaving the conserved function of signal transduction in other, invariant, proteins. The collection of antigen receptors and signaling molecules in B

FIGURE 4-1 **Properties of antibodies and T cell antigen receptors (TCRs).** Antibodies (also called immunoglobulins) may be expressed as membrane receptors or secreted proteins; TCRs only function as membrane receptors. When immunoglobulin (Ig) or TCR molecules recognize antigens, signals are delivered to the lymphocytes by proteins associated with the antigen receptors. The antigen receptors and attached signaling proteins form the B cell receptor (BCR) and TCR complexes. Note that single antigen receptors are shown recognizing antigens, but signaling requires the cross-linking of two or more receptors by binding to adjacent antigen molecules. The important characteristics of these antigen-recognizing molecules are summarized.

Feature or function	Antibody (Immunoglobulin)	T cell receptor (TCR)
Forms of antigens recognized	Macromolecules (proteins, polysaccharides, lipids, nucleic acids), small chemicals Conformational and linear epitopes	Peptides displayed by MHC molecules on APCs Linear epitopes
Diversity	Each clone has a unique specificity; potential for >10^9 distinct specificities	Each clone has a unique specificity; potential for >10^{11} distinct specificities
Antigen recognition is mediated by:	Variable (V) regions of heavy and light chains of membrane Ig	Variable (V) regions of α and β chains
Signaling functions are mediated by:	Proteins (Igα and Igβ) associated with membrane Ig	Proteins (CD3 and ζ) associated with TCR
Effector functions are mediated by:	Constant (C) regions of secreted Ig	TCR does not perform effector functions

lymphocytes is called the **B cell receptor (BCR) complex,** and in T lymphocytes it is called the **T cell receptor (TCR) complex.** When adjacent antigen receptors of lymphocytes bind to two or more antigen molecules, the receptors are pulled together into an aggregate. This process is called cross-linking, and it brings the associated signaling proteins of the receptor complexes into close proximity. When this happens, enzymes attached to the cytoplasmic portions of the signaling proteins catalyze the phosphorylation of other proteins. Phosphorylation triggers complex signaling cascades that culminate in the transcriptional activation of many genes and the production of numerous proteins that mediate the responses of the lymphocytes. We will return to the processes of T and B lymphocyte activation in Chapters 5 and 7, respectively.

Antibodies may be membrane-bound antigen receptors of B cells or secreted proteins, but TCRs exist only as membrane receptors of T cells. Secreted antibodies are present in the blood and mucosal secretions, where they function to neutralize and eliminate microbes and toxins (i.e., they are the effector molecules of humoral immunity). Antibodies also are called **immunoglobulins (Igs),** referring to immunity-conferring proteins with the characteristic electrophoretic mobility of plasma globulins. Secreted antibodies recognize microbial antigens and toxins by their variable domains just like the membrane-bound antigen receptors of B lymphocytes. The constant regions of some secreted antibodies have the ability to bind to other molecules that participate in the elimination of antigens; these molecules include receptors on phagocytes and proteins of the complement system. Thus, antibodies serve different functions at different stages of humoral immune responses: B cell membrane-bound antibodies recognize antigens to initiate the responses, and secreted antibodies neutralize and eliminate microbes and their toxins in the effector phase of humoral immunity. In cell-mediated immunity, the effector function of microbe elimination is performed by T lymphocytes themselves. The antigen receptors of T cells are involved only in antigen recognition and T cell activation, and these proteins do not mediate effector functions and are not secreted.

With this introduction, we proceed to a description of the antigen receptors of lymphocytes—first antibodies and then TCRs.

ANTIBODIES

An antibody molecule is composed of four polypeptide chains, including two identical heavy (H) chains and two identical light (L) chains, with each chain containing one variable region and one constant region (Fig. 4-2). The four chains are assembled to form a Y-shaped molecule. Each light chain is attached to one heavy chain, and the two heavy chains are attached to each other, all by disulfide bonds. A light chain is made up of one V and one C domain, and a heavy chain has one V and three or four C domains. Each domain folds into a characteristic three-dimensional shape, which is called the immunoglobulin (Ig) domain. An Ig domain consists of two layers of β-pleated sheet held together by a disulfide bridge. The adjacent strands of each β-sheet are connected by short loops, and it is these loops in Ig molecules that are the sites of antigen recognition. Ig domains are present in many other proteins in the immune system as well as outside the immune system, and most of these proteins are involved in sensing signals from the environment and from other cells. All these proteins are said to be members of the Ig superfamily, and they may have evolved from a common ancestral gene.

Each variable region of the heavy chain (called V_H) or of the light chain (called V_L) contains three hypervariable regions, or CDRs. Of these three, the greatest variability is in CDR3, which is located at the junction of the V and C regions. As may be predicted from this variability, CDR3 is also the portion of the Ig molecule that contributes most to antigen binding. Regions of antibody molecules are often named based on the properties of proteolytic fragments of immunoglobulins. The fragment of an antibody that contains a whole light chain (with its single V and C domains) attached to the V and first C domains of a heavy chain contains the portion of the antibody required for antigen recognition and is therefore called Fab (fragment antigen binding). The remaining heavy chain C domains make up the Fc region, with Fc referring to fragment crystalline (so named because this fragment tends to crystallize in solution). In each Ig molecule, there are two identical Fab regions that bind antigen and one Fc region that is responsible for most of the biologic activity and effector functions of the antibodies. (As will be seen

Crystal structure of secreted IgG

FIGURE 4-2 The structure of antibodies: immunoglobulins G (IgG) and M (IgM). Schematic diagrams of a secreted IgG molecule **(A)** and a molecule of a membrane-bound form of IgM **(B)** are shown, illustrating the domains of the heavy and light chains and the regions of the proteins that participate in antigen recognition and effector functions. N and C refer to the amino-terminal and carboxy-terminal ends of the polypeptide chains, respectively. The crystal structure of a secreted IgG molecule **(C)** illustrates the domains and their spatial orientation. In the crystal structure, the heavy chains are colored *blue* and *red,* and the light chains are colored *green;* carbohydrates are shown in *gray.* (Courtesy of Dr. Alex McPherson, University of California, Irvine.)

later, some antibodies exist as multimers of two or five antibody molecules attached to one another.) Between the Fab and Fc regions of most antibody molecules is a flexible portion called the hinge region. The hinge allows the two antigen-binding Fab regions of each antibody molecule to move independently of each other, enabling them to simultaneously bind antigen epitopes that are separated from one another by varying distances. The C-terminal end of the heavy chain may be anchored in the plasma membrane, as seen in B cell receptors, or it may terminate in a tail piece that lacks the membrane anchor so that the antibody is produced as a secreted protein. Light chains are not attached to cell membranes.

There are two types of light chains, called κ and λ, that differ in their C regions but do not differ in function. Each B cell expresses either κ or λ, but not both. There are five types of heavy chains, called μ, δ, γ, ε, and α, that also differ in their C regions. Each type of light chain may complex with any type of heavy chain in an antibody molecule. Antibodies that contain different heavy chains are said to belong to different **isotypes,** or **classes,** and are named according to their heavy chains (i.e., IgM, IgD, IgG, IgE, and IgA), regardless of the light chain class. Each isotype has distinct physical and biological properties and effector functions (Fig. 4-3). The antigen receptors of naive B lymphocytes, which are mature B cells that have not encountered antigen, are membrane-bound IgM and IgD. After stimulation by antigen and helper T lymphocytes, the antigen-specific clone of B lymphocytes may expand and differentiate into progeny that secrete antibodies. Some of the progeny of IgM- and IgD-expressing B cells may secrete IgM, and other progeny of the same B cells may produce antibodies of other heavy chain classes. This change in Ig isotype production is called **heavy chain class** (or **isotype**) **switching;** its mechanism and importance are discussed in Chapter 7. Although heavy chain C regions may switch during humoral immune responses, each clone of B cells maintains its specificity, because the V regions do not change. The light chain class (i.e., κ or λ) also remains fixed throughout the life of each B cell clone.

Antibodies are capable of binding a wide variety of antigens, including macromolecules and small chemicals. The reason for this is that the antigen-binding regions of antibody molecules form flat surfaces capable of accommodating many different shapes (Fig. 4-4). Antibodies bind to antigens by reversible, noncovalent interactions, including hydrogen bonds and charge interactions. The parts of antigens that are recognized by antibodies are called **epitopes,** or **determinants.** Different antigenic determinants may be recognized based on sequence (linear epitopes) or shape (conformational epitopes). Some of these epitopes are hidden within antigen molecules and are exposed as a result of a physicochemical change.

The strength with which one antigen-binding surface of an antibody binds to one epitope of an antigen is called the **affinity** of the interaction. Affinity often is expressed as the dissociation constant (K_d), which is the molar concentration of an antigen required to occupy half the available antibody molecules in a solution; the lower the K_d, the higher the affinity. Most antibodies produced in a primary immune response have a K_d in the range of 10^{-6} to 10^{-9} M, but with repeated stimulation (e.g., in a secondary immune response) the affinity increases to a K_d of 10^{-8} to 10^{-11} M. This increase in antigen-binding strength is called **affinity maturation;** its mechanisms and importance are discussed in Chapter 7. Each IgG, IgD, and IgE antibody molecule has two antigen-binding sites. Secreted IgA is a dimer and therefore has four antigen-binding sites, and secreted IgM is a pentamer, with 10 antigen-binding sites. Therefore, each antibody molecule can bind 2 to 10 epitopes of an antigen, as long as identical epitopes are present sufficiently close together, e.g., on a cell surface, in an aggregated antigen or in some lipids, polysaccharides, and nucleic acids that contain multiple repeated epitopes. The total strength of binding is much greater than the affinity of a single antigen-antibody bond and is called the **avidity** of the interaction. Antibodies produced against one antigen may bind other, structurally similar, antigens. Such binding to similar epitopes is called a **cross-reaction.**

In B lymphocytes, the Ig molecules are noncovalently attached to two other proteins, called Igα and Igβ, that make up the BCR complex. When the Ig receptor recognizes antigen, Igα and Igβ transmit the signals to the interior of the B cell that

Isotype of antibody	Subtypes	H chain	Serum concentr. (mg/mL)	Serum half-life (days)	Secreted form	Functions
IgA	IgA1,2	α(1 or 2)	3.5	6	Monomer, dimer, trimer **IgA (dimer)**	Mucosal immunity
IgD	None	δ	Trace		None	Naive B cell antigen receptor
IgE	None	ε	0.05	2	Monomer **IgE**	Mast cell activation (immediate hypersensitivity) Defense against helminthic parasites
IgG	IgG1-4	γ (1,2,3 or 4)	13.5	23	Monomer **IgG1**	Opsonization, complement activation, antibody-dependent cell-mediated cytotoxicity, neonatal immunity, feedback inhibition of B cells
IgM	None	μ	1.5	5	Pentamer **IgM**	Naive B cell antigen receptor, complement activation

FIGURE 4-3 Features of the major isotypes (classes) of antibodies. The table summarizes some important features of the major antibody isotypes of humans. Isotypes are classified on the basis of their heavy (H) chains; each isotype may contain either κ or λ light chain. The schematic diagrams illustrate the distinct shapes of the secreted forms of these antibodies. Note that IgA consists of two subclasses, called IgA1 and IgA2, and IgG consists of four subclasses, called IgG1, IgG2, IgG3, and IgG4. (IgG subclasses are given different names in other species, for historical reasons; in mice, they are called IgG1, IgG2a, IgG2b, IgG2c, and IgG3.) The serum concentrations are average values in normal individuals.

Antigen

Antigen

FIGURE 4-4   Binding of an antigen by an antibody. This model of a protein antigen bound to an antibody molecule shows how the antigen-binding site can accommodate soluble macromolecules in their native (folded) conformation. The heavy chains of the antibody are *red,* the light chains are *yellow,* and the antigen is colored *blue.* (Courtesy of Dr. Dan Vaughn, Cold Spring Harbor Laboratory, Cold Spring Harbor, NY.)

initiate the process of B cell activation. These and other signals in humoral immune responses are discussed in Chapter 7.

The realization that one clone of B cells makes an antibody of one specificity has been exploited to produce **monoclonal antibodies,** one of the most important technical advances in immunology, with far-reaching implications for clinical medicine and research. To produce monoclonal antibodies, B cells from an animal immunized with an antigen, which have a short lifespan in vitro, are fused with myeloma cells (tumors of plasma cells), which can be propagated indefinitely in tissue culture. The myeloma cell line is mutated to lack an enzyme, because of which it does not grow in the presence of a certain toxic drug, whereas fused cells do grow because the normal B cells provide the enzyme. Thus, by fusing the two cell populations and selecting them by culture with the drug, it is possible to grow out fused cells derived from the B cells and the myeloma, which are called **hybridomas.** From a population of hybridomas, it is possible to select and clone the continuously growing cells that secrete the antibody of desired specificity; such antibodies are monoclonal antibodies. By this means, monoclonal antibodies against virtually any antigen can be produced. Most of these antibodies are

made by fusing cells from immunized mice with mouse myelomas. Such mouse monoclonal antibodies cannot be injected repeatedly into human subjects, because the human immune system sees the mouse Ig as foreign and mounts an immune response against the injected antibodies. This problem has been overcome by retaining the antigen-binding V regions of the mouse monoclonal antibody and replacing the rest of the Ig with human Ig; such "humanized" antibodies are suitable for administration to people. More recently, monoclonal antibodies have been synthesized by using recombinant DNA technology to clone the DNA encoding human antibodies and by selecting antibodies of desired specificity. Another recent approach is to replace the Ig genes of mice with human antibody genes and then immunize these mice with an antigen to produce specific human antibodies. Monoclonal antibodies are now in widespread use as therapeutic and diagnostic reagents for many diseases in humans.

T CELL RECEPTORS FOR ANTIGENS

The TCR for peptide antigen displayed by MHC molecules is a membrane-bound heterodimer composed of an α chain and a β chain, each chain containing one variable (V) region and one constant (C) region (Fig. 4-5). The V and C regions are homologous to immunoglobulin V and C regions. In the V region of each TCR chain there are three hypervariable, or complementarity-determining, regions. As in antibodies, CDR3 is the most variable among different TCRs. The three-dimensional structure of the TCR is very similar to that of the Fab region of an Ig molecule. Unlike in antibodies, both TCR chains are anchored in the plasma membrane, and TCRs are not produced in a secreted form. Also, TCRs do not undergo class switching or affinity maturation during the life of a T cell clone.

Both the α chain and the β chain of the TCR participate in specific recognition of MHC molecules and bound peptides (Fig. 4-6). One of the remarkable features of T cell antigen recognition that has emerged from x-ray crystallographic analyses of TCRs bound to MHC-peptide complexes is that each TCR recognizes as few as one to three residues of the MHC-associated peptide. We also know that only a few peptides of even complex microbes, called the immunodominant epitopes, are actually recognized by the immune system. This means that T cells can tell the difference between complex microbes on the basis of very few amino acid differences between the immunodominant epitopes of the microbes.

From 5% to 10% of T cells in the body express receptors composed of γ and δ chains, which are structurally similar to the αβ TCR but have very different specificities. The γδ TCR may recognize a variety of protein and nonprotein antigens, usually not displayed by classical MHC molecules. T cells expressing γδ TCRs are abundant in epithelia. This observation suggests that γδ T cells recognize microbes that are commonly encountered at epithelial surfaces, but neither the specificity nor the function of these T cells is well established. Another subpopulation of T cells, comprising less than 5% of all T cells, express markers

FIGURE 4-5   The structure of the T cell antigen receptor (TCR). The schematic diagram of the αβ TCR (*left*) shows the domains of a typical TCR specific for a peptide-MHC complex. The antigen-binding portion of the TCR is formed by the Vα and Vβ domains. N and C refer to the amino-terminal and carboxy-terminal ends of the polypeptides. The ribbon diagram (*right*) shows the structure of the extracellular portion of a TCR as revealed by x-ray crystallography. (From Bjorkman PJ. MHC restriction in three dimensions: a view of T cell receptor/ligand interactions. Cell 89:167-170, 1997. © Cell Press; with permission.)

FIGURE 4-6 **The recognition of a peptide-MHC complex by a T cell antigen receptor.** This ribbon diagram is drawn from the crystal structure of the extracellular portion of a peptide-MHC complex bound to a TCR that is specific for the peptide displayed by the MHC molecule. The peptide can be seen attached to the cleft at the top of the MHC molecule, and one residue of the peptide contacts the V region of a TCR. The structure of MHC molecules and their function as peptide display proteins is described in Chapter 3. β_2m, β_2-microglobulin; MHC, major histocompatibility complex; TCR, T cell receptor. (From Bjorkman PJ: MHC restriction in three dimensions: A view of T cell receptor/ligand interactions. Cell 89:167-170, 1997. © Cell Press; with permission.)

of natural killer (NK) cells and are called NK-T cells. NK-T cells express $\alpha\beta$ TCRs, but they recognize lipid antigens displayed by nonpolymorphic class I MHC–like molecules. The functions of NK-T cells also are not well understood.

The TCR recognizes antigen, but it, like membrane Ig on B cells, is incapable of transmitting signals to the T cell. Associated with the TCR is a complex of proteins, called the CD3 and ζ proteins, that make up the TCR complex (see Fig. 4-1). The CD3 and ζ chains transmit some of the signals that are initiated when the TCR recognizes antigen. In addition, T cell activation requires engagement of the coreceptor molecules,

CD4 or CD8, which recognize nonpolymorphic portions of MHC molecules and also transmit activating signals. The functions of these TCR-associated proteins and co-receptors are discussed in Chapter 5.

The antigen receptors of B and T lymphocytes have many similarities, but they also are different in important ways (Fig. 4-7). Antibodies bind the greatest variety of antigens with the highest affinities, which is why antibodies can bind to and neutralize many different microbes and toxins that may be present at low concentrations in the circulation. The affinity of TCRs is low, which is why the binding of T cells to APCs has to be strengthened by additional cell surface adhesion molecules (see Chapter 5).

Development of Immune Repertoires

Now that we know what the antigen receptors of B and T lymphocytes are composed of and how these receptors recognize antigens, the next question that arises is how the enormous diversity of these receptors is produced. As the clonal selection theory predicted, there are many clones of lymphocytes with distinct specificities, perhaps as many as 10^9, and these clones arise before encounter with antigen. There are not enough genes in the human genome for every possible receptor to be encoded by a different gene. In fact, the immune system has developed mechanisms for generating extremely diverse repertoires of B and T lymphocytes, and the generation of diverse receptors is intimately linked to the process of lymphocyte maturation. In the remainder of this chapter we discuss the way in which mature B and T lymphocytes with their highly variable antigen receptors are produced.

MATURATION OF LYMPHOCYTES

The maturation of lymphocytes from bone marrow stem cells consists of three types of processes: proliferation of immature cells, expression of antigen receptor genes, and selection of lymphocytes that express useful antigen receptors (Fig. 4-8). These events are common to B and T lymphocytes, even though B lymphocytes mature in the bone marrow and T lymphocytes mature in the thymus.

Feature	Antigen-binding molecule	
	Immunoglobulin (Ig)	T cell receptor (TCR)
Antigen binding	Made up of three CDRs in V_H and three CDRs in V_L	Made up of three CDRs in $V\alpha$ and three CDRs in $V\beta$
Structure of antigens bound	Linear and conformational determinants of macromolecules and small chemicals	Only 1 to 3 amino acid residues of a peptide and polymorphic residues of an MHC molecule
Affinity of antigen binding	K_d 10^{-7} to 10^{-11} M; average affinity of Igs increases during immune response	K_d 10^{-5} to 10^{-7} M; no change during immune responses
On-rate and off-rate	Rapid on-rate, variable off-rate	Slow on-rate, slow off-rate
Accessory molecules involved in binding	None	CD4 or CD8 simultaneously binds MHC molecule

FIGURE 4-7 **Features of antigen recognition by immunoglobulins (Igs) and T cell antigen receptors (TCRs).** A summary is presented of the important similarities and differences of Ig and TCR molecules, the antigen receptors of B and T lymphocytes, respectively.

Each of the three processes that occur during lymphocyte maturation plays a special role in the generation of the lymphocyte repertoire.

Immature lymphocytes undergo tremendous proliferation at several stages during their maturation. The generation of useful antigen receptor genes is an inefficient process involving random genetic recombination events (discussed later), and the process fails more often than not in the developing lymphocytes. Therefore, the proliferation of developing lymphocytes is necessary to ensure that an adequate number of cells will ultimately express useful antigen receptors and mature into functionally competent lymphocytes. Survival and proliferation of the earliest lymphocyte precursors are stimulated mainly by the growth factor, interleukin-7 (IL-7), which is produced by stromal cells in the bone marrow and the thymus. IL-7 maintains and expands the number of

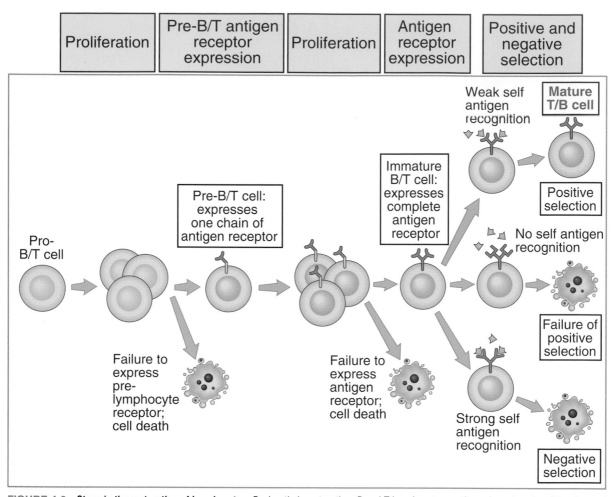

FIGURE 4-8 **Steps in the maturation of lymphocytes.** During their maturation, B and T lymphocytes go through cycles of proliferation and expression of receptor chains by gene recombination. Cells that fail to express useful receptors die by apoptosis, because they do not receive necessary survival signals. At the end of the process, the cells undergo positive and negative selection. The lymphocytes shown may be B or T cells.

lymphocyte progenitors (mainly T cell progenitors in humans, and both B and T cell precursors in mice) before they express antigen receptors, thus generating a large pool of cells in which diverse antigen receptors may be produced. After antigen receptor proteins are expressed, these receptors take over the function of delivering the signals for proliferation, ensuring that only the clones with intact receptors are selected to expand.

Antigen receptors are encoded by several gene segments that are separate from one another in the germline and recombine during lymphocyte maturation. Diversity is generated during this recombination process mainly by varying the nucleotide sequences at the site of recombination. The expression of diverse antigen receptors is the central event in lymphocyte maturation and is described in the next section.

Maturing lymphocytes are selected at multiple steps during their maturation to preserve the useful specificities. Selection is based on the expression of intact antigen receptor components and what they recognize. Prelymphocytes that fail to express antigen receptors die by apoptosis (see Fig. 4-8). Immature T cells are selected to recognize self MHC molecules in the thymus; this process is called **positive selection.** After they mature and enter peripheral tissues, these T cells need to recognize the same MHC molecules to be activated. The basis for positive selection is that antigen receptors on developing lymphocytes recognize MHC molecules in the thymus and deliver signals for the survival and proliferation of the cells, ensuring that cells with the correct (self MHC-restricted) antigen receptors complete the maturation process. Immature B and T lymphocytes are also selected against high-affinity recognition of self antigens present in the bone marrow and thymus, respectively. This process, called **negative selection,** eliminates potentially dangerous lymphocytes that may be capable of reacting against self antigens that are present throughout the body, including in the generative lymphoid organs.

The processes of B and T lymphocyte maturation and selection share some important features but also differ in many respects. We start with the central event that is common to both lineages, namely, the recombination and expression of antigen receptor genes.

PRODUCTION OF DIVERSE ANTIGEN RECEPTORS

The expression of B and T lymphocyte antigen receptors is initiated by somatic recombination of gene segments that code for the variable regions of ·the receptors, and diversity is generated during this process. Hematopoietic stem cells in the bone marrow as well as early lymphoid progenitors contain Ig and TCR genes in their inherited, or germline, configuration. In this configuration, Ig heavy chain and light chain loci and the TCR α chain and β chain loci each contain multiple variable region (V) genes, numbering up to a few hundred, and one or a few constant region (C) genes (Fig. 4-9). Between the V and C genes are several small stretches of nucleotides, which are called joining (J) and diversity (D) gene

segments. (All antigen receptor gene loci contain V, J, and C genes, but only the Ig heavy chain and TCR β loci also contain D gene segments.) The commitment of a lymphocyte progenitor to become a B lymphocyte is associated with recombination of one Ig V_H gene segment with one D and one J segment, the segments being selected randomly (Fig. 4-10). Thus, the committed but still developing B cell now has a recombined V-D-J gene in the heavy chain locus. This gene is transcribed, and in the primary RNA, the VDJ complex is spliced onto the first C region RNA, which happens to encode the μ chain, to form the complete μ mRNA. This μ mRNA is translated to produce the μ heavy chain, which is the first Ig protein synthesized during B cell maturation. A similar sequence of DNA recombination and RNA splicing leads to production of a light chain in B cells and of the TCR α and β chains in T lymphocytes.

The somatic recombination of V and J, or V, D, and J, gene segments is mediated by a group of enzymes collectively called the **VDJ recombinase.** The lymphoid-specific component of the VDJ recombinase, which is composed of the recombinase-activating gene (RAG)-1 and RAG-2 proteins, recognizes DNA sequences that flank all antigen receptor V, D, and J gene segments. As a result of this recognition, the recombinase brings the V, D, and J segments close together and cleaves the DNA at specific sites. The DNA breaks are then repaired by ligases, producing a full-length recombined V-J or V-D-J gene without the intervening DNA segments (see Fig. 4-10). The lymphoid-specific component of the VDJ recombinase is expressed only in immature B and T lymphocytes. Although the same enzymes can mediate recombination of all Ig and TCR genes, intact Ig heavy and light chain genes are expressed only in B cells, and TCR α and β genes are expressed only in T cells. The mechanisms responsible for this lineage specificity of receptor expression are not known.

Diversity of antigen receptors is produced by the use of different combinations of V, D, and J gene segments in different clones of lymphocytes (called combinatorial diversity) and even more by changes in nucleotide sequences introduced at the junctions of V, D, and J gene segments (called junctional diversity) (Fig. 4-11). Combinatorial

FIGURE 4-9   The germline organization of antigen receptor gene loci. In the germline, inherited antigen receptor gene loci contain coding segments (exons, shown as blocks of various sizes) that are separated by segments that are not expressed (introns, shown as *lines*). Each Ig heavy chain constant (C) region and TCR C region consists of multiple exons that encode the domains of the C regions; the organization of the Cμ exon in the Ig heavy chain locus is shown as an example. The diagrams illustrate the antigen receptor gene loci in humans; the basic organization is the same in all species, although the precise order and number of gene segments may vary. The sizes of the segments and the distances between them are not drawn to scale. L, leader sequence (a small stretch of nucleotides that encodes a peptide that guides proteins through the endoplasmic reticulum and is cleaved from the mature proteins); C, constant; D, diversity; J, joining; V, variable.

diversity is limited by the number of available V, D, and J gene segments, but junctional diversity is almost unlimited. This junctional diversity is produced by three types of sequence changes, each of which generates more sequences than are present in the germline genes. First, exonucleases may remove nucleotides from V, D, and J gene segments at the time of recombination, and if the resulting recombined sequences do not contain stop or nonsense codons, many different and new sequences may be produced. Second, a

FIGURE 4-10 Recombination and expression of immunoglobulin (Ig) genes. The expression of an Ig heavy chain involves two gene recombination events (D-J joining, followed by joining of a V region to the DJ complex, with deletion and loss of intervening gene segments). The recombined gene is transcribed, and the VDJ segment is spliced onto the first heavy chain RNA (which is μ), to give rise to the μ mRNA. The mRNA is translated to produce the μ heavy chain protein. The recombination of other antigen receptor genes, that is, the Ig light chain and the TCR α and β chains, follows essentially the same sequence, except that in loci lacking D segments (Ig light chains and TCR α), a V gene recombines directly with a J gene segment. TCR, T cell receptor.

	Immunoglobulin		T cell receptor	
	Heavy chain	κ	α	β
Number of V gene segments	~100	35	54	67
Number of diversity (D) gene segments	27	0	0	2
Number of joining (J) gene segments	6	5	61	4

Mechanism

Combinatorial diversity:

Number of possible V-(D)-J combinations — Ig: ~10^6   TCR: ~3×10^6

Junctional diversity:

Removal of nucleotides

Addition of nucleotides (N-region or P-nucleotides)

Total potential repertoire with junctional diversity — Ig: ~10^11   TCR: ~10^16

FIGURE 4-11   Mechanisms of diversity in antigen receptors. Diversity in immunoglobulins and T cell receptors (TCRs) is produced by random combinations of V, D, and J gene segments, which is limited by the numbers of these segments, and by removal and addition of nucleotides at the V-J or V-D-J junctions, which is almost unlimited. Both mechanisms maximize diversity in the CDR3 regions of the antigen receptor proteins. The estimated contributions of these mechanisms to the potential size of the mature B and T cell repertoires are shown. Also, diversity is increased by the ability of different Ig heavy and light chains, or different TCR α and β chains, to associate in different cells, forming different receptors (not shown). Although the upper limit on the number of Ig and TCR proteins that may be expressed is very large, it is estimated that each individual contains on the order of only 10^7 clones of B cells and T cells with distinct specificities and receptors; in other words, only a fraction of the potential repertoire may actually be expressed. Ig, immunoglobulin. (Adapted from Davis MM, Bjorkman PJ: T-cell antigen receptor genes and T-cell recognition. Nature 334:395-402, 1988. © 1988, Macmillan Magazines Ltd; with permission.)

lymphocyte-specific enzyme called terminal deoxyribonucleotidyl transferase (TdT) catalyzes the random addition of nucleotides that are not parts of germline genes to the sites of V(D)J recombination, forming so-called N regions. Third, during an intermediate stage in the process of V(D)J recombination, before breaks in the DNA are repaired, overhanging DNA sequences may be generated that are then filled in by "P-nucleotides," introducing even more variability at the sites of recombination. As a result of these mechanisms, the nucleotide sequence at the site of V(D)J recombination in antibody or TCR molecules made by one clone of lymphocytes differs from the sequence at the V(D)J site of antibody or TCR molecules made by every other clone. These junctional sequences encode the amino acids of the CDR3 loop, which was mentioned earlier as the most variable of the CDRs and the one most important for antigen recognition. Thus, junctional diversity maximizes the variability in the antigen-binding regions of antibodies and TCRs. In the process of creating junctional diversity, many genes may be produced that cannot code for proteins and are therefore useless. This is a price the immune system pays for generating tremendous diversity. The

risk of producing nonfunctional genes also is why the process of lymphocyte maturation contains several checkpoints at which only cells with useful receptors are selected to survive.

MATURATION AND SELECTION OF B LYMPHOCYTES

The maturation of B lymphocytes occurs mainly in the bone marrow (Fig. 4-12). Progenitors committed to the B cell lineage proliferate, giving rise to a large number of precursors of B cells, called **pro-B cells.** In the next stage of maturation, called **pre-B cells,** Ig genes in the heavy chain locus of one chromosome recombine and give rise to the μ heavy chain protein. Most of this protein remains in the cytoplasm, and cytoplasmic μ is the hallmark of pre-B cells. Some of the μ protein is expressed on the cell surface in association with two other, invariant, proteins that together are called the surrogate light chain, because they resemble light chains and they associate with a heavy chain. The μ chain and surrogate light chain associate with the Igα and Igβ signaling molecules to form the pre-B cell receptor (pre-BCR) complex. It is not clear what, if

	Stem cell	Pro-B	Pre-B	Immature B	Mature B
Ig DNA, RNA	Germline DNA	Germline DNA	Recombined H chain gene (VDJ); μ mRNA	Recombined H chain gene, κ or λ genes; μ and κ or λ mRNA	Alternative splicing of primary transcript to form Cμ and Cδ mRNA
Ig expression	None	None	Cytoplasmic μ and pre-B receptor–associated μ	Membrane IgM (μ+κ or λ light chain)	Membrane IgM and IgD

FIGURE 4-12 Steps in the maturation and selection of B lymphocytes. The maturation of B lymphocytes proceeds through sequential steps, each of which is characterized by particular changes in Ig gene expression and in the patterns of Ig protein expression. At the pro-B cell and pre-B cell stages, failure to express functional antigen receptors (Ig heavy chain and Ig light chain, respectively) results in death of the cells by a default pathway of apoptosis.

anything, the pre-BCR recognizes, and simply the assembly of the components of this complex may deliver signals that promote the survival and proliferation of the cells on which the pre-B cell receptor is expressed. This is the first checkpoint in B cell development, and it selects and expands all the pre-B cells that express a functional μ heavy chain. If the μ chain protein is not produced, perhaps because of faulty recombination of the μ gene, the cell cannot be selected, and it dies by programmed cell death (apoptosis).

The μ protein and the pre-BCR complex signal two other processes. One process shuts off recombination of Ig heavy chain genes on the second chromosome, because of which each B cell can express Ig from only one of the two inherited parental alleles. This process is called **allelic exclusion,** and it helps ensure that each cell can express receptors of a single specificity. A second signal triggers recombination at the Ig light chain locus, first κ and then λ. Whichever functional light chain is produced associates with the μ chain to form the complete membrane-associated IgM antigen receptor. This receptor again delivers signals that promote survival and proliferation, thus preserving and expanding cells that express complete antigen receptors (the second checkpoint during maturation). Signals from the antigen receptor shut off production of the recombinase enzyme and further recombination at unrecombined light chain loci. As a result, each B cell produces either one κ or λ light chain from one of the inherited parental alleles. The presence of two sets of light chain genes simply increases the chance of completing successful gene recombination and receptor expression. The IgM-expressing B lymphocyte is the **immature B cell.** Its further maturation may occur in the bone marrow or after it leaves the bone marrow and enters the spleen. The final maturation step involves coexpression of IgD with IgM, which occurs because the recombined VDJ heavy chain RNA may be spliced onto the Cμ RNA or the Cδ RNA, giving rise to a μ or δ mRNA, respectively. We know that the ability of B cells to respond to antigens develops together with the coexpression of IgM and IgD, but why both classes of receptor are needed is not known. The IgM+IgD+ cell is the **mature B cell,** able to respond to antigen in peripheral lymphoid tissues.

The B cell repertoire is further shaped by negative selection. In this process, if an immature B cell binds an antigen in the bone marrow with high affinity, further maturation is stopped. The B cell either dies by apoptosis, or it may reactivate the V(D)J recombinase enzyme, generate a second light chain, and change the specificity of the antigen receptor (a process called receptor editing). The antigens most commonly found in the bone marrow are self antigens that are abundantly expressed throughout the body (i.e., are ubiquitous), such as blood proteins, and membrane molecules common to all cells. Therefore, negative selection eliminates potentially dangerous cells that can recognize and react against ubiquitous self antigens.

The process of Ig gene recombination is random and cannot be inherently biased toward recognition of microbes, yet the receptors that are produced are able to recognize the antigens of the large number and variety of microbes that the immune system must defend against. It is likely that the repertoire of B lymphocytes is generated randomly, selected positively for expression of intact receptors, and selected negatively against strong recognition of self antigens. What is left after these selection processes is the collection of mature B cells able to recognize all the microbial antigens that may be encountered.

Most mature B cells are follicular B cells. Marginal zone B cells develop from the same progenitors (pro-B cells) as do follicular B cells, whereas B-1 cells may develop earlier and from different precursors. The roles of these B cell subsets in humoral immunity will be described in Chapter 7.

MATURATION AND SELECTION OF T LYMPHOCYTES

The process of T lymphocyte maturation has some unique features, which are largely related to the specificity of different subsets of T cells for peptides displayed by different classes of MHC molecules. T cell progenitors migrate from the bone marrow to the thymus, where the entire process of maturation occurs (Fig. 4-13). The most immature progenitors are called **pro-T cells** or **double-negative T cells** because they do not express CD4 or CD8. These cells expand in number mainly under the influence of IL-7 produced in the thymus. Some of the progeny of double-negative cells undergo TCR β gene recombination, mediated by

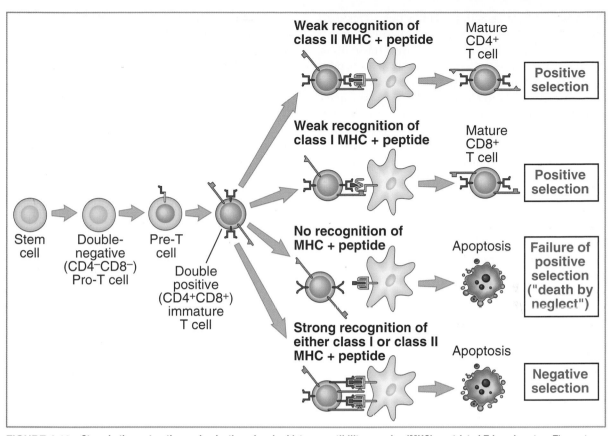

FIGURE 4-13 **Steps in the maturation and selection of major histocompatibility complex (MHC)–restricted T lymphocytes.** The maturation of T lymphocytes in the thymus proceeds through sequential steps that are often defined by the expression of the CD4 and CD8 coreceptors. The TCR β chain is first expressed at the double-negative pre-T cell stage, and the complete TCR is expressed in double-positive cells. Maturation culminates in the development of CD4+ and CD8+ single-positive T cells. As in B cells, failure to express antigen receptors at any stage leads to death of the cells by apoptosis.

the V(D)J recombinase. (The γδ T cells undergo similar recombination involving the TCR γ and δ loci, but they are a distinct lineage, and they will not be discussed further.) If successful VDJ recombination takes place on one chromosome and a β chain protein is synthesized, it is expressed on the surface in association with an invariant protein called pre-Tα, to form the pre-TCR complex of **pre-T cells.** If the complete β chain is not produced in a pro-T cell, that cell dies. The pre-TCR complex delivers intracellular signals in response to assembly alone or the recognition of some unknown ligand. These signals promote survival, proliferation, and TCR α gene recombination, and inhibit VDJ recombination in the second TCR β chain locus (allelic exclusion), much like the signals from the pre-BCR complex in developing B cells. Failure to express the α chain and the complete TCR again results in death of the cell. The surviving cells express both the CD4 and CD8 co-receptors, and these cells are called **double-positive T cells** (or double-positive thymocytes).

Different clones of double-positive T cells express different αβ TCRs. If the TCR of a T cell recognizes an MHC molecule in the thymus, which has to be a self MHC molecule displaying a self peptide, that T cell is selected to survive. T cells that do not recognize an MHC molecule in the thymus die by apoptosis; these T cells would not be useful because they would be incapable of seeing MHC-displayed cell-associated antigens in that individual. This preservation of self MHC–restricted (i.e., useful) T cells is the process of **positive selection.** During this process, T cells whose TCRs recognize class I MHC–peptide complexes preserve the expression of CD8, the coreceptor that binds to class I MHC, and lose expression of CD4, the coreceptor specific for class II MHC molecules. Conversely, if a T cell recognizes class II MHC–peptide complexes, that cell maintains expression of CD4 and loses expression of CD8. Thus, what emerges are **single-positive T cells,** which are either CD8+ class I MHC restricted or CD4+ class II MHC restricted. During positive selection, the T cells also become functionally segregated: The CD8+ T cells are capable of becoming CTLs on activation, and the CD4+ cells are helper cells. How the functional segregation accompanies coreceptor expression is not known.

Immature, double-positive T cells whose receptors strongly recognize MHC-peptide complexes in the thymus undergo apoptosis. This is the process of **negative selection,** and it serves to eliminate T lymphocytes that could react in a harmful way against self proteins that are expressed in the thymus. Some of these self proteins are present throughout the body, and others are tissue proteins that are expressed in thymic epithelial cells by special mechanisms, which are discussed in Chapter 9 in the context of self-tolerance. It may seem surprising that both positive selection and negative selection are mediated by recognition of the same set of self MHC–self peptide complexes in the thymus. (Note that the thymus can contain only self MHC molecules and self peptides; microbial peptides are concentrated in peripheral lymphoid tissues and tend not to enter the thymus.) The likely explanation for these distinct outcomes is that if the antigen receptor of a T cell recognizes a self MHC–self peptide complex with low avidity, the result is positive selection, whereas high-avidity recognition leads to negative selection. High-avidity recognition happens if the self peptide is present in the thymus and if the T cell expresses a TCR that has a high affinity for that self peptide. In such situations, antigen recognition could lead to harmful immune responses against the self antigen, so the T cell has to be eliminated. Low-avidity recognition of self is unlikely to be harmful. As in the case of B cells, the ability to recognize foreign antigens seems to rely on chance: T cells that weakly recognize self antigens in the thymus may strongly recognize and respond to foreign microbial antigens in the periphery.

SUMMARY

■ In the adaptive immune system, the molecules responsible for specific recognition of antigens are antibodies and T cell antigen receptors.

■ Antibodies (also called immunoglobulins) may be produced as membrane receptors of B lymphocytes and as proteins secreted by antigen-stimulated B cells that have differentiated into antibody-secreting plasma cells. Secreted antibodies are the effector molecules of humoral immunity, capable of neutralizing microbes and microbial toxins and eliminating them by activating various effector mechanisms.

■ TCRs are membrane receptors and are not secreted.

■ The core structure of antibodies consists of two heavy chains and two light chains forming a disulfide-linked complex. Each chain consists of a variable (V) region, which is the portion that recognizes antigen, and a constant (C) region, which provides structural stability and, in heavy chains, performs the effector functions of antibodies.

■ T cell receptors consist of an α chain and a β chain. Each chain contains one V region and one C region, and both chains participate in the recognition of antigens, which for most T cells are peptides displayed by MHC molecules.

■ The V regions of Ig and TCR molecules contain hypervariable segments, also called complementarity-determining regions, which are the regions of contact with antigens.

■ The genes that encode antigen receptors consist of multiple segments that are separate in the germline and are brought together during the maturation of lymphocytes. In B cells, the Ig gene segments undergo recombination as the cells mature in the bone marrow, and in T cells the TCR gene segments undergo recombination during maturation in the thymus.

■ Receptors of different specificities are generated in part by different combinations of V, D, and J gene segments. The process of recombination introduces variability in the nucleotide sequences at the sites of recombination by adding or removing nucleotides from the junctions. The result of this introduced variability is the development of a diverse repertoire of lymphocytes, in which clones of cells with different antigen specificities express receptors that differ in sequence and recognition, and most of the differences are concentrated at the regions of gene recombination.

■ During their maturation, lymphocytes undergo alternating cycles of proliferation and antigen receptor expression and traverse several checkpoints at which they are selected such that only cells with complete functional antigen receptors are preserved and expanded. In addition, T lymphocytes are positively selected to recognize peptide antigens displayed by self MHC molecules.

■ Immature lymphocytes that strongly recognize self antigens are negatively selected and prevented from completing their maturation, thus eliminating cells with the potential of reacting in harmful ways against self tissues.

REVIEW QUESTIONS

1 *What are the functionally distinct domains (regions) of antibody and TCR molecules? What features of the amino acid sequences in these regions are important for their functions?*

2 *What are the differences in the types of antigens recognized by antibodies and TCRs?*

3 *What mechanisms contribute to the diversity of antibody and TCR molecules? Which of these mechanisms contributes the most to the diversity?*

4 *What are some of the checkpoints during lymphocyte maturation that ensure survival of the useful cells?*

5 *What is the phenomenon of negative selection, and what is its importance?*

Chapter 5

CELL-MEDIATED IMMUNE RESPONSES

Activation of T Lymphocytes by Cell-Associated Microbes

Cell-mediated immunity is the arm of the adaptive immune response whose role is to combat infections by intracellular microbes. This type of immunity is mediated by T lymphocytes. Two types of infections may lead to microbes finding a haven inside cells, from where they have to be eliminated by cell-mediated immune responses (Fig. 5-1). First, microbes are ingested by phagocytes as part of the early defense mechanisms of innate immunity, but some of these microbes have evolved to resist the microbicidal activities of phagocytes. Many pathogenic intracellular bacteria and protozoa are able to survive, and even replicate, in the vesicles of phagocytes. Some of these phagocytosed microbes may enter the cytoplasm of infected cells and multiply in this compartment, using the nutrients of the infected cells. Cytoplasmic microbes are protected from microbicidal mechanisms, because these mechanisms are confined to vesicular compartments (where they cannot damage the host cells). Second, viruses may bind to receptors on a wide variety of cells and are able to infect and replicate in the cytoplasm of these cells. These cells often do not possess intrinsic mechanisms for destroying the viruses. The elimination of microbes that are able to live in phagocytic vesicles or in the cytoplasm of infected cells is the main function of the T cell arm of adaptive immunity. CD4+ helper T lymphocytes also help B cells to produce antibodies. A common feature of all these reactions is that to perform their functions T lymphocytes have to interact with other cells, which may be phagocytes,

Intracellular microbes	Examples
(A) Phagocyte — Phagocytosed microbes that survive within phagolysosomes — Microbes that escape from phagolysosomes into cytoplasm	Intracellular bacteria: Mycobacteria *Listeria monocytogenes* *Legionella pneumophila* Fungi: *Cryptococcus neoformans* Protozoa: *Leishmania* *Trypanosma cruzi*
(B) Non-phagocytic cell (e.g., epithelial cell) — Virus — Cellular receptor for virus — Microbes that infect nonphagocytic cells	Viruses: All Rickettsiae: All Protozoa: *Plasmodium falciparum* *Cryptosporidium parvum*

FIGURE 5-1 Types of intracellular microbes combated by T cell–mediated immunity. A, Microbes may be ingested by phagocytes and survive within vesicles (phagolysosomes) or escape into the cytoplasm where they are not susceptible to the microbicidal mechanisms of the phagocytes. **B,** Viruses may bind to receptors on many cell types, including nonphagocytic cells, and replicate in the cytoplasm of the infected cells. Some viruses establish latent infections, in which viral proteins are produced in infected cells *(not shown).*

infected host cells, or B lymphocytes. Recall that the specificity of T cells for peptides displayed by major histocompatibility complex (MHC) molecules ensures that the T cells can see and respond to only antigens associated with other cells (see Chapters 3 and 4). This chapter discusses the way in which T lymphocytes are activated by recognition of cell-associated antigens and other stimuli. We address the following questions:

• What signals are needed to activate T lymphocytes, and what cellular receptors are used to sense and respond to these signals?
• How are the few naive T cells specific for any microbe converted into the large number of effector T cells that have specialized functions and the ability to eliminate diverse microbes?
• What molecules are produced by T lymphocytes that mediate their communications with other cells, such as macrophages and B lymphocytes?

After the description of how T cells recognize and respond to the antigens of cell-associated microbes, in

Chapter 6 we will discuss how these T cells function to eliminate the microbes.

Phases of T Cell Responses

The responses of T lymphocytes to cell-associated microbial antigens consist of a series of sequential steps that result in an increase in the number of antigen-specific T cells and the conversion of naive T cells to effector cells (Fig. 5-2). As we have discussed in previous chapters, naive T lymphocytes constantly recirculate through peripheral lymphoid organs searching for foreign protein antigens. Naive T cells express antigen receptors and other molecules that make up the machinery of antigen recognition, but naive lymphocytes are incapable of performing the effector functions required for eliminating microbes. To perform these functions, the naive T cells have to differentiate into effector cells, and this process is initiated by antigen recognition. The protein antigens of microbes are transported from the portals of entry of

| Antigen recognition | Activation | Clonal expansion | Differentiation | | Effector functions |

FIGURE 5-2 Steps in the activation of T lymphocytes. Naive T cells recognize major histocompatibility complex (MHC)-associated peptide antigens displayed on antigen-presenting cells (APCs) and other signals *(not shown)*. The T cells respond by producing cytokines, such as IL-2, and expressing receptors for these cytokines, leading to an autocrine pathway of cell proliferation. The result is clonal expansion of the T cells. Some of the progeny differentiate into effector cells, which serve various functions in cell-mediated immunity, and memory cells, which survive for long periods. (The effector functions of T lymphocytes are described in Chapter 6.) CTL, cytotoxic T lymphocyte; IL-2, interleukin-2; IL-2R, interleukin-2 receptor.

the microbes to the same peripheral lymphoid organs through which naive T cells recirculate. In these organs, the antigens are processed and displayed by MHC molecules on dendritic cells, the antigen-presenting cells (APCs) that are the most efficient stimulators of naive T cells (see Chapter 3). Naive T cells enter lymph nodes from the circulation, and then rapidly move around in the nodes, scanning the surfaces of dendritic cells for the presence of antigen. When a T cell recognizes antigen, the cell transiently stops moving and initiates its activation program. Thus, naive T lymphocytes first encounter protein antigens in the peripheral lymphoid

organs. At the same time as the T cells are seeing antigen, they receive additional signals in the form of microbial products or molecules expressed by APCs during innate immune reactions to the microbes.

On activation by antigen and other stimuli, the antigen-specific T cells begin to secrete **cytokines**, whose multiple functions in cell-mediated immunity are described later in this chapter. Some cytokines stimulate the proliferation of the antigen-specific T cells, resulting in a rapid increase in the number of antigen-specific lymphocytes—a process called **clonal expansion.** A fraction of these activated lymphocytes undergo the process of **differentiation**, which results in the conversion of naive T cells, whose function is to recognize microbial antigens, into a population of effector T cells, whose function is to eliminate microbes. Some effector T cells may remain in the lymph node, where they function to eradicate infected cells in the lymph node or to provide signals to B cells that promote antibody responses against the microbes. Other effector T cells leave the lymphoid organs where they differentiated from naive T cells, enter the circulation, and migrate to any site of infection, where they can eradicate the infection (see Chapter 6). Some of the progeny of the T cells that have proliferated in response to antigen develop into **memory T cells,** which are long-lived and functionally inactive and circulate for months or years, ready to rapidly respond to repeat exposures to the same microbe. As effector T cells eliminate the infectious agent, the stimuli that triggered T cell expansion and differentiation also are eliminated. As a result, the greatly expanded clone of antigen-specific lymphocytes dies, thereby returning the system to its basal resting state. This sequence of events is common to CD4+ T lymphocytes and CD8+ T lymphocytes, although, as we will see later, there are important differences in the properties and effector functions of CD4+ and CD8+ cells.

With this overview, we proceed to a description of the stimuli that are required for T cell activation and regulation. We then describe the biochemical signals that are generated by antigen recognition and are translated into the biologic responses of the lymphocytes. We conclude with a discussion of the functional responses of T cells, and the generation of effector cells that eliminate cell-associated microbes.

Antigen Recognition and Costimulation

The initiation of T cell responses requires multiple receptors on the T cells recognizing ligands on APCs: The TCR recognizes MHC-associated peptide antigens, CD4 or CD8 co-receptors recognize the MHC molecules, adhesion molecules strengthen the binding of T cells to APCs, and receptors for costimulators recognize second signals provided by the APCs (Fig. 5-3). The molecules other than antigen receptors that are involved in T cell responses to antigens sometimes are called **accessory molecules** of T lymphocytes. Accessory molecules are invariant among all T cells. Their functions fall into two categories: signaling and adhesion. Different accessory molecules bind to different ligands, and each of these interactions plays a distinct and complementary role in the process of T cell activation.

RECOGNITION OF MAJOR HISTOCOMPATIBILITY COMPLEX–ASSOCIATED PEPTIDES

The T cell receptor for antigen (the TCR) and the CD4 or CD8 co-receptor together recognize the complex of peptide antigens and MHC molecules on APCs, and this recognition provides the first, or initiating, signal for T cell activation (Fig. 5-4). As we discussed in Chapter 3, when protein antigens are ingested by APCs from the extracellular milieu into vesicles, these antigens are processed into peptides that are displayed by class II MHC molecules. By contrast, protein antigens that are present in the cytoplasm are processed into peptides that are displayed

---

FIGURE 5-3   **Ligand-receptor pairs involved in T cell activation. A,** The major surface molecules of CD4+ T cells involved in the activation of these cells (the receptors), and the molecules on APCs (the ligands) recognized by the receptors, are shown. CD8+ T cells use most of the same molecules, except that the TCR recognizes peptide–class I MHC complexes, and the co-receptor is CD8, which recognizes class I MHC. Immunoreceptor tyrosine-based activation motifs (ITAMs) are the regions of signaling proteins that are phosphorylated on tyrosine residues and become docking sites for other signaling molecules (see Fig. 5-9). CD3 is composed of three polypeptide chains, named δ, ε, and γ, arranged in two pairs (δε and γε); we show CD3 as three protein chains. **B,** The important properties are summarized of the major "accessory" molecules of T cells, so called because they participate in responses to antigens but are not the receptors for antigen. CTLA-4 (CD152) is a receptor for B7 molecules that delivers inhibitory signals; its role in shutting off T cell responses is described in Chapter 9. VLA molecules are integrins involved in leukocyte binding to endothelium (see Fig. 6-3, Chapter 6). APC, antigen-presenting cell; ICAM-1, intercellular adhesion molecule-1; LFA-1, leukocyte function–associated antigen-1; MHC, major histocompatibility complex; TCR, T cell receptor; VLA, very late antigen.

Ⓐ

Receptors of CD4+ helper T lymphocyte

Ligands on class II MHC expressing APC

Signal transduction — CD4

Antigen recognition — TCR

Peptide

Class II MHC

Signal transduction — CD3 — ITAM — ζ — CD28 — B7-1/B7-2

Adhesion — LFA-1 — ICAM-1

Ⓑ

T cell accessory molecule	Function	Ligand	
		Name	Expressed on
CD3	Signal transduction by TCR complex	None	
ζ	Signal transduction by TCR complex	None	
CD4	Signal transduction	Class II MHC	Antigen-presenting cells
CD8	Signal transduction	Class I MHC	Antigen-presenting cells, CTL target cells
CD28	Signal transduction (costimulation)	B7-1/B7-2	Antigen-presenting cells
CTLA-4	Signal transduction (negative regulation)	B7-1/B7-2	Antigen-presenting cells
LFA-1	Adhesion	ICAM-1	Antigen-presenting cells, endothelium
VLA-4	Adhesion	VCAM-1	Endothelium

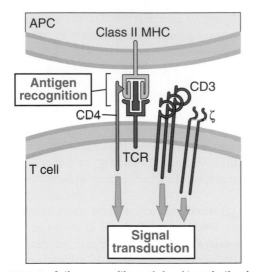

FIGURE 5-4   Antigen recognition and signal transduction during T cell activation. Different T cell molecules recognize antigen and deliver the signal to the interior of the cell as a result of antigen recognition. Note that two or more TCRs need to be cross-linked to initiate signals, but only a single TCR is shown for simplicity. The CD3 and ζ proteins are noncovalently attached to the TCR α and β chains by interactions between charged amino acids in the transmembrane domains of these proteins *(not shown)*. The figure illustrates a CD4+ T cell; the same interactions are involved in the activation of CD8+ T cells, except that the co-receptor is CD8 and the TCR recognizes a peptide-class I MHC complex. APC, antigen-presenting cell; MHC, major histocompatibility complex; TCR, T cell receptor.

by class I MHC molecules. The TCR expressed on most T cells consists of an α chain and a β chain, both of which participate in antigen recognition (see Chapter 4). (A small subset of T cells expresses TCRs composed of γ and δ chains, as discussed in Chapter 4.) The TCR of a peptide antigen–specific T cell recognizes the displayed peptide and simultaneously recognizes residues of the MHC molecule that are located around the peptide-binding cleft. Every mature MHC-restricted T cell expresses either CD4 or CD8, both of which are called co-receptors because they function with the TCR to bind MHC molecules. At the time when the TCR is recognizing the peptide-MHC complex, CD4 or CD8 recognizes the class II or class I MHC molecule, respectively, at a site separate from the peptide-binding cleft. Thus, CD4+ T cells—which function as cytokine-producing helper cells—recog-

nize microbial antigens that are ingested from the extracellular milieu and are displayed by class II MHC molecules, and CD8+ T cells—which function as cytotoxic T lymphocytes (CTLs)—recognize peptides derived from cytoplasmic microbes displayed by class I MHC molecules. The specificity of CD4 and CD8 for different classes of MHC molecules and the distinct pathways of processing of vesicular and cytosolic antigens ensure that the "correct" T cells respond to different microbes (see Fig. 3-15, Chapter 3). Two or more TCRs and co-receptors need to be engaged simultaneously to initiate the T cell response, because only if multiple TCRs and co-receptors are brought together can appropriate biochemical signaling cascades be activated (discussed later in the chapter). Therefore, any one T cell can respond only if it encounters an array of peptide-MHC complexes on an APC. Also, each T cell needs to engage antigen (i.e., MHC-peptide complexes) for a long period, at least several minutes, or multiple times to generate enough biochemical signals to initiate a response. Once these conditions are achieved, the T cell begins its activation program.

The biochemical signals that lead to T cell activation are triggered by a set of proteins that are linked to the TCR to form the TCR complex and by the CD4 or CD8 co-receptor (see Fig. 5-4). Different T cells must possess antigen receptors that are variable enough to recognize diverse antigens and other molecules that serve the conserved signaling roles and do not need to be variable. In lymphocytes, these two types of functions, antigen recognition and signaling, are segregated into different sets of molecules. The TCR recognizes antigens, but it is not able to transmit biochemical signals to the interior of the cell. The TCR is noncovalently associated with a complex of three proteins that make up CD3 and with a homodimer of another signaling protein called the ζ chain. The TCR, CD3, and ζ chain make up the TCR complex. In the TCR complex, the function of antigen recognition is performed by the variable TCR α and β chains, whereas the conserved signaling function is performed by the attached CD3 and ζ proteins. The mechanisms of signal transduction by these proteins of the TCR complex are discussed later in the chapter.

T cells can also be activated experimentally by molecules that bind to the TCRs of many or all clones of

T cells, regardless of the peptide-MHC specificity of the TCR. These polyclonal activators of T cells include antibodies specific for the TCR or associated CD3 proteins, polymeric carbohydrate-binding proteins such as phytohemagglutinin, and certain microbial proteins called superantigens. Polyclonal activators often are used as experimental tools to study T cell responses and in clinical settings to test for T cell function or to prepare metaphase spreads for chromosomal analyses. Microbial superantigens may cause serious disease by inducing excessive cytokine release from many T cells.

ROLE OF ADHESION MOLECULES IN T CELL RESPONSES

Adhesion molecules on T cells recognize their ligands on APCs and stabilize the binding of the T cells to the APCs. Most TCRs bind the peptide-MHC complexes for which they are specific with low affinity. A possible reason for this weak recognition is that T cells are positively selected during their maturation by weak recognition of self antigens, and their ability to recognize foreign microbial peptides is fortuitous and not predetermined (see Chapter 4). (Recall that this type of selection is inevitable, because the thymus, where T cells mature, cannot possibly contain the entire universe of microbial peptides, and the antigens that maturing T cells can encounter in the thymus are self antigens.) To induce a productive response, the binding of T cells to APCs must be stabilized for a sufficiently long period that the necessary signaling threshold is achieved. This stabilization function is performed by adhesion molecules on the T cells whose ligands are expressed on APCs. The most important of these adhesion molecules belong to the family of heterodimeric (two-chain) proteins called **integrins.** The major T cell integrin involved in binding to APCs is leukocyte function–associated antigen-1 (LFA-1), whose ligand on APCs is called intercellular adhesion molecule-1 (ICAM-1).

Integrins play an important role in enhancing T cell responses to microbial antigens. On resting naive T cells, which are cells that have not previously recognized and been activated by antigen, the LFA-1 integrin is in a low-affinity state. If a T cell is exposed to chemokines produced as part of the innate immune response to infection, that T cell's LFA-1 molecules are converted to a high-affinity state and cluster together within minutes (Fig. 5-5). As a result, T cells bind strongly to APCs at sites of infection. Antigen recognition by a T cell also increases the affinity of that cell's LFA-1. Therefore, once a T cell sees antigen, it increases the strength of its binding to the APC presenting that antigen, providing a positive feedback loop. Thus, integrin-mediated adhesion is critical for the ability of T cells to bind to APCs displaying microbial antigens.

Integrins also play an important role in directing the migration of effector T cells from the circulation to sites of infection. This process is described in Chapter 6.

ROLE OF COSTIMULATION IN T CELL ACTIVATION

The full activation of T cells is dependent on the recognition of costimulators on APCs (Fig. 5-6). We have previously referred to costimulators as "second signals" for T cell activation (see Chapters 2 and 3). The name **costimulator** derives from the fact that these molecules provide stimuli to T cells that function together with stimulation by antigen. The best-defined costimulators for T cells are two related proteins called B7-1 (CD80) and B7-2 (CD86), both of which are expressed on APCs and whose expression is greatly increased when the APCs encounter microbes. These B7 proteins are recognized by a receptor called CD28, which is expressed on virtually all T cells. Signals from CD28 on T cells binding to B7 on APCs work together with signals generated by binding of the TCR and co-receptor to peptide-MHC complexes on the same APCs. CD28-mediated signaling is essential for initiating the responses of naive T cells; in the absence of CD28-B7 interactions, engagement of the TCR alone is unable to activate the T cells. The requirement for costimulation ensures that naive T lymphocytes are activated fully by microbial antigens, and not by harmless foreign substances, because, as stated previously, microbes stimulate the expression of B7 costimulators on APCs.

Another set of molecules that participate in increasing costimulatory signals for T cell responses are CD40

FIGURE 5-5 **Regulation of integrin avidity.** Integrins are present in a low-affinity state in resting T cells. Chemokines produced by APCs and signals induced by the TCR when it recognizes antigen both act on integrins and lead to their clustering and to conformational changes that increase the affinity of the integrins for their ligands. As a result, the integrins bind with high avidity to their ligands on APCs and thus promote T cell activation. APC, antigen-presenting cell; TCR, T cell receptor.

ligand (CD154) on the T cells and CD40 on APCs. These molecules do not directly enhance T cell activation. Instead, CD40L expressed on an antigen-stimulated T cell binds to CD40 on APCs and activates the APCs to express more B7 costimulators and to secrete cytokines, such as interleukin-12 (IL-12), that enhance T cell differentiation. Thus, the CD40L-CD40 interaction promotes T cell activation by making APCs better at stimulating T cells.

The role of costimulation in T cell activation explains an old observation that we have mentioned in earlier chapters. Protein antigens, such as those used in vaccines, fail to elicit T cell–dependent immune responses unless these antigens are administered with substances that activate APCs, including dendritic cells and macrophages (and possibly B cells as well). Such substances are called **adjuvants,** and they function mainly by inducing the expression of costimulators on APCs and by stimulating the APCs to secrete cytokines that activate T cells. Most adjuvants are

products of microbes (e.g., killed mycobacteria) or substances that mimic microbes. Thus, adjuvants convert inert protein antigens into mimics of pathogenic microbes.

Understanding the nature and biology of costimulators is an evolving story, and much remains to be learned about the regulation and functions of this family of proteins. These issues are of practical importance because enhancing the expression of costimulators may be useful for stimulating T cell responses (e.g., against tumors), and blocking costimulators may be a strategy for inhibiting unwanted responses. Agents that block B7:CD28 are used in the treatment of rheumatoid arthritis and other inflammatory diseases, and antibodies to block CD40:CD40L interactions are being tested in inflammatory diseases and in transplant recipients to reduce or prevent graft rejection.

Proteins homologous to CD28 also are critical for limiting and terminating immune responses. Thus, different members of the CD28 family are

FIGURE 5-6 **The role of costimulation in T cell activation.** Resting APCs, which have not been exposed to microbes or adjuvants, may present peptide antigens, but they do not express costimulators and are unable to activate naive T cells. As shown by some experimental studies, T cells that recognize antigen without costimulation may become unresponsive to subsequent exposure to antigen; this state of unresponsiveness is called *anergy*. Microbes, and cytokines produced during innate immune responses to microbes, induce the expression of costimulators, such as B7 molecules, on the APCs. The B7 costimulators are recognized by the CD28 receptor on naive T cells, providing "signal 2"; in conjunction with antigen recognition ("signal 1"), this recognition initiates T cell responses. APC, antigen-presenting cell; IL, interleukin.

involved in activating and inhibiting T cells. The prototypes of the inhibitory receptors are CTLA-4, which, like CD28, recognizes B7 on APCs, and PD-1, which recognizes different but related ligands on many cell types. Both are induced in activated T cells, and genetic deletion of these molecules in mice results in excessive lymphocyte expansion and autoimmune disease. CTLA-4 also is involved in inhibiting responses to some tumors, and PD-1 inhibits responses to some infections and allows the infections to become chronic. Many fundamental questions about when these inhibitory pathways become active, how the choice between activation and inhibition is determined, and how these inhibitory receptors work to shut off lymphocytes, remain to be answered.

STIMULI FOR THE ACTIVATION OF CD8+ T CELLS

The activation of CD8+ T cells is stimulated by recognition of class I MHC–associated peptides and requires costimulation and/or helper T cells (Fig. 5-7). The responses of CD8+ T cells have some features that make them different from responses of other T lymphocytes. An unusual feature of CD8+ T cell activation is that its initiation often requires that cytoplasmic antigen from one cell (e.g., a virus-infected cell) has to be cross-presented by dendritic cells (see Fig. 3-5, Chapter 3). Another characteristic of CD8+ T cells is that their differentiation into CTLs may require the concomitant activation of CD4+ helper T cells. When virus-infected cells are ingested by host dendritic cells and the viral

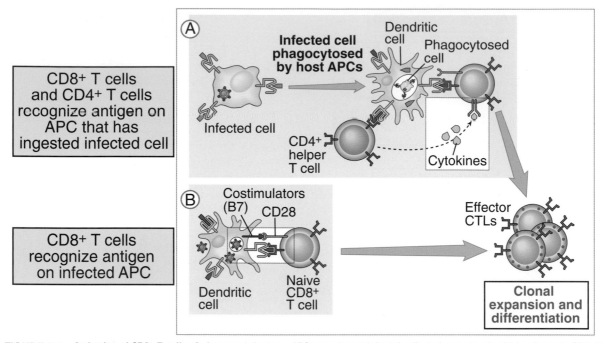

FIGURE 5-7   Activation of CD8+ T cells. A, In some infections, APCs may ingest infected cells and present microbial antigens to CD8+ T cells and to CD4+ helper T cells. The helper T cells then produce cytokines that stimulate the expansion and differentiation of the CD8+ T cells. It also is thought that helper cells may activate APCs to make them competent at stimulating CD8+ T cells *(not shown).* **B,** A CD8+ T cell recognizes class I MHC–associated peptides and receives costimulatory signals if an APC harbors a cytoplasmic microbe. APC, antigen-presenting cell; CTLs, cytotoxic T lymphocytes; MHC, major histocompatibility complex.

antigens are cross-presented by the APCs, the same APC may present antigens from the cytosol in complexes with class I MHC molecules and from vesicles in complex with class II MHC molecules. Thus, both CD8+ T cells and CD4+ T cells specific for viral antigens are activated near one another. The CD4+ T cells may produce cytokines or membrane molecules that help to activate the CD8+ T cells. This requirement for helper T cells in CD8+ T cell responses is the likely explanation for the defective CTL responses to many viruses in patients infected with the human immunodeficiency virus (HIV), which kills CD4+ but not CD8+ T cells. CTL responses to some viruses do not appear to require help from CD4+ T cells, for reasons that are not known.

Now that we have described the stimuli that are required to activate naive T lymphocytes, we next consider the biochemical pathways triggered by antigen recognition and other stimuli.

Biochemical Pathways of T Cell Activation

On recognition of antigens and costimulators, T cells express proteins that are involved in proliferation, differentiation, and effector functions of the cells (Fig. 5-8). Naive T cells that have not encountered antigen (so-called resting cells) have a low level of protein synthesis. Within minutes of antigen recognition, new gene transcription and protein synthesis are seen in the activated T cells. The functions of many of these newly expressed proteins have been mentioned earlier.

The biochemical pathways that link antigen recognition with T cell responses consist of the activation of enzymes, recruitment of adapter proteins, and production of active transcription factors (Fig. 5-9). These biochemical pathways are initiated by physically bringing together multiple TCRs ("cross-linking"), and they occur at or near the TCR com-

FIGURE 5-8 **Proteins produced by antigen-stimulated T cells.** Antigen recognition by T cells results in the synthesis and expression of a variety of proteins, examples of which are shown. The kinetics of production of these proteins are approximations and may vary in different T cells and with different types of stimuli. The possible effects of costimulation on the patterns or kinetics of gene expression are not shown. IFN-γ, interferon-γ; IL, interleukin; IL-2R, IL-2 receptor.

Gene product	Time of expression
Transcription factors 　c-Fos 　c-Myc	Minutes Hours
Membrane effector molecules 　CD40 ligand 　Fas ligand	Hours Hours
Cytokines 　IL-2 　IFN-γ 　IL-4	Hours Hours to days Hours to days
Cytokine receptors 　IL-2R	Hours

eral ring. This ordered redistribution of signaling and adhesion molecules is thought to be responsible for optimal induction of activating signals in the T cell. The region of contact between the APC and T cell, including the redistributed membrane proteins, is called the **immunologic synapse.** Although the synapse was first described as the site of transduction of activating signals, it may serve other functions. Some effector molecules and cytokines may be secreted through this region, ensuring that they do not diffuse away but are targeted to the APC. Enzymes that serve to degrade or inhibit signaling molecules also are recruited to the synapse, so it may be involved in terminating lymphocyte activation.

The clustering of CD4 or CD8 co-receptors activates a protein tyrosine kinase called Lck that is noncovalently attached to the cytoplasmic tails of these co-receptors. As we discussed in Chapter 4 and earlier in this chapter, several transmembrane signaling proteins are associated with the TCR, including the CD3 and ζ chains. CD3 and ζ contain tyrosine-rich motifs, called **immunoreceptor tyrosine-based activation motifs (ITAMs),** that are critical for signaling. Lck, which is carried near the TCR complex by the CD4 or CD8 molecules, phosphorylates tyrosine residues contained within the ITAMs of the ζ and CD3 proteins. The phosphorylated ITAMs of the ζ chain become docking sites for a tyrosine kinase called ZAP-70 (ζ-associated protein of 70 kD), which also is phosphorylated by Lck and thereby made enzymatically active. The active ZAP-70 then phosphorylates various adapter proteins and enzymes, which assemble near the TCR complex and mediate additional signaling events. Three major signaling pathways linked to ζ chain phosphorylation and ZAP-70 are the calcium-NFAT pathway, the Ras/Rac–MAP kinase pathway, and the PKCθ–NF-κB pathway, discussed next.

Nuclear factor of activated T cells (NFAT) is a transcription factor whose activation is dependent on Ca^{2+} ions. The calcium-NFAT pathway is initiated by ZAP-70–mediated phosphorylation and activation of an enzyme called phospholipase Cγ (PLCγ), which catalyzes the hydrolysis of a plasma membrane inositol phospholipid called phosphatidylinositol 4,5-bisphosphate (PIP_2). One byproduct of PLCγ-mediated PIP_2 breakdown, called inositol 1,4,5-triphosphate (IP_3), stimulates release of Ca^{2+} ions from the endoplas-

plexes. Multiple TCRs and co-receptors are brought together when they bind MHC-peptide complexes that are near one another on the surface of APCs. In addition, there is an orderly redistribution of other proteins in both the APC and T cell membranes at the point of cell-to-cell contact, such that the TCR complex, CD4/CD8 co-receptors, and CD28 coalesce to the center and the integrins move to form a periph-

FIGURE 5-9   Signal transduction pathways in T lymphocytes. Antigen recognition by T cells induces early signaling events, which include tyrosine phosphorylation of molecules of the TCR complex and the recruitment of adapter proteins to the site of T cell antigen recognition. These early events lead to the activation of several biochemical intermediates, which in turn activate transcription factors that stimulate transcription of genes whose products mediate the responses of the T cells. The possible effects of costimulation on these signaling pathways are not shown. PLCγ1 refers to the γ1 isoform of phosphatidylinositol-specific phospholipase C. AP-1, activating protein-1; APC, antigen-presenting cell; GTP/GDP, guanosine triphosphate/guanosine diphosphate; ITAM, immunoreceptor tyrosine-based activation motif; NFAT, nuclear factor of activated T cells; PKC, protein kinase C; TCR, T cell receptor.

mic reticulum, thereby raising the cytoplasmic Ca^{2+} concentration. In response to the elevated calcium, a plasma membrane calcium channel is opened, leading to the influx of extracellular Ca^{2+} into the cell, which sustains the elevated Ca^{2+} concentration for hours. Cytoplasmic Ca^{2+} binds a protein called calmodulin, and the Ca^{2+}–calmodulin complex activates a phosphatase called calcineurin. This enzyme removes phosphates from NFAT, which resides in the cytoplasm. Once dephosphorylated, NFAT is able to migrate into the nucleus, where it binds to and activates the promoters of several genes, including the genes encoding the T cell growth factor interleukin-2 (IL-2) and components of the IL-2 receptor. A drug called **cyclosporine** binds to and inhibits the activity of calcineurin and thus inhibits the production of cytokines by T cells.

This agent is widely used as an immunosuppressive drug to prevent graft rejection; its introduction was one of the major factors in the success of organ transplantation (see Chapter 10).

The **Ras/Rac–MAP kinase pathways** include the guanosine triphosphate (GTP) binding Ras and Rac proteins, several adapter proteins, and a cascade of enzymes that eventually activate one of a family of mitogen-activated protein (MAP) kinases. These pathways are initiated by ZAP-70–dependent phosphorylation and accumulation of adapter proteins at the plasma membrane, leading to the recruitment of Ras or Rac, and their activation by exchange of bound guanosine diphosphate (GDP) with GTP. Ras•GTP and Rac•GTP initiate different enzyme cascades, leading to the activation of distinct MAP kinases. The terminal MAP kinases in these pathways, called extracellular signal–regulated kinase (ERK) and c-Jun amino-terminal (N-terminal) kinase (JNK), promote the expression of a protein called c-Fos and the phosphorylation of another protein called c-Jun. c-Fos and phosphorylated c-Jun combine to form the transcription factor AP-1 (activating protein-1), which enhances the transcription of several T cell genes.

The third major pathway involved in TCR signaling consists of activation of the θ isoform of the serine-threonine kinase called **protein kinase C (PKCθ)** and activation of the transcription factor **nuclear factor-κB (NF-κB)**. PKC is activated by diacylglycerol, which, like IP$_3$, is generated by phospholipase C–mediated hydrolysis of membrane inositol lipids. PKCθ acts via adapter proteins that are recruited to the TCR complex to activate NF-κB. NF-κB exists in the cytoplasm of resting T cells in an inactive form, bound to an inhibitor called IκB. TCR-induced signals, downstream of PKCθ, activate a kinase that phosphorylates IκB and targets it for destruction. As a result, NF-κB is released and moves to the nucleus, where it promotes the transcription of several genes.

A fourth pathway of signal transduction involves a lipid kinase called **phosphatidylinositol-3 (PI-3) kinase,** which phosphorylates membrane PIP$_2$ to generate PIP$_3$. This phospholipid ultimately activates a serine-threonine kinase called Akt, which has many roles, including stimulating expression of anti-apoptotic proteins and thus promoting survival of antigen-stimulated T cells. The PI-3 kinase/Akt pathway is triggered not only by the TCR but also by CD28 and IL-2 receptors.

The various transcription factors we have mentioned, including NFAT, AP-1, and NF-κB, stimulate transcription and subsequent production of cytokines, cytokine receptors, cell cycle inducers, and effector molecules such as CD40L (see Fig. 5-8). All of these signals are initiated by antigen recognition, because binding of the TCR and co-receptors to antigen (peptide-MHC complexes) is necessary to assemble the signaling molecules and initiate their enzymatic activity.

As stated earlier, recognition of costimulators, such as B7 molecules, by their receptor (i.e., CD28) is essential for full T cell responses. The biochemical signals transduced by CD28 on binding to B7 costimulators are less defined than are TCR-triggered signals. It is likely that CD28 engagement amplifies some TCR signals and initiates a distinct set of signals that complement TCR signals.

Now that we have described the stimuli and biochemical pathways in T cell activation, we end with a discussion of how T cells respond to antigens and differentiate into effector cells capable of combating microbes.

Functional Responses of T Lymphocytes to Antigen and Costimulation

The recognition of antigen and costimulators by T cells initiates an orchestrated set of responses that culminate in the expansion of the antigen-specific clones of lymphocytes and the differentiation of the naive T cells into effector cells and memory cells (see Fig. 5-2). Many of the responses of T cells are mediated by cytokines that are secreted by the T cells and act on the T cells themselves and on many other cells involved in immune defenses. In the following section each component of the biologic responses of T cells is discussed.

SECRETION OF CYTOKINES AND EXPRESSION OF CYTOKINE RECEPTORS

In response to antigen and costimulators, T lymphocytes, especially CD4$^+$ T cells, rapidly secrete

Ⓐ General properties of cytokines

Property	Mechanism
Produced transiently in response to antigen	TCR signal and costimulation induce cytokine gene transcription
Usually acts on same call that produces the cytokine (autocrine) or nearby cells (paracrine)	T cell activation induces expression of both cytokines and high-affinity receptors for cytokines
Pleiotropism: each cytokine has multiple biological actions	Many different cell types may express receptors for a particular cytokine
Redundancy: multiple cytokines may share the same or similar biological activities	Many cytokines use same conserved signaling pathways

Ⓑ Biologic actions of selected T cell cytokines

Cytokine	Principal action	Cellular source(s)
Interleukin-2 (IL-2)	Survival, proliferation and differentiation of effector and regulatory T cells	CD4+ and CD8+ T cells
IL-4	B cell switching to IgE	CD4+ T cells, mast cells
IL-5	Activation of eosinophils	CD4+ T cells, mast cells
Interferon-γ (IFN-γ)	Activation of macrophages	CD4+ and CD8+ T cells, natural killer cells
TGF-β	Inhibition of T cell activation; differentiation of regulatory T cells	CD4+ regulatory T cells; many other cell types

FIGURE 5-10 Properties of the major cytokines produced by CD4+ helper T lymphocytes. A, The general properties of all cytokines and the mechanisms responsible for these properties are summarized. **B,** The effector functions of selected cytokines involved in T cell–mediated immunity are summarized. TGF-β functions mainly as an inhibitor of immune responses; its role is discussed in Chapter 9. The cytokines of innate immunity are shown in Figure 2-13. IgE, immunoglobulin E; TCR, T cell receptor; TGF-β, transforming growth factor-β.

several different cytokines that have diverse activities (Fig. 5-10). Cytokines are a large group of proteins that function as mediators of immunity and inflammation. We have already discussed cytokines in innate immune responses, which are produced mainly by macrophages (see Chapter 2). In adaptive immunity, cytokines are secreted by T cells. These proteins share some important properties (see Fig. 5-10A), although different cytokines have distinct activities and play different roles in immune responses (see Fig. 5-10B).

The first cytokine to be produced by CD4+ T cells, within 1 to 2 hours after activation, is IL-2. (The term *interleukin* refers to the fact that many of these proteins are produced by leukocytes and act on leukocytes.) Activation also rapidly enhances the ability of T cells to bind and respond to IL-2, by increasing the expression of the IL-2 receptor (Fig. 5-11). The high-affinity receptor for IL-2 is a three-chain molecule. Naive T cells express two signaling chains of this receptor but do not express the chain that enables the receptor to bind IL-2 with high

FIGURE 5-11 **The role of interleukin-2 (IL-2) and IL-2 receptors in T cell proliferation.** Naive T cells express the low-affinity IL-2 receptor (IL-2R) complex, made up of the β and γc chains (γc designates the common γ chain—so called because it is a component of the receptors for several cytokines). On activation by antigen recognition and costimulation, the cells produce IL-2 and express the α chain of the IL-2R, which associates with the β and γc chains to form the high-affinity IL-2 receptor. Binding of IL-2 to its receptor initiates proliferation of the T cells that recognized the antigen. APC, antigen-presenting cell.

affinity. Within hours after activation by antigens and costimulators, the T cells produce the third chain of the receptor and now the complete IL-2 receptor is able to bind IL-2 strongly. Thus, IL-2 produced by antigen-stimulated T cells preferentially binds to and acts on the same T cells. The principal actions of IL-2 are to stimulate survival and proliferation of T cells; for this reason IL-2 is also called T cell growth factor. (As we will see in Chapter 9, IL-2 also is essential for the maintenance of regulatory T cells and thus for controlling immune responses.) IL-2 stimulates T cells to enter the cell cycle and begin to divide, resulting in an increase in the number of the antigen-specific T cells. Differentiated effector CD4+ T cells produce

many other cytokines, and the functions of some of the major ones are described later.

CD8+ T lymphocytes that recognize antigen and costimulators do not appear to secrete large amounts of IL-2, yet, as we shall see later, these lymphocytes proliferate prodigiously during immune responses. It is possible that antigen recognition and costimulation are able to drive the proliferation of CD8+ T cells without a requirement for much IL-2.

CLONAL EXPANSION

Within 1 or 2 days after activation, T lymphocytes begin to proliferate, resulting in expansion of

antigen-specific clones. This expansion helps the adaptive immune response to keep pace with rapidly dividing microbes and quickly provides a large pool of antigen-specific lymphocytes from which effector cells can be generated to combat infection. The magnitude of clonal expansion is remarkable, especially for CD8+ T cells. For instance, before infection, the frequency of CD8+ T cells specific for any one microbial protein antigen is about 1 in 10^5 or 10^6 lymphocytes in the body. At the peak of some viral infections, which may be within a week after the infection, as many as 10% to 20% of all of the lymphocytes in the lymphoid organs may be specific for that virus. This means that the antigen-specific clones have increased by more than 100,000-fold, with an estimated doubling time of about 6 hours. Several features of this clonal expansion are surprising. First, this enormous expansion of T cells specific for a microbe is not accompanied by a detectable increase in "bystander" cells that do not recognize that microbe. Second, even in infections with complex microbes that contain many protein antigens, a majority of the expanded clones are specific for only a few, and often less than five, immunodominant peptides of that microbe. The expansion of CD4+ T cells appears to be much less than that of CD8+ cells, probably on the order of 100-fold to 1000-fold. This difference in the magnitude of clonal expansion of CD8+ T cells and CD4+ T cells may reflect differences in their functions. CD8+ CTLs are effector cells that themselves kill infected cells, and many CTLs may be needed to kill large numbers of infected cells. By contrast, each CD4+ effector cell secretes cytokines that activate many other effector cells, as described later, so a relatively small number of cytokine producers may be all that is needed.

DIFFERENTIATION OF NAIVE T CELLS INTO EFFECTOR CELLS

The progeny of antigen-stimulated proliferating T cells begin to differentiate into effector cells that function to eradicate infections. This process of differentiation is the result of changes in gene expression (e.g., the activation of genes encoding cytokines [in CD4+ and CD8+ T cells] or cytotoxic proteins [in CD8+ CTLs]). It begins in concert with clonal expansion, and differentiated effector cells appear within 3 or 4 days

after exposure to microbes. These cells leave the peripheral lymphoid organs and migrate to the site of infection. Here the effector cells again encounter the microbial antigens that stimulated their development. On recognition of antigen, the effector cells respond in ways that serve to eradicate the infection. Effector cells of the CD4+ and CD8+ populations perform different functions, and are best described separately.

CD4+ helper T cells differentiate into effector cells that respond to antigen by producing surface molecules and cytokines that function to activate phagocytes and B lymphocytes (Fig. 5-12). The most important cell surface protein involved in the effector function of CD4+ T cells is CD40 ligand (CD40L). The CD40L gene is transcribed in CD4+ T cells in response to antigen recognition and costimulation, and the result is that CD40L is expressed on helper T cells after activation. It binds to its receptor, CD40, which is expressed mainly on macrophages, B lymphocytes, and dendritic cells. Engagement of CD40 activates these cells, and thus CD40L is an important participant in the activation of macrophages and B lymphocytes by helper T cells (see Chapters 6 and 7). As discussed earlier, the interaction of CD40L on T cells with CD40 on dendritic cells stimulates the expression of costimulators on these APCs and the production of T cell–activating cytokines, thus providing a positive feedback (amplification) mechanism for APC-induced T cell activation.

The analysis of cytokine production by helper T cells has answered a long-standing question in immunology. It has been known for many years that the immune system responds very differently to different microbes. For instance, intracellular microbes such as mycobacteria are ingested by phagocytes but resist intracellular killing. The adaptive immune response to such microbes results in the activation of the phagocytes to kill the ingested microbes. In striking contrast, helminthic parasites are too large to be phagocytosed, and the immune response to helminths is dominated by the production of immunoglobulin E (IgE) antibodies and the activation of eosinophils. IgE antibody binds to the helminths, and eosinophils and other leukocytes destroy the helminths. Both types of immune responses are dependent on CD4+ helper T cells, but for many years it was not clear how the CD4+

FIGURE 5-12 **The molecules involved in the effector functions of CD4+ helper T cells.** CD4+ T cells that have differentiated into effector cells express CD40L and secrete cytokines. CD40L binds to CD40 on macrophages or B lymphocytes, and cytokines bind to their receptors on the same cells. The combination of signals delivered by CD40 and cytokine receptors activates macrophages in cell-mediated immunity **(A)** and activates B cells to produce antibodies in humoral immune responses **(B)**. IL, interleukin.

helper cells are able to stimulate such distinct immune effector mechanisms. This puzzle was answered by the discovery of functionally distinct subpopulations of CD4+ effector T cells that are distinguished by the cytokines they produce, as described next.

CD4+ helper T cells may differentiate into subsets of effector cells that produce distinct sets of cytokines and perform different functions (Fig. 5-13). The subsets that were defined first are called T_H1 cells and T_H2 cells (for type 1 helper T cells and type 2 helper T cells); more recently, a third population has been identified and called T_H17 cells because its signature cytokine is IL-17. (Regulatory T cells are yet another subset of CD4+ T cells. Because their role

is in suppressing immune responses, we will discuss them in Chapter 9, in the context of immunologic tolerance [unresponsiveness].) T_H1 and T_H2 cells may be distinguished not only by the cytokines they produce but also by the cytokine receptors and adhesion molecules they express (Fig. 5-13B). Comparable data are not yet available for the T_H17 subset. It also is likely that many activated CD4+ T cells produce various mixtures of cytokines and therefore cannot be readily classified into these subsets.

T_H1 cells stimulate phagocyte-mediated ingestion and killing of microbes, a key component of cell-mediated immunity (Fig. 5-14). The most important cytokine produced by T_H1 cells is **interferon-γ**

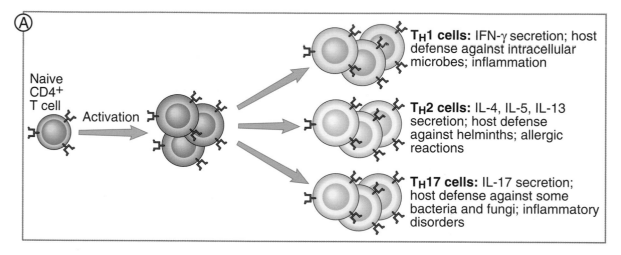

(B) Property	T$_H$1	T$_H$2	T$_H$17
Principal cytokines produced	IFN-γ	IL-4, IL-5, IL-13	IL-17, IL-22
Antibody isotypes stimulated	Complement and Fc receptor-binding IgG subclasses such as IgG2a (mouse)	IgE; IgG1 (mouse), IgG4 (humans)	?
Macrophage activation	Classical (microbial killing)	Alternative (tissue repair)	?
Dominant leukocytes recruited	Monocytes	Eosinophils	Neutrophils, monocytes

FIGURE 5-13 The development and characteristics of subsets of CD4+ helper T lymphocytes. A, A naive CD4+ T cell may differentiate into subsets that produce different cytokines and perform different effector functions. **B,** The major differences between T$_H$1, T$_H$2, and T$_H$17 subsets of helper T cells are summarized. Note that many helper T cells may not be readily classified into these distinct and polarized subsets. Classical macrophage activation refers to the acquisition of microbicidal functions (and the capacity to damage tissues), and alternative macrophage activation results in activities that promote tissue repair and remodeling. These pathways of macrophage activation are described in Chapter 6. GM-CSF, granulocyte macrophage colony-stimulating factor; IFN, interferon; IL, interleukin.

APC

Naive CD4+ T cell

Microbes

Proliferation and differentiation

IFN-γ

T_H1 cells

B cell

IFN-γ

Macrophage activation (enhanced microbial killing)

Complement binding and opsonizing antibodies

Fc receptor

Opsonization and phagocytosis

FIGURE 5-14   The functions of T_H1 cells. T_H1 cells produce the cytokine interferon-γ (IFN-γ), which activates phagocytes to kill ingested microbes and stimulates the production of antibodies that promote the ingestion of microbes by the phagocytes. APC, antigen-presenting cell.

(IFN-γ), so called because it was discovered as a cytokine that inhibited (or interfered with) viral infection. IFN-γ is a potent activator of macrophages. (The type I IFNs [Chapter 2] are much more potent anti-viral cytokines than is IFN-γ.) IFN-γ also stimulates the production of antibody isotypes that promote the phagocytosis of microbes, because these antibodies bind directly to phagocyte Fc receptors, and they acti-

vate complement, generating products that bind to phagocyte complement receptors. (These functions of antibodies are described in Chapter 8.) IFN-γ also stimulates the expression of class II MHC molecules and B7 costimulators on macrophages and dendritic cells, and this action of IFN-γ may serve to amplify T cell responses.

T_H2 cells stimulate phagocyte-independent, eosinophil-mediated immunity, which is especially effective against helminthic parasites (Fig. 5-15). T_H2 cells produce IL-4, which stimulates the production of IgE antibodies, and IL-5, which activates eosinophils. IgE activates mast cells and binds to eosinophils. T_H2 cells also produce IL-5, which activates eosinophils. These IgE-dependent, mast cell– and eosinophil-mediated reactions are important in killing helminthic parasites. In addition, some of the cytokines produced by T_H2 cells, such as IL-4 and IL-13, promote the expulsion of parasites from mucosal organs and inhibit the entry of microbes by stimulating mucus secretion. This type of host defense sometimes is called "barrier immunity" because it blocks the entry of microbes at mucosal barriers. The cytokines of T_H2 cells also activate macrophages. Unlike T_H1-mediated activation, which stimulates the ability of macrophages to kill ingested microbes, T_H2-mediated macrophage activation enhances other functions, such as synthesis of extracellular matrix proteins involved in tissue repair. This type of response has been called "alternative" macrophage activation. Some of the cytokines produced by T_H2 cells, such as IL-4, IL-10, and IL-13, inhibit the microbicidal activities of macrophages and thus suppress T_H1 cell–mediated immunity. Therefore, the efficacy of cell-mediated immune responses against a microbe may be determined by a balance between the activation of T_H1 and T_H2 cells in response to that microbe. We will return to this concept and its importance in infectious diseases in Chapter 6.

T_H17 cells secrete the cytokines IL-17 and IL-22 and are the principal mediators of inflammation in a number of immunologic reactions (Fig. 5–16). This subset was discovered because of its role in animal models of diseases such as multiple sclerosis, inflammatory bowel disease, and rheumatoid arthritis, and is increasingly being implicated in these diseases in humans. Studies in experimental models suggest that T_H17 cells also are involved in defense against some bacterial and fungal infections.

The development of T_H1, T_H2, and T_H17 subsets is not a random process but is regulated by the stimuli that naive CD4+ T cells receive when they encounter microbial antigens (Fig. 5–17). T_H1 differentiation is driven by a combination of the cytokines IL-12 and IFN-γ. In response to many bacteria and viruses, dendritic cells and macrophages produce a cytokine called IL-12, and NK cells produce IFN-γ. When naive T cells recognize the antigens of these microbes, the T cells also are exposed to IL-12 and

FIGURE 5-15 **The functions of T$_H$2 cells.** T$_H$2 cells produce the cytokines IL-4, which stimulates the production of immunoglobulin E (IgE) antibody, and IL-5, which activates eosinophils. IgE participates in the activation of mast cells by protein antigens and coats helminthes, and eosinophils destroy the helminthes. T$_H$2 cells stimulate the production of other antibody isotypes that may neutralize microbes and toxins but do not opsonize microbes for phagocytosis or activate complement by the classical pathway. APC, antigen-presenting cell; IL, interleukin.

FIGURE 5-16 **The functions of T$_H$17 cells.** T$_H$17 cells produce the cytokines IL-17, which induces production of chemokines and other cytokines from various cells, and these recruit neutrophils (and monocytes, not shown) into the site of inflammation. Some of the cytokines made by T$_H$17 cells, notably IL-22, function to maintain epithelial barrier function in the intestinal tract and other tissues.

IFN-γ. These two cytokines activate transcription factors that promote the differentiation of the T cells to the T_H1 subset. T_H1 cells produce IFN-γ, which not only activates macrophages to kill the microbes but also promotes more T_H1 development. This sequence illustrates an important principle that has been mentioned in earlier chapters: The innate immune response—in this case, IL-12 production by APCs and IFN-γ production by NK cells—influences the nature of the subsequent adaptive immune response, driving it toward T_H1 cells.

FIGURE 5-17 The development of T_H1, T_H2, and T_H17 effector cells. After activation by antigen and costimulators, naive helper T cells may differentiate into different subsets under the influence of cytokines produced at the site of activation. Cytokines that induce T_H1 development include IL-12 (and IL-18), which are produced by microbe-activated antigen-presenting cells (APCs), such as dendritic cells and macrophages. Interferon-γ (IFN-γ) made by natural killer (NK) cells or by the responding T cells themselves also is critical for T_H1 development. T_H2 cells are induced by IL-4, which may be produced by the T cells themselves and by other cells, such as mast cells. T_H17 differentiation is triggered by TGF-β, which can be made by many cell types, in the presence of inflammatory cytokines such as IL-6, IL-1, and IL-23, which may be produced by APCs. The major transcription factors that are involved in helper T cell differentiation are shown; these include T-bet (for T_H1 cells), GATA-3 (for T_H2 cells), and RORγt (for T_H17 cells). Other transcription factors that control these differentiation pathways include cytokine-activated STAT proteins (STAT, "signal transducers and activators of transcription"); these are not shown.

The development of T_H2 cells is stimulated by the cytokine IL-4 (see Fig. 5-17). On face value, this is puzzling, because the main source of IL-4 is T_H2 cells—so how could the cytokine induce the cells that produce it? It appears that if an infectious microbe does not elicit IL-12 production by APCs, as may be the case with helminths, the T cells themselves produce IL-4. Also, helminths may activate cells of the mast cell lineage to secrete IL-4. In antigen-stimulated T cells, IL-4 activates transcription factors that promote differentiation to the T_H2 subset.

The development and maintenance of T_H17 cells (see Fig. 5–17) require inflammatory cytokines such as IL-6 and IL-1 (produced by macrophages and dendritic cells); IL-23 (which is related to IL-12 and made by the same cells); and TGF-β (particularly in mice). Defining the stimuli for development of this T cell subset is an area of active investigation.

The differentiation of CD4+ helper T cells into T_H1, T_H2, and T_H17 subsets is an excellent example of the specialization of adaptive immunity, illustrating how immune responses to different types of microbes are designed to be most effective against these microbes. Furthermore, once one of these populations develops from antigen-stimulated helper T cells, it produces cytokines that enhance the differentiation of T cells toward that subset and inhibits development of the other populations. This "cross-regulation" may lead to increasing polarization of the response toward one population. There is emerging evidence that some differentiated CD4+ T cells can convert from one subset into another, under certain conditions, but the extent or significance of such inter-conversion is unknown.

CD8+ T lymphocytes activated by antigen and costimulators differentiate into CTLs that are able to kill infected cells expressing the antigen. Effector CTLs kill infected cells by secreting proteins that create pores in the membranes of the infected cells and induce DNA fragmentation and apoptotic death of these cells. The differentiation of naive CD8+ T cells into effector CTLs is accompanied by the synthesis of the molecules that kill infected cells. The mechanisms of CTL-mediated killing are discussed in more detail in Chapter 6.

DEVELOPMENT OF MEMORY T LYMPHOCYTES

A fraction of antigen-activated T lymphocytes differentiates into long-lived memory cells. Memory cells survive even after the infection is eradicated and antigen as well as the innate immune reaction to the infectious pathogen are no longer present. These memory T cells can be found in lymphoid organs, in mucosal tissues, and in the circulation. Memory T cells require signals delivered by certain cytokines, including IL-7, in order to stay alive. We do not know what factors determine whether the progeny of antigen-stimulated lymphocytes will differentiate into effector cells or memory cells. Memory T cells do not continue to produce cytokines or kill infected cells, but they may do so rapidly on encountering the antigen that they recognize. Thus, memory cells are a pool of lymphocytes waiting for the infection to return. A subset of memory T cells, called central memory cells, populate lymphoid organs and are responsible for rapid clonal expansion after re-exposure to antigen. Another subset, called effector memory cells, localize in mucosal tissue and mediate rapid effector functions on reintroduction of antigen to these sites.

DECLINE OF THE IMMUNE RESPONSE

Because of the remarkable expansion of antigen-specific lymphocytes at the peak of an immune response, it is predictable that once the response is over, the system has to return to its steady state, called homeostasis, so that it is prepared to respond to the next infectious pathogen. During the response, the survival and proliferation of T cells are maintained by antigen, costimulatory signals from CD28, and cytokines such as IL-2. Once an infection is cleared and the stimuli for lymphocyte activation disappear, many of the cells that had proliferated in response to antigen are deprived of these survival signals. As a result, these cells die by a process of apoptosis (programmed cell death). The response subsides within 1 or 2 weeks after the infection is eradicated, and the only sign that a T cell–mediated immune response had occurred is the pool of surviving memory lymphocytes.

Numerous mechanisms ensure the generation of a useful T cell response, despite several obstacles. First, naive T cells have to find the antigen. This problem is solved by APCs that capture the antigen and concentrate it in specialized lymphoid organs in the regions through which naive T cells recirculate. Second, the correct type of T lymphocytes (i.e., CD4+ helper T cells or CD8+ CTLs) must respond to antigens from the extracellular and intracellular compartments. This

selectivity is determined by the specificity of the CD4 and CD8 co-receptors for class II and class I MHC molecules, and by the segregation of extracellular (vesicular) and intracellular (cytoplasmic) protein antigens for display by class II and class I MHC molecules, respectively. Third, T cells must interact with antigen-bearing APCs long enough to be activated. This is accomplished by adhesion molecules that stabilize T cell binding to APCs. Fourth, T cells should respond to microbial antigens but not to harmless proteins. This preference for microbes is maintained because T cell activation requires costimulators that are induced on APCs by microbes. Finally, antigen recognition by a small number of T cells must lead to a response that is large enough to be effective. This is accomplished by several amplification mechanisms that are induced by microbes and by activated T cells themselves and lead to enhanced T cell activation.

SUMMARY

- T lymphocytes are the cells of cell-mediated immunity, the arm of the adaptive immune system that combats intracellular microbes, which may be microbes that are ingested by phagocytes and live within these cells or microbes that infect non-phagocytic cells.

- The responses of T lymphocytes consist of sequential phases: recognition of cell-associated microbes by naive T cells, expansion of the antigen-specific clones by proliferation, and differentiation of some of the progeny into effector cells and memory cells.

- T cells use their antigen receptors to recognize peptide antigens displayed by MHC molecules on antigen-presenting cells (which accounts for the specificity of the ensuing response) and polymorphic residues of the MHC molecules (accounting for the MHC restriction of T cell responses).

- Antigen recognition by the TCR triggers signals that are delivered to the interior of the cells by molecules associated with the TCR (the CD3 and ζ chains) and by the co-receptors, CD4 and CD8, which recognize class II and class I MHC molecules, respectively.

■ The binding of T cells to APCs is enhanced by adhesion molecules, notably the integrins, whose affinity for their ligands is increased by chemokines produced in response to microbes and by antigen recognition by the TCR.

■ APCs exposed to microbes or to cytokines produced as part of the innate immune reactions to microbes express costimulators that are recognized by receptors on T cells and deliver necessary "second signals" for T cell activation.

■ The biochemical signals triggered in T cells by antigen recognition and costimulation result in the activation of various transcription factors that stimulate the expression of genes encoding cytokines, cytokine receptors, and other molecules involved in T cell responses.

■ In response to antigen recognition and costimulation, T cells secrete cytokines, of which some induce proliferation of the antigen-stimulated T cells and others mediate the effector functions of T cells.

■ CD4+ helper T cells may differentiate into subsets of effector cells that produce restricted sets of cytokines and perform different functions. T_H1 cells, which produce IFN-γ, activate phagocytes to eliminate ingested microbes, and stimulate the production of opsonizing and complement-binding antibodies. T_H2 cells, which produce IL-4 and IL-5, stimulate IgE production and activate eosinophils, which function mainly in defense against helminths. T_H17 cells, which produce IL-17, are implicated in several inflammatory diseases and may play a role in defense against bacterial infections.

■ CD8+ T cells recognize peptides of intracellular (cytoplasmic) protein antigens and may require help from CD4+ T cells to differentiate into effector CTLs. The function of CTLs is to kill cells producing cytoplasmic microbial antigens.

REVIEW QUESTIONS

1 *What are the components of the TCR complex? Which of these components are responsible for antigen recognition and which for signal transduction?*

2 *What are some of the accessory molecules that T cells use to initiate their responses to antigens, and what are the functions of these molecules?*

3 *What is costimulation? What is the physiologic significance of costimulation? What are some of the ligand-receptor pairs that are involved in costimulation?*

4 *Summarize the links between antigen recognition, the major biochemical signaling pathways in T cells, and the production of transcription factors.*

5 *What is the principal growth factor for T cells? Why do antigen-specific T cells expand more than other ("bystander") T cells on exposure to an antigen?*

6 *What are the major subsets of CD4+ helper T cells, and how do they differ?*

7 *What signals are required to induce the responses of CD8+ T cells?*

EFFECTOR MECHANISMS OF CELL-MEDIATED IMMUNITY

Eradication of Intracellular Microbes

The specialized immune mechanisms that function to eradicate intracellular microbes constitute cell-mediated immunity. The effector phase of cell-mediated immunity is carried out by T lymphocytes, and antibodies play no role in eradicating infections by microbes that are living inside host cells. The phases of cell-mediated immunity consist of the activation of naive T cells to proliferate and to differentiate into effector cells and the elimination of cell-associated microbes by the actions of these effector T cells. In Chapter 3 we described the function of major histocompatibility complex (MHC) molecules in displaying the antigens of intracellular microbes for recognition by T lymphocytes, and in Chapter 5 we discussed the way in which naive T cells recognize these antigens in lymphoid organs and develop into effector cells. In this chapter, we will address the following questions:

- How do effector T lymphocytes locate intracellular microbes at any site in the body?
- How do effector T cells eradicate infections by these microbes?

Types of Cell-Mediated Immunity

There are two types of cell-mediated immune reactions designed to eliminate different types of intracellular microbes: CD4+ helper T cells activate phagocytes to destroy microbes residing in the vesicles of these phagocytes, and CD8+ cytotoxic T lymphocytes (CTLs) kill any cell containing

FIGURE 6-1 **Cell-mediated immunity against intracellular microbes. A,** Effector T cells of the CD4+ T$_H$1 subset recognize the antigens of microbes ingested by phagocytes and activate the phagocytes to kill the microbes and induce inflammation. Phagocyte activation and inflammation are responses to cytokines produced by the T cells (discussed later). CD8+ T lymphocytes also produce cytokines that elicit the same reactions, but CD8+ T cells recognize microbial antigens in the cytoplasm of infected cells *(not shown)*. **B,** CD8+ CTLs kill infected cells with microbes in the cytoplasm. CTLs, cytotoxic T lymphocytes.

microbes or microbial proteins in the cytoplasm, thereby eliminating the reservoir of infection (Fig. 6-1). This separation of the effector functions of T lymphocytes is not absolute. Some CD4+ T cells are capable of killing infected macrophages, and CD8+ T cells activate macrophages to eliminate phagocytosed microbes. Nevertheless, phagocyte activation, which is the principal function of CD4+ T cells in cell-mediated immunity, and CD8+ T cell-mediated killing of infected cells are fundamentally different immune reactions and are described separately.

Microbial infections may occur anywhere in the body, and some infectious pathogens are able to infect and live within host cells. Pathogenic microbes that infect and survive inside host cells include (1) many bacteria and some protozoa that are ingested by phagocytes but resist the killing mechanisms of these phagocytes and live in vesicles or cytoplasm, and (2) viruses that infect phagocytic and nonphagocytic cells and live and replicate in the cytoplasm of these cells (see Fig. 5-1, Chapter 5). Effector T cells whose function is to eradicate these microbes are generated from naive T cells that were stimulated by microbial antigens in lymph nodes and spleen (see Chapter 5). The differentiated effector T cells then migrate to the site of infection. Phagocytes at these sites that have ingested the microbes into intracellular vesicles display peptide fragments of microbial proteins attached to class II MHC molecules for recognition by CD4+ effector T cells. Peptide antigens derived from microbes living in the cytoplasm of infected cells are displayed by class I MHC molecules for recognition by CD8+ effector T cells. Antigen recognition by the effector T cells then activates them to perform their task of eliminating the infectious pathogens. Thus, in cell-mediated immunity, T cells recognize protein antigens at two stages: naive T cells recognize antigens in lymphoid tissues and respond by proliferating and by differentiating into effector cells, and effector T cells recognize the same antigens anywhere in the body and respond by eliminating these microbes (Fig. 6-2).

In the remainder of this chapter, we will describe first how differentiated effector T cells locate microbes in tissues and then how CD4+ and CD8+ T cells eliminate these microbes.

Migration of Effector T Lymphocytes to Sites of Infection

Effector T cells migrate to sites of infection because these lymphocytes express high levels of adhesion

FIGURE 6-2 **The induction and effector phases of cell-mediated immunity.** (1) *Induction of response:* Naïve CD4+ T cells and CD8+ T cells recognize peptides that are derived from protein antigens and presented by antigen-presenting cells in peripheral lymphoid organs. The T lymphocytes are stimulated to proliferate and differentiate, and effector cells enter the circulation. (2) *Migration of effector T cells and other leukocytes to site of antigen:* Effector T cells and other leukocytes migrate through blood vessels in peripheral tissues by binding to endothelial cells that have been activated by cytokines produced in response to infection in these tissues. (3) *T cell effector functions:* CD4+ T cells activate phagocytes to destroy microbes and CD8+ cytotoxic T lymphocytes (CTLs) kill infected cells.

Within figure:

IL-12

Induction of response

Antigen recognition in lymphoid organs

CD4+ T cells

CD8+ T cells

CD4+ effector T cells (TH1 cells)

CD8+ T cells (CTLs)

T cell expansion and differentiation

Differentiated effector T cells enter circulation

Migration of effector T cells and other leukocytes to site of antigen

Cells with intracellular microbes

Effector T cells encounter antigens in peripheral tissues

Activation of effector T cells

IFN-γ

T cell effector functions

Macrophage activation ⇒ killing of phagocytosed microbes

CTL killing of target cell

FIGURE 6-3   Migration of naive and effector T lymphocytes. A, Naive T lymphocytes home to lymph nodes as a result of L-selectin and integrin binding to their ligands on high endothelial venules (HEVs). Chemokines expressed in lymph nodes bind to receptors on naive T cells, enhancing integrin-dependent adhesion and migration through the HEV. Activated T lymphocytes, including effector cells, home to sites of infection in peripheral tissues, and this migration is mediated by E-selectin and P-selectin, integrins, and chemokines secreted at inflammatory sites. **B,** The functions of the principal T cell homing receptors and their ligands are shown. ICAM-1, intercellular adhesion molecule-1; LFA-1, leukocyte function–associated antigen-1; VCAM-1, vascular cell adhesion molecule-1; VLA-4, very late antigen 4.

molecules and chemokine receptors that bind to ligands expressed or displayed on endothelium after exposure to microbes and in response to chemokines produced at the site. The process of differentiation of naive T lymphocytes into effector cells is accompanied by changes in the profiles of adhesion molecules and chemokine receptors that are expressed on these cells (Fig. 6-3). Activated T cells decrease expression of the receptor for the chemokines that are produced in the T cell zones of lymph nodes and at the same time increase expression of the receptor for a phospholipid, sphingosine 1-phosphate, that is present at high concentrations in the blood. As a result, the activated T lymphocytes are induced to migrate out of the lymph nodes. The migration of activated T cells into peripheral tissues is controlled by the same interactions that are involved in the migration of other leukocytes into tissues (see Chapter 2, Fig. 2-7). To summarize the key points, activated T cells express high levels of the glycoprotein ligands for E- and P-selectins and the high-affinity forms of the integrins LFA-1 (leukocyte function–associated antigen-1) and VLA-4 (very late antigen-4, so called because it, as well as other similar integrins, appear later than LFA-1 during the course of T cell activation). The endothelium at the site of infection is exposed to cytokines such as tumor necrosis factor (TNF) and interleukin-1 (IL-1), which act on the endothelial cells to increase expression of E- and P-selectins as well as ligands for integrins, especially ICAM-1 (intercellular adhesion molecule-1, the ligand for LFA-1) and VCAM-1 (vascular cell adhesion molecule-1, the ligand for the VLA-4 integrin). Effector T cells that are passing through the blood vessels at the infection site bind first to the selectins, leading to rolling interactions. Effector T cells also express receptors for chemokines that are produced by macrophages and endothelial cells at these inflammatory sites and are displayed on the surface of the endothelium. The rolling T cells recognize these chemokines, leading to increased binding affinity of the integrins for their ligands and firm adhesion of the T cells to the endothelium. After the effector T lymphocytes are arrested on the endothelium, the chemokines that were produced by macrophages in adjacent tissues stimulate the motility of the adherent leukocytes. The net result of the adhesion and chemokine-mediated attraction is that the T cells migrate out of the blood vessels to the site of infection.

After activation, T cells decrease expression not only of receptors for chemokines produced in lymph nodes but also of L-selectin, the adhesion molecule that mediates naive T cell migration into lymph nodes. Therefore, activated T cells tend to stay out of normal lymph nodes. Some microbes, however, frequently infect phagocytes within lymph nodes. In such instances, an inflammatory response to the microbes in the lymph nodes leads to expression of adhesion molecules and production of chemokines as at any site of inflammation, thereby attracting effector T cells into the lymph nodes.

The homing of effector T cells to a site of infection is independent of antigen recognition, but lymphocytes that recognize microbial antigens are preferentially retained at the site (Fig. 6-4). Because the homing of effector T cells to sites of infection is dependent on adhesion molecules and chemokines, and not on antigen recognition, all effector T cells present in the blood that were generated in response to different microbial infections can enter the site of any infection. This nonselective migration presumably maximizes the ability of effector lymphocytes to search out the microbes they can specifically recognize and eliminate. The same lack of selectivity, however, creates a problem: How are lymphocytes specific for a microbe able to focus on those microbes long enough to perform their function? A likely answer is that an effector T lymphocyte that has left the circulation and entered a tissue specifically recognizes microbial antigen, and the cell is again activated. One consequence of activation is an increase in the expression and binding affinity of VLA integrins on the T

T cell molecules involved in homing	Endothelial cell molecules	Function of receptor: ligand pair
Naive T cells L-selectin	L-selectin ligand	Adhesion of naive T cells to high endothelial venule (HEV) in lymph node
LFA-1 (β2-integrin)	ICAM-1	Stable arrest on HEV
CCR7	CCL19 or CCL21	Activation of integrins and chemotaxis
Activated (effector and memory) T cells E- and P-selectin ligand	E- or P-selectin	Initial weak adhesion of effector and memory T cells to cytokine activated endothelium at peripheral site of infection
LFA-1 (β2-integrin) or VLA-4 (β1 integrin)	ICAM-1 or VCAM-1	Stable arrest on cytokine activated endothelium at peripheral site of infection
CXCR3, others	CXCL10, others	Activation of integrins and chemotaxis

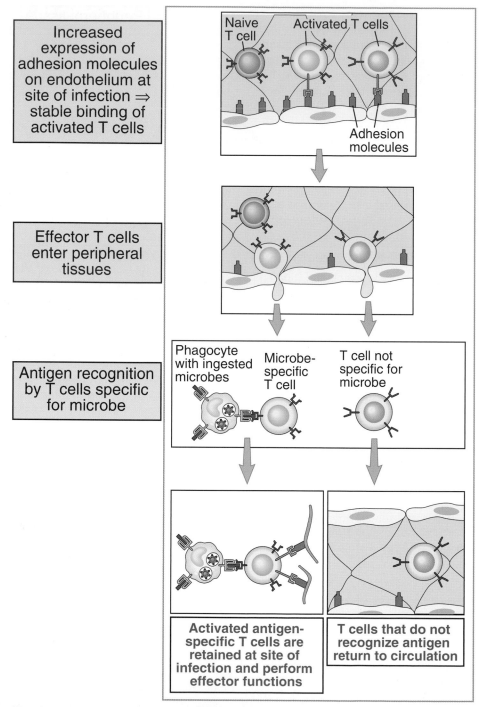

FIGURE 6-4   Migration and retention of effector T cells at sites of infection. Effector T cells migrate to sites of infection by using receptors to bind to ligands that are induced on endothelium by cytokines produced during innate immune reactions to microbes. T cells that recognize microbial antigens in extravascular tissues are retained at these sites by integrin-mediated adhesion to the extracellular matrix. These antigen-specific T cells perform their effector function of eradicating the infection, whereas T cells that do not see antigen return through lymphatic vessels to the circulation.

cells. Some of these integrins specifically bind to molecules present in the extracellular matrix, such as hyaluronic acid and fibronectin. Therefore, the antigen-stimulated lymphocytes adhere firmly to the tissue near the antigen, so the cells stay long enough to respond to the microbe and eradicate the infection. Lymphocytes that enter the tissue but do not recognize an antigen are not activated to adhere. They may enter lymphatic vessels draining the tissue and return to the circulation, prepared to home to another site of infection in search of the microbial antigen for which they are specific.

The net result of this sequence of cell migration and retention is that effector T lymphocytes, which were produced in the peripheral lymphoid organs in response to an infection, are able to locate that infectious microbe at any site in the body. These effector lymphocytes are activated by the microbe and respond in ways that eliminate the microbe. In contrast with the activation of naive T cells, which requires antigen presentation and costimulation by dendritic cells, differentiated effector cells appear to be less dependent on costimulation than are naive cells. Therefore, the proliferation and differentiation of naive T cells are confined to lymphoid organs, where dendritic cells display antigens, but the functions of effector T cells may be directed at any host cell displaying microbial antigens, not just dendritic cells.

Because CD4+ helper T lymphocytes and CD8+ CTLs employ some distinct mechanisms to combat infections, we will discuss the effector mechanisms of these lymphocyte classes individually. We conclude by describing how the two classes of lymphocytes may cooperate to get rid of intracellular microbes.

Effector Functions of CD4+ Helper T Lymphocytes

Cell-mediated immunity was discovered as a form of immunity to an intracellular bacterial infection that could be transferred from immune animals to naive animals by cells (now known to be T lymphocytes) but not by serum antibodies (Fig. 6-5). It was known from the earliest studies that the specificity of cell-mediated immunity against different microbes was a function of the lymphocytes, but the elimination of the microbes was a function of activated macrophages. The roles of T lymphocytes and phagocytes in cell-mediated immunity are now well understood.

In cell-mediated immunity, CD4+ T lymphocytes of the T_H1 subset activate macrophages that have phagocytosed microbes, resulting in increased microbicidal activities of the phagocytes and killing of the ingested microbes. The ability of T cells to activate macrophages is dependent on antigen recognition, accounting for the specificity of the reaction. Essentially, the same reaction may be elicited by injecting a microbial protein into the skin of an individual who has been immunized against the microbe by prior infection or vaccination. This reaction is called **delayed-type hypersensitivity (DTH)**, because it occurs 24 to 48 hours after an immunized individual is challenged with a microbial protein (i.e., the reaction is delayed), and because it reflects an increased sensitivity to antigen challenge. The delay occurs because it takes 24 to 48 hours for circulating effector T lymphocytes to home to the site of antigen challenge, respond to the antigen at this site, and induce a detectable reaction. DTH reactions are manifested by infiltrates of T cells and blood monocytes into the tissues, edema and fibrin deposition caused by increased vascular permeability in response to cytokines produced by CD4+ T cells, and tissue damage induced by the products of macrophages activated by T cells (Fig. 6-6). DTH reactions often are used to determine if people have been previously exposed to and have responded to an antigen. For instance, a DTH reaction to a mycobacterial antigen, PPD (purified protein derivative), is an indicator of a T cell response to the mycobacteria. This is the basis for the PPD skin test, which frequently is used to detect past or active mycobacterial infection.

In another form of cell-mediated immunity, CD4+ T cells of the T_H17 subset induce the production of chemokines that recruit neutrophils and monocytes, and anti-microbial proteins that attack bacteria and fungi. This T cell subset contributes to eradication of extracellular bacterial and fungal infections, and also to inflammation in autoimmune and other immune-mediated diseases. A characteristic feature of all these T_H17-mediated reactions is the abundance of inflammatory leukocytes, notably neutrophils.

In the following discussion, we describe how T lymphocytes activate macrophages and how the macrophages eliminate phagocytosed microbes.

T CELL–MEDIATED MACROPHAGE ACTIVATION

Effector T lymphocytes of the T_H1 subset that recognize macrophage-associated antigens activate the macrophages by CD40 ligand–CD40 interac-

FIGURE 6-5 **Cell-mediated immunity to an intracellular bacterium, *Listeria monocytogenes*.** In this experiment, a sample of lymphocytes or serum (a source of antibodies) was taken from a mouse that had previously been exposed to a sublethal dose of *Listeria* organisms (immune mouse) and transferred to a normal (naive) mouse, and the recipient of the "adoptive transfer" was challenged with the bacteria. The numbers of bacteria were measured in the spleen of the recipient mouse to determine if the transfer had conferred immunity. Protection against bacterial challenge (seen by reduced recovery of live bacteria) was induced by the transfer of immune lymphoid cells, now known to be T cells **(A)**, but not by the transfer of serum **(B)**. The bacteria were killed in vitro by activated macrophages but not by T cells **(C)**. Therefore, protection is dependent on antigen-specific T lymphocytes, but bacterial killing is the function of activated macrophages.

tions and by secreting the macrophage-activating cytokine interferon-γ **(IFN-γ)** (Fig. 6-7). As we discussed in Chapter 3, macrophages ingest microbes into intracellular vesicles, called phagosomes, that fuse with lysosomes to form phagolysosomes. The microbial proteins in these vesicles are processed, and a few microbial peptides are displayed by class II MHC molecules on the surface of the macrophages. Effector CD4+ T cells specific for these peptides recognize the class II–associated peptides. The T cells respond by expressing on their surface the effector molecule CD40 ligand (CD40L or CD154), which binds to the

CD40 receptor that is expressed on macrophages. At the same time, the effector T cells, being of the TH1 subset, secrete the macrophage-activating cytokine IFN-γ, which binds to its receptors on macrophages. Binding of IFN-γ to its receptor functions together with engagement of CD40 to trigger biochemical signaling pathways that lead to the production of several transcription factors. These transcription factors turn on the transcription of genes that encode lysosomal proteases and enzymes that stimulate the synthesis of microbicidal reactive oxygen species and nitric oxide. The requirement for the membrane-associated CD40L-

Perivascular
cell infiltrates

Vessel with activated
endothelial cells

Activated lymphocytes
and macrophages

FIGURE 6-6 **The morphology of a delayed-type hypersensitivity (DTH) reaction.** In an individual previously exposed to an antigen, skin challenge with that antigen elicits a DTH reaction. Histopathologic examination of the reaction shows perivascular mononuclear cell infiltrates in the dermis **(A)**. At higher magnification, the infiltrate is seen to consist of activated lymphocytes and macrophages surrounding small blood vessels in which the endothelial cells are activated **(B)**. (Courtesy of Dr. J. Faix, Department of Pathology, Stanford University School of Medicine, Palo Alto, California.)

CD40 interaction ensures that macrophages that are in direct contact with T cells are the ones that are activated best. The macrophages that contact T cells also are the macrophages that are presenting antigens of phagocytosed microbes, and these are the phagocytes that need to be activated. The net result of CD40L- and IFN-γ–mediated activation is that macrophages become strongly microbicidal and can destroy most ingested microbes.

The interaction between macrophages and T lymphocytes is an excellent example of bidirectional interactions between cells of the innate and adaptive immune systems (i.e., macrophages and T lymphocytes) (Fig. 6-8). Macrophages that have encountered microbes produce the cytokine IL-12. IL-12 stimulates the differentiation of naive CD4+ T cells to the T_H1 subset, which produces IFN-γ on encountering macrophage-associated microbial antigens; IL-12 also increases the amount of IFN-γ produced by these T cells. The IFN-γ then activates the phagocytes to kill the ingested microbes, thus completing the circle. IFN-γ also stimulates more IL-12 production, thus amplifying the response.

CD4+ T lymphocytes perform functions in addition to macrophage activation in cell-mediated immune reactions. Antigen-stimulated CD4+ T cells of the T_H1 subset secrete cytokines such as TNF, which act on vascular endothelium to increase the expression of adhesion molecules and production of chemokines. T_H17 cells may secrete chemokines that attract neutrophils and monocytes. As a result, more T cells and other leukocytes are recruited to the site of infection. In this manner, the T cell response is amplified, and additional phagocytes are called in to assist in eradicating the infection. This T cell–stimulated cellular infiltration, along with an accompanying vascular reaction, is typical of inflammation. Inflammation is a component of T cell–mediated reactions, such as DTH, and also is seen in innate immune reactions to microbes (see Chapter 2). In addition to their role in helping macrophages eradicate phagocytosed microbes, CD4+ T cells help CD8+ T cells to differentiate into active CTLs and help B lymphocytes to differentiate into antibody-producing cells (see Chapters 5 and 7).

CD8+ T lymphocytes that recognize class I MHC–associated microbial peptides on macrophages also are able to activate macrophages to kill intracellular microbes. Recall that class I MHC–associated peptides are produced from cytoplasmic proteins, which may be derived from phagocytosed microbes (and, of course, from infection of nonphagocytic cells). Some microbes are ingested by macrophages into vesicles, and the microbes or their proteins pass through the membranes of the vesicles into the cytoplasm, where they are processed into class I MHC–binding peptides. In such infections, CD8+ T cells also func-

FIGURE 6-7 Activation of macrophages by T lymphocytes. Effector T lymphocytes recognize the antigens of ingested microbes on macrophages. In response to this recognition, the T lymphocytes express CD40L, which engages CD40 on the macrophages, and the T cells secrete interferon-γ (IFN-γ), which binds to IFN-γ receptors on the macrophages. This combination of signals activates the macrophages to produce microbicidal substances that kill the ingested microbes. Activated macrophages also secrete cytokines that induce inflammation—tumor necrosis factor (TNF), interleukin-1 (IL-1), chemokines—and activate T cells (IL-12), and they express more MHC molecules and costimulators, which enhance T cell responses. The illustration shows a CD4+ T cell recognizing class II MHC–associated peptides and activating the macrophage, but the same reaction may be elicited by a CD8+ T cell that recognizes class I MHC–displayed peptides derived from cytoplasmic microbial antigens. MHC, major histocompatibility complex.

FIGURE 6-8 Cytokine-mediated interactions between T lymphocytes and macrophages in cell-mediated immunity. APCs that encounter microbes secrete the cytokine IL-12, which stimulates naive CD4+ T cells to differentiate into IFN-γ–secreting T$_H$1 cells and enhances IFN-γ production. IFN-γ activates the macrophages to kill ingested microbes. APC, antigen-presenting cell; IFN, interferon; IL, interleukin.

tion to activate the macrophages, by essentially the same mechanism as that used by CD4+ cells, namely, CD40L- and IFN-γ–mediated activation. Macrophage activation is not useful for defense against microbes, such as viruses, that live and replicate only in the cytoplasm, because the microbicidal mechanisms of macrophages are largely limited to vesicles. Obviously, macrophage activation also is of little value for eliminating viral infections of cells other than these phagocytes.

ELIMINATION OF MICROBES BY ACTIVATED MACROPHAGES

Macrophage activation leads to the expression of enzymes that catalyze the production of microbicidal substances in phagosomes and phagolysosomes (see Fig. 6-7). We described the microbicidal mechanisms of activated phagocytes in Chapter 2, when we discussed the role of phagocytes in innate immunity (see Fig. 2-9, Chapter 2). To reiterate the key points, the major microbicidal substances produced in the lysosomes of macrophages are reactive oxygen species (ROS), nitric oxide (NO), and proteolytic enzymes. These mechanisms are activated in innate immunity when macrophages encounter microbes. As described previously, effector T_H1 cells are potent activators of the same microbicidal mechanisms in cell-mediated immunity. Cell-mediated immunity is critical for host defense in two situations: when macrophages are not activated by the microbes themselves (i.e., when innate immunity is ineffective) and when pathogenic microbes have evolved to resist the defense mechanisms of innate immunity. In these situations, the additional macrophage activation by T cells changes the balance between microbes and host defense in favor of the macrophages, thus serving to eradicate intracellular infections.

The substances that are toxic to microbes may injure normal tissues if they are released into the extracellular milieu, because these substances do not distinguish between microbes and host cells. This is the reason for tissue injury (a reflection of "hypersensitivity") in DTH reactions, which often accompany protective cell-mediated immunity. It is also the reason why prolonged macrophage activation in chronic cell-mediated immune reactions is associated with considerable injury to adjacent normal tissues. For instance, in mycobacterial infections, which are difficult to eradicate, much of the pathologic process is caused by a sustained T cell and macrophage response that attempts to wall off the bacteria. Histologically, such chronic cell-mediated immune responses often appear as granulomas, which are collections of activated lymphocytes and macrophages around the microbe with fibrosis and tissue necrosis.

Activated macrophages serve several roles, in addition to killing microbes, that are important in cell-mediated immunity (see Fig. 2-8, Chapter 2). Activated macrophages secrete cytokines, including TNF, IL-1, and chemokines, which stimulate the recruitment of neutrophils, monocytes, and effector T lymphocytes to the site of infection. Macrophages produce other cytokines, such as platelet-derived growth factor, that stimulate the growth and activities of fibroblasts and endothelial cells, helping to repair tissue after the infection is cleared. Macrophage activation also leads to the increased expression of class II MHC molecules and costimulators on these cells, thereby enhancing their antigen-presenting function, which promotes T cell activation and amplifies the cell-mediated immune reaction.

ROLE OF T_H2 CELLS IN CELL-MEDIATED IMMUNITY

The T_H2 subset of CD4+ T lymphocytes stimulates eosinophil-rich inflammation and also functions to limit the injurious consequences of macrophage activation. When differentiated T_H2 cells recognize antigens, the cells produce the cytokines IL-4 and IL-5 (as well as IL-10, which is also produced by many other cell populations). IL-4 stimulates the production of IgE antibody, and IL-5 activates eosinophils. This reaction is important for defense against helminthic infections, because helminths are killed by the granule proteins of activated eosinophils and by IgE-mediated mast cell activation, which releases mediators that are toxic to parasites or promote their expulsion from the gut.

Several cytokines produced by T_H2 cells, including IL-4, IL-10, and IL-13, inhibit the microbicidal activities of macrophages. IL-4 and IL-13 also can activate macrophages to express mannose receptors and IL-13 acts on fibroblasts to increase collagen synthesis and fibrosis. This type of macrophage response is called alternative macrophage activation, to distinguish it from classical activation, which enhances microbicidal functions. Alternative macrophage activation mediated by T_H2 cytokines may play a role in tissue repair and may contribute to tissue damage in the setting of chronic parasitic infections and allergic diseases.

The relative activation of T_H1 and T_H2 cells in response to an infectious microbe may determine the outcome of the infection (Fig. 6-9). For instance, the protozoal parasite *Leishmania major* lives inside macrophages, and its elimination requires the activation of the macrophages by *L. major*–specific T_H1 cells. Most inbred strains of mice make an effective T_H1 response to the parasite and are thus able to eradicate the infection. In some inbred mouse strains, however, the response to *L. major* is dominated by T_H2 cells, and these mice succumb to the infection. *Mycobacterium leprae,* the bacterium that causes leprosy, is a pathogen for humans that also lives inside macro-

Infection	Response	Outcome
Leishmania major	Most mouse strains: T$_H$1 $\Rightarrow$ BALB/c mice: T$_H$2 $\Rightarrow$	Recovery Disseminated infection
Mycobacterium leprae	Some patients: T$_H$1 $\Rightarrow$ Some patients: Defective T$_H$1 or dominant T$_H$2 $\Rightarrow$	Tuberculoid leprosy Lepromatous leprosy (high bacterial count)

FIGURE 6-9 **The balance between T$_H$1 and T$_H$2 cell activation determines the outcome of intracellular infections.** Naive CD4+ T lymphocytes may differentiate into T$_H$1 cells, which activate phagocytes to kill ingested microbes, and T$_H$2 cells, which inhibit macrophage activation. The balance between these two subsets may influence the outcome of infections, as illustrated by *Leishmania* infection in mice and leprosy in humans. IFN, interferon; IL, interleukin; TNF, tumor necrosis factor.

phages and may be eliminated by cell-mediated immune mechanisms. Some persons infected with *M. leprae* are unable to eradicate the infection, which, if left untreated, will progress to the classic destructive lesions of lepromatous leprosy. By contrast, in other patients, the bacteria induce strong cell-mediated immune responses with activated T cells and macrophages around the infection and few surviving microbes; this form of less destructive disease is called tuberculoid leprosy. Some studies have shown that the tuberculoid form is associated with the activation of *M. leprae*–specific T$_H$1 cells, whereas the destructive lepromatous form is associated with a defect in T$_H$1 cell activation or a dominant T$_H$2 response. The same principle, that the T cell cytokine response to an infectious pathogen is an important determinant of the outcome of the infection, may be true for many other infectious diseases.

As we mentioned earlier, activated macrophages are best at killing microbes that are confined to vesicles, and microbes that directly enter the cytoplasm (e.g., viruses) or escape from phagosomes into the cytoplasm (e.g., some phagocytosed bacteria) are relatively resistant to the microbicidal mechanisms of phagocytes. Eradication of such pathogens requires the second major effector mechanism of cell-mediated immunity, namely, cytotoxic T lymphocytes (CTLs).

Effector Functions of CD8+ Cytotoxic T Lymphocytes

CD8+ CTLs recognize class I MHC–associated peptides on infected cells and kill those cells, thereby eliminating the reservoir of infection (Fig. 6-10). The sources of class I–associated peptides are protein antigens synthesized in the cytoplasm and protein antigens of phagocytosed microbes that escape from phagocytic vesicles into the cytoplasm (see Chapter 3). Differentiated CD8+ CTLs recognize class I MHC–peptide complexes on the surface of infected cells by their T cell receptor (TCR) and by the CD8 co-receptor. (These infected cells also are called "targets" of CTLs, because they are destined to be killed by the CTLs.) CTLs adhere tightly to their target cells, mainly by virtue of integrins on the CTLs binding to ligands on the infected cells. The antigen receptors and co-receptors of the CTL cluster at the site of contact with the target cell, forming an immunologic synapse (see Chapter 5). The CTLs are activated by antigen recognition and firm adhesion; at this stage in their lives, the CTLs do not require costimulation or T cell help for activation. Therefore, differentiated CTLs are able to kill any infected cell in any tissue.

Antigen recognition by effector CTLs results in the activation of signal transduction pathways that lead to the exocytosis of the contents of the CTL's granules to the region of contact with the targets. CTLs kill target cells mainly as a result of delivery of granule proteins into the target cells. Two types of granule proteins that are critical for killing are granzymes and perforin. **Granzymes** are enzymes that cleave and thereby activate enzymes called caspases that are present in the cytoplasm of target cells, and the active caspases induce apoptosis. (Caspases are so named because they are cysteine proteases that cleave proteins at aspartic acid residues; their major function is to induce apoptosis.) **Perforin** is necessary for delivery of granzymes into the cytoplasm of the target cell. Perforin and granzymes may enter the target cells by receptor-mediated endocytosis, both proteins bound to a sulfated glycoprotein called serglycin. Perforin may then insert into endosomal membranes and facilitate the movement of granzymes through these membranes and into the cytoplasm. Activated CTLs also express a membrane protein called Fas ligand, which binds to a death-inducing receptor, called Fas (CD95), on target cells (see Chapter 9, Fig. 9-6). Engagement of Fas activates caspases and induces target cell apoptosis; this pathway of CTL killing does not require granule exocytosis and is probably a minor pathway. The net result of these effector mechanisms of CTLs

FIGURE 6-10 Mechanisms of killing of infected cells by CD8+ cytotoxic T lymphocytes (CTLs). CTLs recognize class I MHC–associated peptides of cytoplasmic microbes in infected cells and form tight adhesions ("conjugates") with these cells. Adhesion molecules, such as integrins, stabilize the binding of the CTLs to infected cells *(not shown)*. The CTLs are activated to release ("exocytose") their granule contents toward the infected cell (referred to as "targets" of CTL killing). The granule contents are taken into the target cell by receptor-mediated endocytosis, and granzymes are released into the cytoplasm by a perforin-dependent mechanism. Granzymes then induce apoptosis.

FIGURE 6-11 Cooperation between CD4+ and CD8+ T cells in the eradication of intracellular infections. In a macrophage infected by an intracellular bacterium, some of the bacteria are sequestered in vesicles (phagosomes) and others may escape into the cytoplasm. CD4+ T cells recognize antigens derived from the vesicular microbes and activate the macrophage to kill the microbes in the vesicles. CD8+ T cells recognize antigens derived from the cytoplasmic bacteria and are needed to kill the infected cell, thus eliminating the reservoir of infection. CTL, cytotoxic T lymphocyte; IFN, interferon; TNF, tumor necrosis factor.

is that the infected cells are killed. Cells that have undergone apoptosis are rapidly phagocytosed and eliminated. The mechanisms that induce fragmentation of target cell DNA, which is the hallmark of apoptosis, also may break down the DNA of microbes living inside the infected cells. Each CTL can kill a target cell, detach, and go on to kill additional targets.

As we mentioned earlier, CD8+ T lymphocytes also secrete the cytokine IFN-γ, which activates macrophages to destroy phagocytosed microbes and enhance the recruitment of additional leukocytes. Thus, CD8+ CTLs, like CD4+ helper cells, contribute to the elimination of microbes ingested by phagocytes.

Although we have described the effector functions of CD4+ T cells and CD8+ T cells separately, it is clear from our discussion that these types of T lymphocytes function cooperatively to eradicate intracellular

microbes (Fig. 6-11). If microbes are phagocytosed and remain sequestered in macrophage vesicles, CD4+ T cells may be adequate to eradicate these infections by secreting IFN-γ and activating the microbicidal mechanisms of the macrophages. If, however, the microbes are able to escape from vesicles into the cytoplasm, they become insusceptible to T cell–mediated macrophage activation, and their elimination requires killing of the infected cells by CD8+ CTLs.

Resistance of Pathogenic Microbes to Cell-Mediated Immunity

Different microbes have evolved diverse mechanisms to resist T lymphocyte–mediated host defense (Fig. 6-12). Many intracellular bacteria, such as *Mycobacterium tuberculosis, Legio1nella pneumo-*

FIGURE 6-12 Evasion of cell-mediated immunity by microbes. Different bacteria and viruses resist the effector mechanisms of cell-mediated immunity by different mechanisms, selected examples of which are shown. ER, endoplasmic reticulum; IFN, interferon; IL, interleukin; TAP, transporter associated with antigen processing.

Microbe	Mechanism	
Mycobacteria	Inhibition of phagolysosome fusion	
Herpes simplex virus (HSV)	Inhibition of antigen presentation: HSV peptide interferes with TAP transporter	
Cytomegalovirus (CMV)	Inhibition of antigen presentation: inhibition of proteasomal activity; removal of class I MHC molecules from endoplasmic reticulum (ER)	
Epstein-Barr virus (EBV)	Inhibition of antigen presentation: inhibition of proteasomal activity	
Epstein-Barr virus (EBV)	Production of IL-10, inhibition of macrophage and dendritic cell activation	
Pox Virus	Inhibition of effector cell activation: production of soluble cytokine receptors	

phila, and *Listeria monocytogenes,* inhibit the fusion of phagosomes with lysosomes and create pores in phagosome membranes, allowing these organisms to escape into the cytoplasm. Thus, these microbes are able to resist the microbicidal mechanisms of phagocytes and survive and even replicate inside phagocytes. Many viruses inhibit class I MHC–associated antigen presentation, by inhibiting production or expression of class I molecules, by blocking transport of antigenic peptides from the cytosol into the endoplasmic reticulum (ER), and by removing newly synthesized class I molecules from the ER. All of these viral mechanisms reduce the loading of class I MHC molecules by viral peptides. The result of this defective loading is reduced surface expression of class I MHC molecules, because empty class I molecules are unstable and are not expressed on the cell surface. It is interesting that natural killer (NK) cells are activated by class I–deficient cells (see Chapter 2). Thus, host defenses have evolved to combat immune evasion mechanisms of microbes: CTLs recognize class I MHC–associated viral peptides, viruses inhibit class I MHC expression, and NK cells recognize the absence of class I MHC molecules. Other viruses produce inhibitory cytokines or soluble ("decoy") cytokine receptors that bind and "sop up" cytokines such as IFN-γ, thereby reducing the amount of cytokines available to trigger cell-mediated immune reactions. Some viruses evade elimination and establish chronic infections by stimulating expression of the inhibitory receptor PD-1 (see Chapter 5) on CD8+ T cells and thus inhibiting the effector functions of CTLs. Still other viruses directly infect and kill T lymphocytes; the best example of such a virus is human immunodeficiency virus, which is able to survive in infected persons by killing CD4+ T cells. The outcome of infections is influenced by the strength of host defenses and the ability of pathogens to resist these defenses. The same principle is evident when the effector mechanisms of humoral immunity are considered.

One approach for tilting the balance between the host and microbes in favor of protective immunity is to vaccinate individuals to enhance immune responses. The principles underlying vaccination strategies are described at the end of Chapter 8, after the discussion of humoral immunity.

SUMMARY

■ Cell-mediated immunity is the arm of adaptive immunity that eradicates infections by intracellular microbes. Cell-mediated immune reactions are of two types: CD4+ T cells activate macrophages to kill ingested microbes that are able to survive in the vesicles of phagocytes, and CD8+ CTLs kill cells harboring microbes in their cytoplasm, thereby eliminating reservoirs of infection.

■ Effector T cells are generated in peripheral lymphoid organs, mainly lymph nodes draining sites of microbe entry, by the activation of naive T lymphocytes. The effector T cells are able to migrate to any site of infection.

■ The migration of effector T cells is controlled by adhesion molecules and chemokines. Various adhesion molecules are induced on the T cells after activation and bind to their ligands, which themselves are induced on endothelial cells by microbes and by cytokines produced during innate immune responses to microbes. The migration of T cells is independent of antigen, but cells that recognize microbial antigens in tissues are retained at these sites.

■ Effector cells of the T$_H$1 subset of CD4+ T cells recognize the antigens of microbes that have been ingested by macrophages. These T cells express CD40 ligand and secrete IFN-γ, which function cooperatively to activate macrophages. T$_H$17 cells may enhance leukocyte recruitment and inflammation.

■ Activated macrophages produce substances, including reactive oxygen species, nitric oxide, and lysosomal enzymes, that kill ingested microbes. Macrophages also produce cytokines that induce inflammation and other cytokines that promote fibrosis and tissue repair.

■ Effector CD4+ T cells of the T$_H$2 subset stimulate eosinophilic inflammation and inhibit the microbicidal functions of activated macrophages. Eosinophils are important in host defense against helminthic parasites. The balance between activation of T$_H$1 and T$_H$2 cells determines the outcomes of many infections, with T$_H$1 cells promoting and T$_H$2 cells suppressing defense against intracellular microbes.

■ CD8$^+$ T cells differentiate into CTLs that kill infected cells, mainly by inducing DNA fragmentation and apoptosis. CD4$^+$ and CD8$^+$ T cells often function cooperatively to eradicate intracellular infections.

■ Many pathogenic microbes have evolved mechanisms to resist cell-mediated immunity. These mechanisms include inhibiting phagolysosome fusion, escaping from the vesicles of phagocytes, inhibiting the assembly of class I MHC–peptide complexes, and producing inhibitory cytokines or decoy cytokine receptors.

REVIEW QUESTIONS

1 *What are the types of T lymphocyte–mediated immune reactions that eliminate microbes that are sequestered in the vesicles of phagocytes and microbes that live in the cytoplasm of infected host cells?*

2 *Why do differentiated effector T cells (which have been activated by antigen) migrate preferentially to tissues that are sites of infection and not to lymph nodes?*

3 *What are the mechanisms by which T cells activate macrophages, and what are the responses of macrophages that result in the killing of ingested microbes?*

4 *What are the roles of T$_H$1 and T$_H$2 cells in defense against intracellular microbes and helminthic parasites?*

5 *How do CD8$^+$ CTLs kill cells infected with viruses?*

6 *What are some of the mechanisms by which intracellular microbes resist the effector mechanisms of cell-mediated immunity?*

Chapter 7

HUMORAL IMMUNE RESPONSES

Activation of B Lymphocytes and Production of Antibodies

Humoral immunity is mediated by antibodies and is the arm of the adaptive immune response that functions to neutralize and eliminate extracellular microbes and microbial toxins. Humoral immunity is more important than cellular immunity in defending against microbes with capsules rich in polysaccharides and lipids, and against polysaccharide and lipid toxins. The reason for this is that B cells respond to, and produce antibodies specific for, many types of molecules, but T cells, the mediators of cellular immunity, recognize and respond only to protein antigens. Antibodies are produced by B lymphocytes and their progeny. Naive B lymphocytes recognize antigens but do not secrete antibodies, and activation of these cells stimulates their differentiation into antibody-secreting plasma cells. In this chapter, we describe the process and mechanisms of B cell activation and antibody production, focusing on the following questions:

- How are receptor-expressing B lymphocytes activated and converted to antibody-secreting cells?
- How is the process of B cell activation regulated so that the most useful types of antibodies are produced in response to different types of microbes?

Chapter 8 describes how the antibodies that are produced during humoral immune responses function to defend individuals against microbes and toxins.

FIGURE 7-1   Phases of humoral immune responses. Naive B lymphocytes recognize antigens, and under the influence of helper T cells and other stimuli *(not shown),* the B cells are activated to proliferate, giving rise to clonal expansion, and to differentiate into antibody-secreting plasma cells. Some of the activated B cells undergo heavy chain isotype switching and affinity maturation, and some become long-lived memory cells.

Phases and Types of Humoral Immune Responses

Naive B lymphocytes express two classes of membrane-bound antibodies, IgM (immunoglobulin M) and IgD, that function as the receptors for antigens. These naive B cells are activated by antigens and by other signals that are discussed later in the chapter. The activation of B lymphocytes results in the proliferation of antigen-specific cells, called **clonal expansion,** and in their differentiation into effector cells, called **plasma cells,** that actively secrete antibodies (Fig. 7-1). The secreted antibodies have the same specificity as that of the naive B cell membrane receptors that recognized antigen to initiate the response. One activated B cell may generate up to 4000 plasma cells, which can produce up to 10^{12} antibody molecules per day. In this way, humoral immunity can

keep pace with rapidly proliferating microbes. During their differentiation, some B cells may begin to produce antibodies of different heavy chain isotypes (or classes), which mediate different effector functions and are specialized to combat different types of microbes. This process is called **heavy chain isotype (class) switching.** Repeated exposure to a protein antigen results in the production of antibodies with increasing affinity for the antigen. This process is called **affinity maturation,** and it leads to the production of antibodies with improved capacity to bind to and neutralize microbes and their toxins.

Antibody responses to different antigens are classified as T-dependent or T-independent, based on the requirement for T cell help. B lymphocytes recognize and are activated by a wide variety of different chemical structures, including proteins, polysaccharides, lipids, and small chemicals. Protein antigens are processed in antigen-presenting cells (APCs) and recognized by helper T lymphocytes, which play an important role in B cell activation and induce heavy chain isotype switching and affinity maturation. (The designation *helper* came from the discovery that some T cells stimulate, or help, B lymphocytes to produce antibodies.) In the absence of T cell help, protein antigens elicit weak or no antibody responses. Therefore, protein antigens, and the antibody responses to these antigens, are called "T-dependent." Polysaccharides, lipids, and other nonprotein antigens stimulate antibody production without the involvement of helper T cells. Therefore, these nonprotein antigens, and the antibody responses to them, are called "T-independent." The antibodies produced in response to T-independent antigens show relatively little heavy chain isotype switching and affinity maturation.

Different subsets of B cells respond preferentially to protein and nonprotein antigens (Fig. 7-2).

A majority of B cells are called **follicular B cells** because they reside in the follicles of lymphoid organs. These follicular B cells make the bulk of T-dependent, class-switched, and high-affinity antibody responses to protein antigens and give rise to long-lived plasma cells. **Marginal zone B cells,** which are located in the marginal zones of the splenic white pulp, respond to blood-borne polysaccharide antigens, and **B-1 B cells** respond to nonprotein antigens in the mucosal tissues and peritoneum. Marginal zone and B-1 B cells express antigen receptors of limited diversity and make predominantly IgM responses, which lack many of the features of T-dependent antibody responses to protein antigens.

Antibody responses to the first and subsequent exposures to an antigen, called primary and secondary responses, differ quantitatively and qualitatively (Fig. 7-3). The amounts of antibody produced after the first encounter with an antigen (i.e., primary responses) are smaller than the amounts of antibody

FIGURE 7-2 **Subsets of B cells.** Follicular B cells make T-dependent responses to protein antigens, and marginal zone and B-1 B cells account for most of the T-independent antibody responses. In mice it has been shown that B-1 B cells arise earlier in development, from progenitors in the fetal liver, and follicular and marginal zone B cells arise later, from bone marrow precursors. Comparable differences in the origins of these subsets have not been defined in humans. Note also that the distinctions in the type of response are not absolute—follicular B cells can make T-independent responses and marginal zone B cells can make some T-dependent responses. Ig, immunoglobulin.

FIGURE 7-3 **Features of primary and secondary antibody responses.** Primary and secondary antibody responses differ in several respects, illustrated schematically in **A** and summarized in **B**. In a primary response, naive B cells in peripheral lymphoid tissues are activated to proliferate and differentiate into antibody-secreting cells and memory cells. Some antibody-secreting plasma cells may migrate to and survive in the bone marrow for long periods. In a secondary response, memory B cells are activated to produce larger amounts of antibodies, often with more heavy chain class switching and affinity maturation. Many of the features of secondary responses (e.g., heavy chain isotype switching, affinity maturation) are seen mainly in responses to protein antigens, because these changes in B cells are stimulated by helper T cells and only proteins activate T cells. The kinetics of the responses may vary with different antigens and types of immunization. Ig, immunoglobulin.

produced on repeated immunization (i.e., secondary responses). With protein antigens, secondary responses also show increased heavy chain isotype switching and affinity maturation, because repeated stimulation by an antigen leads to increases in the numbers of helper T lymphocytes.

With this introduction, we proceed to a discussion of B cell activation and antibody production, beginning with the responses of B cells to the initial encounter with antigen.

Stimulation of B Lymphocytes by Antigen

Humoral immune responses are initiated when antigen-specific B lymphocytes in the spleen, lymph nodes, and mucosal lymphoid tissues recognize antigens. Some of the antigens of microbes that enter tissues or are present in the blood are transported to and concentrated in the B cell–rich follicles and marginal zones of the peripheral lymphoid organs. In lymph nodes, macrophages lining the subcapsular sinus may capture antigens and display them to B cells in adjacent follicles. B lymphocytes specific for an antigen use their membrane-bound immunoglobulin (Ig) receptors to recognize the antigen in its native conformation (i.e., without a need for processing). The recognition of antigen triggers signaling pathways that initiate B cell activation. As with T lymphocytes, B cell activation also requires signals in addition to antigen recognition, and many of these second signals are produced during innate immune reactions to microbes. In the following section, we will describe the mechanisms of B cell activation, followed by discussion of the functional consequences of antigen recognition.

ANTIGEN-INDUCED SIGNALING IN B CELLS

Antigen-induced clustering of membrane Ig receptors triggers biochemical signals that are transduced by receptor-associated signaling molecules (Fig. 7-4). The process of B lymphocyte activation is, in principle, similar to the activation of T cells (see Chapter 5). In B cells, Ig receptor–mediated signal transduction requires the bringing together (cross-linking) of two or more receptor molecules. Receptor

cross-linking occurs when two or more antigen molecules in an aggregate, or repeating epitopes of one antigen molecule, bind to adjacent Ig molecules in the membrane of a B cell. Polysaccharides, lipids, and other nonprotein antigens often contain multiple identical epitopes in each molecule and are therefore able to bind to numerous Ig receptors on a B cell at the same time.

Signals initiated by antigen receptor cross-linking are transduced by receptor-associated proteins. Membrane IgM and IgD, the antigen receptors of naive B lymphocytes, have highly variable extracellular antigen-binding regions (see Chapter 4) and short cytoplasmic domains. These membrane receptors recognize antigens but do not themselves transduce signals. The receptors are noncovalently attached to two proteins, called Igα and Igβ, to form the **B cell receptor (BCR) complex** (analogous to the T cell receptor [TCR] complex of T lymphocytes). The cytoplasmic domains of Igα and Igβ contain conserved immunoreceptor tyrosine-based activation motifs (ITAMs), which are found in signaling subunits of many other activating receptors in the immune system (e.g., the CD3 and ζ proteins of the TCR complex; see Chapter 5). When two or more antigen receptors of a B cell are clustered, the tyrosines in the ITAMs of Igα and Igβ are phosphorylated by kinases associated with the BCR complex. These phosphotyrosines become docking sites for adapter proteins that themselves get phosphorylated and then recruit a number of signaling molecules. The components of receptor-induced signaling cascades are not as well understood in B cells as they are in T lymphocytes, but the signaling events are essentially similar in the two lymphocyte populations (see Chapter 5, Fig. 5-9). The net result of receptor-induced signaling in B cells is the activation of transcription factors that turn on genes whose protein products are involved in B cell proliferation and differentiation. Some of the important proteins are described later in this section of the chapter.

THE ROLE OF COMPLEMENT PROTEINS IN B CELL ACTIVATION

B lymphocytes express a receptor for a protein of the complement system that provides signals for

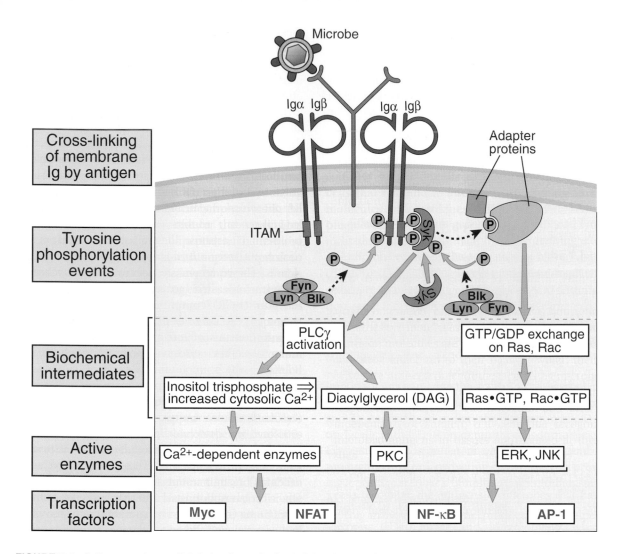

FIGURE 7-4 **Antigen receptor–mediated signal transduction in B lymphocytes.** Cross-linking of immunoglobulin (Ig) receptors of B cells by antigen triggers biochemical signals that are transduced by the Ig-associated proteins Igα and Igβ. These signals induce early tyrosine phosphorylation events, activation of various biochemical intermediates and enzymes, and activation of transcription factors. Similar signaling events are seen in T cells after antigen recognition. Note that signaling requires cross-linking of at least two Ig receptors by antigens, but only a single receptor is shown for simplicity. AP-1, activating protein-1; GDP, guanosine diphosphate; GTP, guanosine triphosphate; ITAM, immunoreceptor tyrosine-based activation motif; NFAT, nuclear factor of activated T cells; NF-κB, nuclear factor-κB; PKC, protein kinase C; PLCγ, phospholipase C-γ.

the activation of the cells (Fig. 7-5). The complement system is a collection of plasma proteins that are activated by microbes and by antibodies attached to microbes and whose function as effector mechanisms of host defense is well known (see Chapter 8). When the complement system is activated by a microbe, the microbe becomes coated with breakdown products of the most abundant complement protein, C3. One of these breakdown products is a fragment called C3d. B lymphocytes express a receptor, called the type 2 complement receptor (CR2, or CD21), that binds C3d. B cells that are specific for a microbe's antigens recognize lates B cell proliferation and Ig secretion, thus promoting antibody responses against microbes.

FUNCTIONAL CONSEQUENCES OF ANTIGEN-MEDIATED B CELL ACTIVATION

The consequences of B cell activation by antigen (and second signals) are to initiate B cell proliferation and differentiation and to prepare the B cells to interact with helper T lymphocytes (if the antigen is a protein) (Fig. 7-6). The activated B lymphocytes enter the cell cycle and begin to proliferate, resulting in expansion of the antigen-specific clones. The cells may also begin to synthesize more IgM and to produce some of this IgM in a secreted form. Thus, antigen stimulation induces the early phase of the humoral immune response. This response is greatest when the antigen is multivalent, cross-links many antigen receptors, and activates complement strongly; all of these features are typically seen with polysaccharides and other T-independent antigens (which are discussed in detail later in the chapter). Most soluble protein antigens do not contain multiple identical epitopes, are not capable of cross-linking many receptors on B cells, and, by themselves, typically do not stimulate high levels of B cell proliferation and differentiation. However, protein antigens do induce signals in B lymphocytes that lead to important changes in the cells that enhance their ability to interact with helper T lymphocytes. B cell activation leads to increased expression of B7 costimulators, which provide second signals for T cell activation and may function to amplify helper T cell responses, and to the expression of receptors for cytokines, which are the secreted mediators of helper T cell functions. Activated B cells also reduce their expression of receptors for chemokines that are produced in lymphoid follicles and whose function is to keep the B cells in these follicles. As a result, the activated B cells migrate out of the follicles and toward the anatomic compartment where helper T cells are concentrated.

So far we have described how B lymphocytes recognize antigens and receive the signals that initiate humoral immune responses. As stated at the outset, antibody responses to protein antigens require the participation of helper T cells. In the next section we describe the interactions of helper T cells with B lymphocytes in antibody responses to T-dependent

FIGURE 7-5 The role of the complement protein C3d in B cell activation. Activation of complement by microbes leads to the binding of a complement breakdown product, C3d, to the microbes. The B cell simultaneously recognizes a microbial antigen (by the immunoglobulin [Ig] receptor) and bound C3d (by the CR2 receptor). CR2 is attached to a complex of proteins (CD19, CD81) that are involved in delivering activating signals to the B cell.

the antigen by their Ig receptors and simultaneously recognize the bound C3d by the CR2 receptor. Engagement of CR2 greatly enhances antigen-dependent activation responses of B cells. Thus, complement proteins provide second signals for B cell activation, functioning in concert with antigen (which is "signal 1") to initiate B cell proliferation and differentiation. This role of complement in humoral immune responses again illustrates an idea we have mentioned previously—that microbes or innate immune responses to microbes provide signals in addition to antigen that are necessary for lymphocyte activation. In humoral immunity, complement activation is the relevant innate immune response and C3d is the second signal for B lymphocytes, analogous to the costimulators of APCs for T lymphocytes.

B cell responses may be enhanced not only by recognition of complement proteins but also by microbial products engaging Toll-like receptors (TLRs) on the B cells. B lymphocytes, like dendritic cells and other leukocytes, express numerous TLRs (Chapter 2). Recognition of microbial products by these TLRs stimu-

B cell response to antigen	Significance
Entry into cell cycle, mitosis	Clonal expansion
Increased expression of cytokine receptors	Ability to respond to cytokines produced by helper T cells
Migration out of lymphoid follicles	Interaction with helper T cells
Secretion of low levels of IgM	Early phase of humoral immune response

FIGURE 7-6 **Functional consequences of immunoglobulin (Ig)-mediated B cell activation.** The activation of B cells by antigen in lymphoid organs initiates the process of B cell proliferation and IgM secretion and "prepares" the B cell to activate helper T cells and respond to T cell help by stimulating migration of the B cells toward the T cell–rich zones of the lymphoid organs.

protein antigens. Responses to T-independent antigens are discussed at the end of the chapter.

The Function of Helper T Lymphocytes in Humoral Immune Responses to Protein Antigens

For a protein antigen to stimulate an antibody response, B lymphocytes and helper T lymphocytes specific for that antigen must come together in lymphoid organs and interact in a way that stimulates B cell proliferation and differentiation. We know that this process works very efficiently, because protein antigens elicit excellent antibody responses within 3 to 7 days of antigen exposure. The efficiency of the process raises many questions. How do B cells and T cells specific for epitopes of the same antigen find one another, considering that both types of lymphocytes specific for any one antigen are rare, probably less than 1 in 100,000 of all of the lymphocytes in the body? How do helper T cells specific for an antigen interact with B cells specific for the same antigen and not with irrelevant B cells? What signals are delivered by helper T cells that stimulate not only the secretion of antibody but also the special features of the antibody response to proteins, namely, heavy chain isotype switching and affinity maturation? As is apparent in the discussion that follows, the answers to these questions are now well understood.

FIGURE 7-7   The interactions of helper T cells and B cells in lymphoid tissues. CD4+ helper T cells recognize processed protein antigens displayed by dendritic cells and are activated to proliferate and differentiate into effector cells. These effector T cells begin to migrate toward lymphoid follicles. Naive B lymphocytes, which reside in the follicles, recognize antigens in this site and are activated to migrate out of the follicles. The two cell populations come together at the edges of the follicles and interact. APC, antigen-presenting cell.

ACTIVATION AND MIGRATION OF HELPER T CELLS

Helper T cells that have been activated to differentiate into effector cells interact with antigen-stimulated B lymphocytes at the edges of lymphoid follicles in the peripheral lymphoid organs (Fig. 7-7). Naive CD4+ helper T lymphocytes are stimulated to proliferate and differentiate into cytokine-producing effector cells as a result of recognizing antigens on APCs, mainly dendritic cells, in the lymphoid organs. The process of T cell activation was described in Chapter 5. To reiterate the important points, the initial activation of T cells requires antigen recognition and costimulation. The antigens that stimulate CD4+ helper T cells are derived from extracellular microbes and proteins that are processed and displayed bound to class II major histocompatibility complex (MHC) molecules of APCs in the T cell–rich zones of peripheral lymphoid tissues. T cell activation is induced best by microbial antigens, and by protein antigens that are administered with adjuvants, which stimulate the expression of costimulators on APCs. The CD4+ T cells may differentiate into effector cells capable of producing various cytokines; the T_H1, T_H2, and T_H17

subsets described in Chapter 5 are examples of such differentiated effector cells. Differentiated effector T cells begin to migrate out of their normal sites of residence. As discussed in Chapter 6, some of these T lymphocytes enter the circulation, find microbial antigens at distant sites, and eradicate the microbes by the reactions of cell-mediated immunity. Other differentiated helper T cells migrate toward the edges of lymphoid follicles at the same time as antigen-stimulated B lymphocytes within the follicles are beginning to migrate outward. This directed migration of the B and T cells toward one another depends on changes in the expression of certain chemokine receptors on the activated lymphocytes. Upon activation, T cells reduce expression of the chemokine receptor CCR7, which recognizes chemokines produced in T cell zones, and increase expression of the chemokine receptor CXCR5, which promotes migration into B cell follicles. B cells, upon activation, undergo precisely the opposite changes, decreasing CXCR5 and increasing CCR7 expression. As a result, antigen-activated B and T cells migrate toward one another and meet at the edges of lymphoid follicles. The next step in their interaction occurs here.

PRESENTATION OF ANTIGENS BY B LYMPHOCYTES TO HELPER T CELLS

B lymphocytes that bind protein antigens by their specific antigen receptors endocytose these antigens, process them in endosomal vesicles, and display class II MHC–associated peptides for recognition by CD4+ helper T cells (Fig. 7-8). The membrane Ig of B cells is a high-affinity receptor that enables a B cell to specifically bind a particular antigen

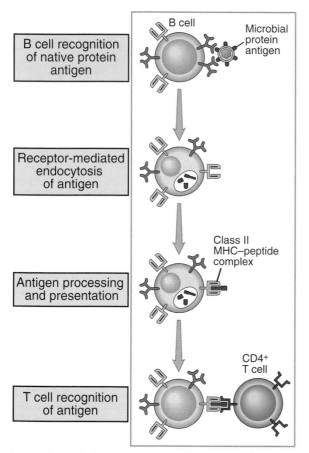

FIGURE 7-8   Antigen presentation by B lymphocytes to helper T cells. B cells specific for a protein antigen bind and internalize that antigen, process it, and present peptides attached to class II major histocompatibility complex (MHC) molecules to helper T cells. The B cells and helper T cells are specific for the same antigen, but the B cells recognize native (conformational) epitopes and the helper T cells recognize peptide fragments of the antigen. B cells also express costimulators (e.g., B7 molecules) that play a role in T cell activation.

even when the extracellular concentration of the antigen is very low. In addition, antigen bound by membrane Ig is endocytosed very efficiently and is delivered to the intracellular endosomal vesicles where proteins are processed into peptides that bind to class II MHC molecules (see Chapter 3). Therefore, B lymphocytes are very efficient APCs for the antigens they specifically recognize. Note that any one B cell may bind a conformational epitope of a protein antigen, internalize and process the protein, and display multiple peptides of that protein for T cell recognition. Therefore, B cells and T cells recognize different epitopes of the same protein antigen. Because B cells present the antigen for which they have specific receptors, and helper T cells specifically recognize peptides derived from the same antigen, the ensuing interaction remains antigen specific. As we mentioned earlier, antigen-activated B lymphocytes also express costimulators, such as B7 molecules, that stimulate the helper T cells that recognize antigen displayed by the B cells. B cells are capable of activating previously differentiated effector T cells but are inefficient at initiating the responses of naive T cells.

MECHANISMS OF HELPER T CELL–MEDIATED ACTIVATION OF B LYMPHOCYTES

Helper T lymphocytes that recognize antigen presented by B cells activate the B cells by expressing CD40 ligand (CD40L) and by secreting cytokines (Fig. 7-9). The process of helper T cell–mediated B lymphocyte activation is analogous to the process of T cell–mediated macrophage activation in cell-mediated immunity (see Chapter 6). CD40L on activated helper T cells binds to CD40 expressed on B lymphocytes. Engagement of CD40 delivers signals to the B cells that stimulate proliferation (clonal expansion) and the synthesis and secretion of antibodies. At the same time, cytokines produced by the helper T cells bind to cytokine receptors on B lymphocytes and stimulate more B cell proliferation and Ig production. The requirement for the CD40L-CD40 interaction ensures that only T and B lymphocytes in physical contact engage in productive interactions. As we described previously, the antigen-specific lymphocytes are the ones that physically interact, thus ensuring that the antigen-specific B cells also are the ones

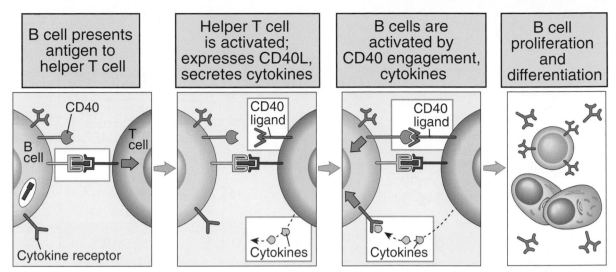

FIGURE 7-9 **Mechanisms of helper T cell–mediated activation of B lymphocytes.** Helper T cells recognize peptide antigens presented by B cells and costimulators (e.g., B7 molecules) on the B cells. The helper T cells are activated to express CD40 ligand (CD40L) and secrete cytokines, both of which bind to their receptors on the same B cells and activate the B cells.

that are activated. Helper T cell signals also stimulate heavy chain isotype switching and affinity maturation, which typically are seen in antibody responses to T-dependent protein antigens.

HEAVY CHAIN ISOTYPE (CLASS) SWITCHING

Helper T cells stimulate the progeny of IgM and IgD–expressing B lymphocytes to produce antibodies of different heavy chain isotypes (classes) (Fig. 7-10). Different antibody isotypes perform different functions and, therefore, the process of isotype switching broadens the functional capabilities of humoral immune responses. For instance, an important defense mechanism against the extracellular stages of most bacteria and viruses is to coat (opsonize) these microbes with antibodies and cause them to be phagocytosed by neutrophils and macrophages. This reaction is best mediated by antibody classes, such as IgG1 and IgG3 (in humans), that bind to high-affinity phagocyte Fc receptors specific for the γ heavy chain (see Chapter 8). By contrast, helminths are best eliminated by eosinophils, and therefore defense against these parasites involves coating them with antibodies to which eosinophils bind. The antibody class that is

able to do this is IgE, because eosinophils have high-affinity receptors for the Fc portion of the ε heavy chain. Thus, effective host defense requires that the immune system make different antibody isotypes in response to different microbes, even though all naive B lymphocytes specific for all these microbes express antigen receptors of the IgM and IgD isotypes.

Heavy chain isotype switching is induced by a combination of CD40L-mediated signals and cytokines. These signals act on antigen-stimulated B cells and induce switching in some of the progeny of these cells. In the absence of CD40 or CD40L, B cells secrete only IgM and fail to switch to other isotypes, indicating the essential role of this ligand-receptor pair in class switching. A disease called the **X-linked hyper-IgM syndrome** is caused by mutations in the CD40L gene, which is located in the X chromosome, leading to production of nonfunctional forms of CD40L. In this disease, much of the serum antibody is IgM, because of defective heavy chain class switching. Patients also suffer from defective cell-mediated immunity against intracellular microbes, because CD40L is important for T cell–mediated immunity (see Chapter 6). Cytokines influence which heavy chain class an individual B cell and its progeny will switch to.

FIGURE 7-10 Immunoglobulin (Ig) heavy chain isotype (class) switching. Antigen-stimulated B lymphocytes may differentiate into IgM antibody–secreting cells, or, under the influence of CD40 ligand (CD40L) and cytokines, some of the B cells may differentiate into cells that produce different Ig heavy chain isotypes. The principal effector functions of some of these isotypes are listed; all isotypes may function to neutralize microbes and toxins. BAFF is a B cell–activating cytokine that may be involved in switching to IgA in T-independent responses. IFN, interferon; IL, interleukin; TGF, transforming growth factor.

The molecular basis of heavy chain isotype switching is understood quite precisely (Fig. 7-11). IgM-producing B cells, which have not undergone switching, contain in their Ig heavy chain locus a rearranged VDJ gene adjacent to the first constant region cluster, which is C_μ. The heavy chain mRNA is produced by splicing of VDJ RNA to C_μ RNA, and this mRNA is translated to produce the μ heavy chain, which combines with a light chain to give rise to IgM antibody. Thus, the first antibody produced by B cells is IgM. Signals from CD40 and cytokine receptors stimulate transcription through one of the constant regions that is downstream of C_μ. In the intron 5′ of each constant region (except C_δ) is a conserved nucleotide sequence called the switch region. When a downstream constant region becomes transcriptionally active, the switch region 3′ of C_μ recombines with

the switch region 5′ of that downstream constant region, and the intervening DNA is deleted. The enzyme called **activation-induced deaminase (AID)** plays a key role in these events by making nucleotides susceptible to cleavage and thus accessible to recombination. Predictably, CD40 signals induce the expression of AID. This process is called **switch recombination.** It brings the rearranged VDJ adjacent to a downstream C region. The result is that the B cell begins to produce a new heavy chain isotype (which is determined by the C region of the antibody) with the same specificity as that of the original B cell (because specificity is determined by the rearranged VDJ).

Cytokines produced by helper T cells determine which heavy chain isotype is produced by influencing which heavy chain constant region gene

FIGURE 7-11 Mechanism of immunoglobulin (Ig) heavy chain isotype switching. In an IgM-secreting B cell *(left panel),* the primary transcript of the rearranged VDJ heavy chain gene is spliced onto the μ messenger RNA (mRNA) to produce the μ heavy chain and IgM antibody, because the μ gene is closest to the VDJ gene. Signals from helper T cells (CD40 ligation and cytokines) may induce recombination of switch (S) regions such that the rearranged VDJ gene is moved close to a C gene downstream of C_μ. The enzyme activation-induced deaminase (AID) alters nucleotides in the switch regions so that they can be cleaved by other enzymes and joined to downstream switch regions. (Switch recombination is shown by *dashed lines.*) Subsequently, the VDJ primary RNA is spliced onto the RNA from the downstream C gene, producing a heavy chain with a new constant region and thus a new class of Ig. The two *right panels* illustrate how the progeny of an activated B cell may switch to produce two different antibody classes, IgG and IgE. (Exons encoding γ and α heavy chains are not shown for simplicity.)

participates in switch recombination (see Fig. 7-10). For instance, the production of opsonizing antibodies, which bind to phagocyte Fc receptors, is stimulated by interferon (IFN)-γ, the signature cytokine of T$_H$1 cells. These opsonizing antibodies promote phagocytosis, a prelude to microbe killing by phagocytes. IFN-γ also is a phagocyte-activating cytokine, and it stimulates the microbicidal activities of phagocytes. Thus, the actions of IFN-γ on B cells complement the actions of this cytokine on phagocytes. Many bacteria and viruses stimulate T$_H$1 responses, which activate the effector mechanisms that are best at eliminating these microbes. By contrast, switching to the IgE class is stimulated by interleukin (IL)-4, the signature cytokine of T$_H$2 cells. IgE functions to eliminate helminths, acting in concert with eosinophils, which are activated by the second T$_H$2 cytokine, IL-5. Predictably, helminths induce strong T$_H$2 responses. Thus, the nature of the helper T cell response to a microbe guides the subsequent antibody response, making it optimal for combating that microbe. These are excellent examples of how different components of the immune system are regulated coordinately and function together in defense against different types of microbes, and how helper T cells may function as the "master" controllers of immune responses.

The nature of antibody isotypes produced is also influenced by the site of immune responses. For instance, IgA antibody is the major isotype produced in mucosal lymphoid tissues. This is probably because B cells committed to IgA migrate to these tissues, and cytokines that promote switching to IgA are made in mucosal tissues. IgA is the principal antibody isotype that can be actively secreted through mucosal epithelia (see Chapter 8), and this presumably is why mucosal lymphoid tissues are the major sites of IgA production. B-1 B cells also appear to be important sources of IgA antibody in mucosal tissues, especially against nonprotein antigens. The cytokines that drive isotype switching in this B cell subset are not fully defined.

AFFINITY MATURATION

Affinity maturation is the process by which the affinity of antibodies produced in response to a protein antigen increases with prolonged or repeated exposure to that antigen. Because of affinity maturation, the ability of antibodies to bind to a microbe or microbial antigen increases if the infection is persistent or recurrent. This increase in affinity is due to point mutations in the V regions, and particularly in the antigen-binding hypervariable regions, of the antibodies produced (Fig. 7-12). Affinity maturation is seen only in responses to helper T cell–dependent protein antigens, suggesting that helper cells are critical in the process. These findings raise two intriguing questions: How do B cells undergo Ig gene mutations, and how are the high-affinity (i.e., most useful) B cells selected to become progressively more numerous?

Affinity maturation occurs in the germinal centers of lymphoid follicles and is the result of somatic hypermutation of Ig genes in dividing B cells followed by the selection of high-affinity B cells by antigen (Fig. 7-13). Some of the progeny of activated B lymphocytes enter lymphoid follicles and form germinal centers. Within these germinal centers, the B cells proliferate rapidly, with a doubling time of approximately 6 hours, so that one cell may produce about 5000 progeny within a week. (The name "germinal center" came from the morphologic observation that some follicles have central regions that stain lightly because they contain large numbers of dividing cells, once believed to be sites of production of lymphocytes.) During this proliferation, the Ig genes of the B cells undergo numerous point mutations. The enzyme AID, which we mentioned is required for isotype switching, also plays a critical role in somatic mutation by changing nucleotides in the Ig genes and making them susceptible to the mutational machinery. The frequency of Ig gene mutations is estimated to be one in 10^3 base pairs per cell per division, which is a thousand-fold greater than the mutation rate in most other genes. For this reason, Ig mutation is called **somatic hypermutation.** This extensive mutation results in the generation of different B cell clones whose Ig molecules may bind with widely varying affinities to the antigen that initiated the response.

FIGURE 7-12 Affinity maturation in antibody responses. Analysis of several individual antibodies produced by different clones of B cells against one antigen at different stages of primary, secondary, and tertiary immune responses shows that with time and repeated immunization, the antibodies that are produced contain increasing numbers of mutations in their antigen-binding regions (the complementarity-determining regions [CDRs]). The antibodies also show increasing affinities for the antigen, as revealed by the lower dissociation constant (K_d) values at the *right*. These results imply that the mutations are responsible for the increased affinities of the antibodies for the immunizing antigen. Secondary and tertiary responses refer to responses to the second and third immunizations with the same antigen. (Adapted from Berek C, Milstein C: Mutation drift and repertoire shift in the maturation of the immune response. Immunol Rev 96:23-41, 1987, with permission.)

Germinal center B cells die by apoptosis unless they are rescued by antigen recognition or T cell help. At the same time as somatic hypermutation of Ig genes is going on in germinal centers, the antibody that was secreted earlier during the immune response binds residual antigen. The antigen-antibody complexes that are formed may activate complement. These complexes are displayed by cells, called **follicular dendritic cells,** that reside in the germinal center and express receptors for the Fc portions of antibodies and for complement products, both of which help to display the antigen-antibody complexes. Thus, B cells that have undergone somatic hypermutation are given a chance to bind antigen on follicular dendritic cells and be rescued from death. B cells also may bind free antigen, process

it, and present peptides to germinal center helper T cells, which then provide survival signals. As the immune response to a protein antigen develops, and especially with repeated antigen exposure, the amount of antibody produced increases. As a result, the amount of available antigen decreases. The B cells that are selected to survive must be able to bind antigen at lower and lower concentrations, and therefore these are cells whose antigen receptors are of higher and higher affinity. The selected B cells leave the germinal center and secrete antibodies, resulting in increasing affinity of the antibodies produced as the response develops.

The various stages of antibody responses to T cell–dependent protein antigens occur sequentially and in

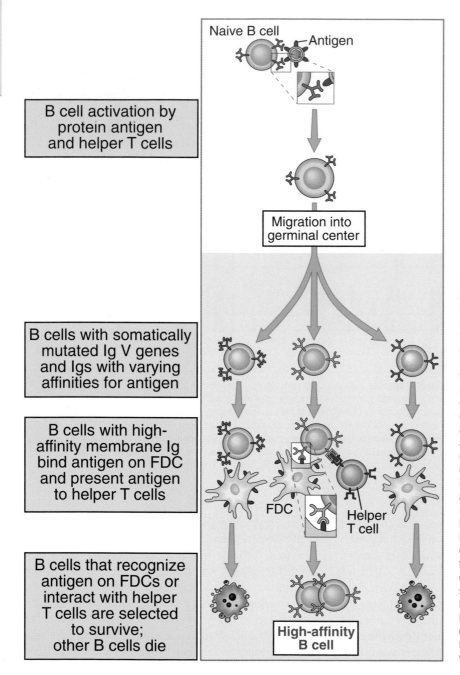

FIGURE 7-13 Selection of high-affinity B cells in germinal centers. Some of the B cells that are activated by antigen, with help from T cells, migrate into follicles to form germinal centers, where they undergo rapid proliferation and accumulate mutations in their immunoglobulin (Ig) V genes. The mutations generate B cells with different affinities for the antigen. Follicular dendritic cells (FDCs) display the antigen, and B cells that recognize the antigen are selected to survive. FDCs display antigens by binding immune complexes to Fc receptors or by binding immune complexes with attached C3b and C3d complement proteins to C3 receptors *(not shown)*. B cells also bind the antigen, process it, and present it to helper T cells in the germinal centers. As more antibody is produced, the amount of available antigen decreases, so the B cells that are selected have to express receptors with higher affinities to bind the antigen. FDCs and germinal center helper T cells express CD40L *(not shown)*, which may be the molecule that delivers survival signals to the B cells.

different anatomic compartments of lymphoid organs (Fig. 7-14). Mature, naive B lymphocytes recognize antigens in lymphoid follicles and migrate out to encounter helper T cells at the edges of the follicles. This interface of the B cell–rich zones and the T cell–rich zones is the site at which B cell proliferation and differentiation into antibody-secreting cells begin. The plasma cells that develop as a consequence of this interaction reside in lymphoid organs, usually outside the B cell–rich follicles, and the antibodies they secrete

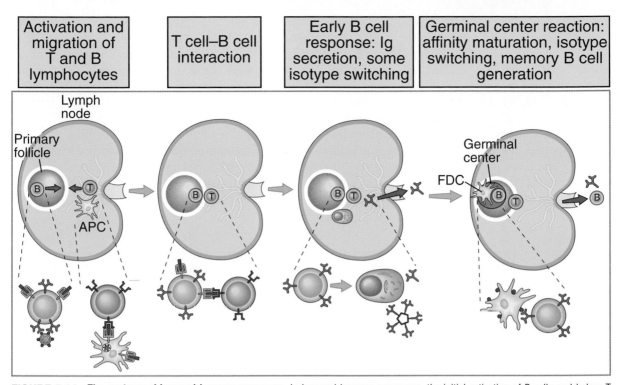

| Activation and migration of T and B lymphocytes | T cell–B cell interaction | Early B cell response: Ig secretion, some isotype switching | Germinal center reaction: affinity maturation, isotype switching, memory B cell generation |

FIGURE 7-14 **The anatomy of humoral immune responses.** In humoral immune responses, the initial activation of B cells and helper T cells occurs in different anatomic compartments of peripheral lymphoid organs. Naive B cells recognize antigens in follicles, and helper T cells recognize antigens in T cell–rich zones outside the follicles. The two cell types interact at the edges of the follicles. The differentiation of B cells into antibody-secreting cells occurs mainly outside lymphoid follicles. Affinity maturation occurs in germinal centers, and heavy chain isotype switching may occur outside follicles or in germinal centers. Some antibody-secreting plasma cells migrate to the bone marrow and continue to produce antibody even after the antigen is eliminated *(not shown)*. Memory B cells develop mainly in the germinal centers and enter the circulation. The illustration shows these reactions in a lymph node, but essentially the same pattern is seen in the spleen. APC, antigen-presenting cell; FDC, follicular dendritic cell; Ig, immunoglobulin.

enter the blood. Heavy chain isotype switching is initiated outside the follicles. Affinity maturation and much more isotype switching occur in germinal centers that are formed in follicles. All of these events may be seen within a week after exposure to antigen. Plasma cells that emerge from the germinal center migrate to the bone marrow, where they may live for months or years, continuing to produce antibodies even after the antigen is eliminated. It is estimated that more than half of the antibodies in the blood of a normal adult are produced by these long-lived plasma cells; thus, circulating antibodies reflect each individual's history of antigen exposure. These antibodies provide a level of immediate protection if the antigen (microbe or toxin) reenters the body. A fraction of the activated B cells, which often are the progeny of isotype-switched high-affinity B cells, do not differentiate into active antibody secretors but instead become **memory cells.** Memory B cells do not secrete antibodies, but they circulate in the blood and reside in various tissues. They survive for months or years in the absence of additional antigen exposure, ready to respond rapidly if the antigen is reintroduced.

Antibody Responses to T-Independent Antigens

Polysaccharides, lipids, and other nonprotein antigens elicit antibody responses without the participation of helper T cells. Recall that these nonprotein antigens cannot bind to MHC molecules, so they cannot be seen by T cells (see Chapter 3). Many bacteria contain polysaccharide-rich capsules, and defense against such bacteria is mediated primarily by antibodies that bind to capsular polysaccharides and target the bacteria for phagocytosis. Despite the importance of antibody responses against such T-independent antigens, very little is known about how these responses are induced. What is known is that antibody responses to T-independent antigens differ in many respects from responses to proteins, and most of these differences are attributable to the roles of helper T cells in antibody responses to proteins (Fig. 7-15). It is thought that because polysaccharide and lipid antigens often contain multivalent arrays of the same epitope, these antigens are able to cross-link many antigen receptors on a specific B cell. This extensive cross-linking may activate the B cells strongly enough to stimulate their proliferation and differentiation without a requirement for T cell help. Naturally occurring protein antigens usually are not multivalent, and this may be why they do not induce full B cell responses by themselves but depend on helper T cells to stimulate antibody production. Also, marginal zone

	Thymus-dependent antigen	Thymus-independent antigen
Chemical nature	Proteins	Polymeric antigens, especially polysaccharides; also glycolipids, nucleic acids
Features of antibody response		
Isotype switching	Yes (IgM → IgG, IgE, IgA)	Little or no; may be some IgG (IgM, IgG)
Affinity maturation	Yes	Little or no
Secondary response (memory B cells)	Yes	Seen only with some antigens

FIGURE 7-15   Features of antibody responses to T-dependent and T-independent antigens. T-dependent antigens (proteins) and T-independent antigens (nonproteins) induce antibody responses with different characteristics, largely reflecting the influence of helper T cells in the responses to protein antigens. Ig, immunoglobulin (class).

B cells in the spleen are the major contributors to T-independent antibody responses to blood-borne antigens, and B-1 B cells make T-independent responses to antigens of microbes in mucosal tissues and microbes that enter the peritoneum.

Regulation of Humoral Immune Responses: Antibody Feedback

After B lymphocytes differentiate into antibody-secreting cells and memory cells, a fraction of these cells survive for long periods, but most of the activated B cells probably die by a process of programmed cell death. This gradual loss of the activated B cells contributes to the physiologic decline of the humoral immune response. B cells also use a special mecha-nism for shutting off antibody production. As IgG antibody is produced and circulates throughout the body, the antibody binds to antigen that is still available in the blood and tissues, forming immune complexes. B cells specific for the antigen may bind the antigen part of the immune complex by their Ig receptors. At the same time, the Fc "tail" of the attached IgG antibody may be recognized by a special type of Fc receptor expressed on B cells called FcγRII (Fig. 7-16). This Fc receptor delivers inhibitory signals that shut off antigen receptor–induced signals, thereby terminating B cell responses. This process, in which antibody bound to antigen inhibits further antibody production, is called **antibody feedback.** It serves to terminate humoral immune responses once sufficient quantities of IgG antibodies have been produced. An

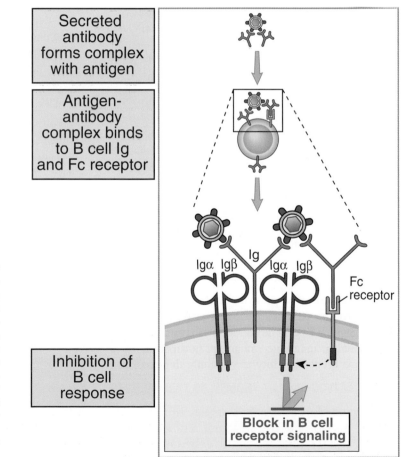

FIGURE 7-16 The mechanism of antibody feedback. Secreted IgG antibodies form immune complexes (antigen-antibody complexes) with residual antigen. The complexes interact with B cells specific for the antigen, with the membrane immunoglobulin (Ig) antigen receptors recognizing epitopes of the antigen and a certain type of Fc receptor (FcγRII) recognizing the bound antibody. The Fc receptors block activating signals from the antigen receptor, thereby terminating B cell activation. The cytoplasmic domain of B cell FcγRII contains an immunoreceptor tyrosine-based inhibition motif (ITIM) that binds enzymes that inhibit antigen receptor–mediated B cell activation.

effective therapy for some inflammatory diseases is the administration of pooled IgG, called intravenous immunoglobulin (IVIG). This treatment was developed empirically. It is now believed that IVIG works by engaging the inhibitory Fc receptor on B cells (and perhaps on dendritic cells), thereby suppressing pathologic immune responses.

SUMMARY

■ Humoral immunity is mediated by antibodies, which bind to extracellular microbes and their toxins, which are thereby neutralized or targeted for destruction by phagocytes and by the complement system.

■ Humoral immune responses to nonprotein antigens are initiated by the recognition of the antigens by specific Ig receptors of naive B cells. The binding of multivalent antigen cross-links Ig receptors of specific B cells, and biochemical signals are delivered to the inside of the B cells by Ig-associated signaling proteins. These signals induce B cell clonal expansion and IgM secretion.

■ Humoral immune responses to a protein antigen, called T-dependent responses, are initiated by binding of the protein to specific Ig receptors of naive B cells in lymphoid follicles. This results in generation of signals that prepare the B cell for interaction with helper T cells. In addition, the B cells internalize and process that antigen and present class II MHC–displayed peptides to helper T cells also specific for the antigen. The helper T cells express CD40L and secrete cytokines, which function together to stimulate high levels of B cell proliferation and differentiation.

■ Heavy chain isotype switching (or class switching) is the process by which the isotype, but not the specificity, of the antibodies produced in response to an antigen changes as the humoral response proceeds. Isotype switching depends on the combination of CD40L and cytokines, both expressed by helper T cells. Different cytokines induce switching to different antibody isotypes, enabling the immune system to respond in the most effective way to different types of microbes.

■ Affinity maturation is the process by which the affinity of antibodies for protein antigens increases with prolonged or repeated exposure to the antigens. The process is initiated by signals from helper T cells, resulting in migration of the B cells into follicles and the formation of germinal centers. Here the B cells proliferate rapidly and their Ig V genes undergo extensive somatic mutations. The antigen complexed with secreted antibody is displayed by follicular dendritic cells in the germinal centers. B cells that recognize the antigen with high affinity are selected to survive, giving rise to affinity maturation of the antibody response.

■ T-dependent humoral responses generate long-lived plasma cells, which home to the bone marrow and secrete antibodies for many years, and long-lived memory B cells, which rapidly respond to reencounter with antigen by proliferation and secretion of high-affinity antibodies.

■ Polysaccharides, lipids, and other nonprotein antigens are called T-independent antigens because they induce antibody responses without T cell help. Most T-independent antigens contain multiple identical epitopes that are able to cross-link many Ig receptors on a B cell, providing signals that stimulate B cell responses even in the absence of helper T cell activation. Antibody responses to T-independent antigens show less heavy chain class switching and affinity maturation than are typical for responses to T-dependent protein antigens.

■ Secreted antibodies form immune complexes with residual antigen and shut off B cell activation by engaging an inhibitory Fc receptor on B cells.

REVIEW QUESTIONS

1 *What are the signals that induce B cell responses to (1) protein antigens and (2) polysaccharide antigens?*

2 *What are some of the differences between primary and secondary antibody responses to a protein antigen?*

3 *How do helper T cells specific for an antigen interact with B lymphocytes specific for the same antigen? Where in a lymph node do these interactions mainly occur?*

4 *What are the mechanisms by which helper T cells stimulate B cell proliferation and differentiation? What are the similarities between these mechanisms and the mechanisms of T cell–mediated macrophage activation?*

5 *What are the signals that induce heavy chain isotype switching, and what is the importance of this phenomenon for host defense against different microbes?*

6 *What is affinity maturation? How is it induced, and how are high-affinity B cells selected to survive?*

7 *What are the characteristics of antibody responses to polysaccharides and lipids? What types of bacteria stimulate mostly these kinds of antibody responses?*

Chapter 8

EFFECTOR MECHANISMS OF HUMORAL IMMUNITY

The Elimination of Extracellular Microbes and Toxins

Humoral immunity is the type of host defense that is mediated by secreted antibodies and is important for protection against extracellular microbes and their toxins. Preventing infection before it becomes established is an important function of the adaptive immune system, and only antibodies mediate this function. Antibodies prevent infections by blocking the ability of microbes to bind to and enter host cells. Antibodies also bind to microbial toxins and stop them from damaging host cells. In addition, antibodies function to eliminate microbes, toxins, and infected cells from the body. Both antibodies and T lymphocytes participate in the destruction of microbes that have colonized and infected hosts. Antibody defenses are the only mechanism of adaptive immunity against extracellular microbes, but antibodies cannot reach microbes that live inside cells. However, humoral immunity is vital even for defense against microbes that live and divide inside cells, such as viruses, because antibodies can bind to these microbes before they enter host cells or during passage from infected to uninfected cells and thus prevent spread of infection. Defects in antibody production are associated with increased susceptibility to infections by many bacteria, viruses, and parasites. Most of the effective vaccines that are currently in use work by stimulating the production of antibodies.

This chapter describes how antibodies function in host defense against infections. We will address the following questions:

- What are the mechanisms used by secreted antibodies to combat different types of infectious agents and their toxins?
- What is the role of the complement system in defense against microbes?
- How do antibodies combat microbes that enter via the gastrointestinal and respiratory tracts?
- How do antibodies protect the fetus and newborn from infections?

Before describing the mechanisms by which antibodies function in host defense, we summarize the features of antibody molecules that are important for these functions.

Properties of Antibodies That Determine Their Effector Functions

Antibodies may function distant from their sites of production. Antibodies are produced after stimulation of B lymphocytes by antigens in peripheral lymphoid organs (i.e., the lymph nodes, the spleen, and mucosal lymphoid tissues). Some of the antigen-stimulated B lymphocytes differentiate into antibody-secreting plasma cells, which synthesize and secrete antibodies of different heavy chain isotypes (classes). These antibodies enter the blood, from where they may reach any peripheral site of infection, and mucosal secretions, where they prevent infections by microbes that try to enter through the epithelia. Thus, antibodies are able to perform their functions throughout the body.

Protective antibodies are produced during the first (primary) response to a microbe and in larger amounts during subsequent (secondary) responses (see Fig. 7-3, Chapter 7). Antibody production begins within the first week after infection or vaccination. Some of the plasma cells migrate to the bone marrow and live in this tissue, continuing to secrete small amounts of antibodies for months or years. If the microbe again tries to infect the host, the continuously secreted antibodies provide immediate protection. Some antigen-stimulated B lymphocytes differentiate into memory cells, which do not secrete antibodies but are ready to respond if the antigen appears again.

On encounter with the microbe, these memory cells rapidly differentiate into antibody-producing cells, providing a large burst of antibody for more effective defense against the infection. A goal of vaccination is to stimulate the development of long-lived plasma cells and memory cells.

Antibodies use their antigen-binding (Fab) regions to bind to and block the harmful effects of microbes and toxins, and they use their Fc regions to activate diverse effector mechanisms that eliminate these microbes and toxins (Fig. 8-1). This spatial segregation of the antigen recognition and effector functions of antibody molecules was introduced in Chapter 4. Antibodies block the infectivity of microbes and the injurious effects of microbial toxins simply by binding to the microbes and toxins, using only their Fab regions to do so. Other functions of antibodies require the participation of various components of host defense, such as phagocytes and the complement system. The Fc portions of immunoglobulin (Ig) molecules, made up of the heavy chain constant regions, contain the binding sites for Fc receptors on phagocytes and for complement proteins. The effective binding of phagocytes and complement to antibodies occurs only after several Ig molecules recognize and become attached to a microbe or microbial antigen. Therefore, even the Fc-dependent functions of antibodies require antigen recognition by the Fab regions. This feature of antibodies ensures that they activate effector mechanisms only when they need to—that is, when they recognize their target antigens.

One type of Fc receptor, called the **neonatal FcR (FcRn)**, is expressed in placenta, in endothelium, and a few other cell types. In the endothelium it plays a special role in protecting IgG antibodies from intracellular catabolism. FcRn is found in the endosomes of endothelial cells, where it binds to IgG that has been taken up by the cells. Once bound to the FcRn, the IgG is recycled back into the circulation, thereby protecting it from lysosomal degradation. This unique mechanism for protecting a blood protein is the reason why IgG antibodies have half-lives of about 3 weeks, much longer than the half-lives of other Ig isotypes. This property of Fc regions of IgG has been exploited to increase the half-lives of other proteins by coupling the proteins to an IgG Fc region. A therapeutic agent

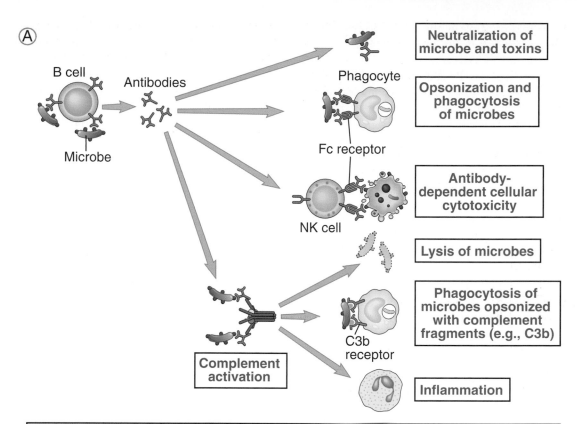

Ⓑ Antibody isotype	Isotype-specific effector functions
IgG	Neutralization of microbes and toxins
	Opsonization of antigens for phagocytosis by macrophages and neutrophils
	Activation of the classical pathway of complement
	Antibody-dependent cellular cytotoxicity mediated by NK cells
	Neonatal immunity: transfer of maternal antibody across placenta and gut
	Feedback inhibition of B cell activation
IgM	Activation of the classical pathway of complement
IgA	Mucosal immunity: secretion of IgA into lumens of gastrointestinal and respiratory tracts, neutralization of microbes and toxins
IgE	Defense against helminths
	Mast cell degranulation (immediate hypersensitivity reactions)

FIGURE 8-1 **The effector functions of antibodies.** Antibodies are produced by the activation of B lymphocytes by antigens and other signals *(not shown)*. Antibodies of different heavy chain classes (isotypes) perform different effector functions, which are illustrated schematically in **A** and summarized in **B**. (Some of the properties of antibodies are listed in Fig. 4-3, Chapter 4.) Ig, immunoglobulin (class); NK, natural killer.

based on this principle is the tumor necrosis factor (TNF) receptor–Fcγ fusion protein, which functions as an antagonist of TNF and is used to treat various inflammatory diseases. By coupling the soluble receptor to the Fc portion of a human IgG molecule, the half-life of the protein becomes much greater than that of the receptor by itself.

Heavy chain isotype (class) switching and affinity maturation enhance the protective functions of antibodies. Isotype switching and affinity maturation are two changes that occur in the antibodies produced by antigen-stimulated B lymphocytes, especially during responses to protein antigens (see Chapter 7). Heavy chain isotype switching results in the production of antibodies with distinct Fc regions, capable of different effector functions (see Fig. 8-1). Thus, by switching to different antibody isotypes in response to various microbes, the humoral immune system is able to engage host mechanisms that are optimal for combating these microbes. The process of affinity maturation is stimulated by prolonged or repeated antigen stimulation, and it leads to the production of antibodies with higher and higher affinities for the antigen. This change increases the ability of antibodies to bind to and neutralize or eliminate microbes, especially if the microbes are persistent or capable of recurrent infections.

With this introduction, we proceed to a discussion of the mechanisms used by antibodies to combat infections. Much of the chapter is devoted to effector mechanisms that are not influenced by anatomic considerations; that is, they may be active anywhere in the body. At the end of the chapter, we describe the special features of antibody functions at particular anatomic locations.

Neutralization of Microbes and Microbial Toxins

Antibodies bind to and block, or neutralize, the infectivity of microbes and the interactions of microbial toxins with host cells (Fig. 8-2). Most microbes use molecules in their envelopes or cell walls to bind to and gain entry into host cells. Antibodies may attach to these microbial envelope or cell wall molecules, thereby preventing the microbes from infecting and colonizing

the host. Neutralization is a very useful defense mechanism because it does not allow an infection to take hold. The most effective vaccines available today work by stimulating the production of neutralizing antibodies, which prevent subsequent infection. Microbes that are able to enter host cells may be released from these infected cells and go on to infect other neighboring cells. Antibodies can neutralize the microbes during their transit from cell to cell and thus limit the spread of infection. If an infectious microbe does colonize the host, its harmful effects may be caused by endotoxins or exotoxins, which often bind to specific receptors on host cells in order to mediate their effects. Antibodies against toxins prevent binding of the toxins to host cells and thus block the harmful effects of the toxins. Emil von Behring's demonstration of this type of humoral immunity mediated by antibodies against diphtheria toxin was the first formal demonstration of immunity against a microbe and the basis for giving von Behring the first Nobel Prize in Medicine in 1901.

Opsonization and Phagocytosis

Antibodies coat microbes and promote their ingestion by phagocytes (Fig. 8-3). The process of coating particles for subsequent phagocytosis is called **opsonization,** and the molecules that coat microbes and enhance their phagocytosis are called **opsonins.** When several antibody molecules bind to a microbe, an array of Fc regions is formed projecting away from the microbe. If the antibodies belong to certain isotypes (IgG1 and IgG3 in humans), their Fc regions bind to a high-affinity receptor for the Fc regions of γ chains, called FcγRI (CD64), which is expressed on neutrophils and macrophages. The phagocyte extends its plasma membrane around the attached microbe and ingests the microbe into a vesicle called a phagosome, which fuses with lysosomes. The binding of antibody Fc tails to FcγRI also activates the phagocytes, because the FcγRI contains a signaling chain that triggers numerous biochemical pathways in the phagocytes. The activated neutrophil or macrophage produces, in its lysosomes, large amounts of reactive oxygen species, nitric oxide, and proteolytic enzymes, all of which combine to destroy the ingested microbe. Antibody-mediated phagocytosis is the major mechanism of defense against encapsulated bacteria,

FIGURE 8-2 **Neutralization of microbes and toxins by antibodies. A,** Antibodies prevent the binding of microbes to cells, thereby blocking the ability of the microbes to infect host cells. **B,** Antibodies inhibit the spread of microbes from an infected cell to an adjacent uninfected cell. **C,** Antibodies block the binding of toxins to cells, thereby inhibiting the pathologic effects of the toxins.

such as pneumococci. The polysaccharide-rich capsules of these bacteria protect the organisms from phagocytosis in the absence of antibody, but opsonization by antibody promotes phagocytosis and destruction of the bacteria. The spleen contains large numbers of phagocytes and is an important site of phagocytic clearance of opsonized bacteria. This is why patients who have undergone splenectomy, for example, for traumatic rupture of the organ, are susceptible to disseminated infections by encapsulated bacteria.

B) Fc receptor	Affinity for Ig	Cell distribution	Function
FcγRI (CD64)	High (K$_d$ ~10^{-9} M); binds IgG1 and IgG3; can bind monomeric IgG	Macrophages, neutrophils; also eosinophils	Phagocytosis; activation of phagocytes
FcγRIIA (CD32)	Low (K$_d$ ~0.6–2.5×10^{-6} M)	Macrophages, neutrophils; eosinophils, platelets	Phagocytosis; cell activation (inefficient)
FcγRIIB (CD32)	Low (K$_d$ ~0.6–2.5×10^{-6} M)	B lymphocytes	Feedback inhibition of B cells
FcγRIIIA (CD16)	Low (K$_d$ ~0.6–2.5×10^{-6} M)	NK cells	Antibody-dependent cellular cytotoxicity (ADCC)
FcεRI	High (K$_d$ ~10^{-10} M); binds monomeric IgE	Mast cells, basophils, eosinophils	Activation (degranulation) of mast cells and basophils

FIGURE 8-3 Antibody-mediated opsonization and phagocytosis of microbes. A, Antibodies of certain IgG subclasses bind to microbes and are then recognized by Fc receptors on phagocytes. Signals from the Fc receptors promote the phagocytosis of the opsonized microbes and activate the phagocytes to destroy these microbes. **B,** The different types of human Fc receptors, and their cellular distribution and functions, are listed. Ig, immunoglobulin; NK, natural killer.

Antibody-Dependent Cellular Cytotoxicity

Natural killer (NK) cells and other leukocytes may bind to antibody-coated cells and destroy these cells (Fig. 8-4). NK cells express an Fc receptor, called FcγRIII (CD16), that binds to arrays of IgG antibodies attached to a cell. As a result of FcγRIII-mediated signals, the NK cells are activated to discharge their granules, which contain proteins that kill the opsonized targets. This process is called **antibody-dependent cellular cytotoxicity (ADCC)**. It is not known if infected cells commonly express surface molecules that may be recognized by antibodies or in which infections this effector mechanism is active. In fact, it is likely that NK cell–mediated ADCC is not as important as phagocytosis of opsonized microbes in defense against most bacterial and viral infections.

IgE- and Eosinophil/Mast Cell– Mediated Reactions

IgE antibodies activate mast cell and eosinophil-mediated reactions that are important in defense

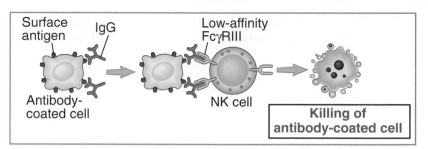

FIGURE 8-4 Antibody-dependent cellular cytotoxicity (ADCC). Antibodies of certain immunoglobulin G (IgG) subclasses bind to cells (e.g., infected cells), and the Fc regions of the bound antibodies are recognized by an Fcγ receptor on natural killer (NK) cells. The NK cells are activated and kill the antibody-coated cells.

against helminthic parasites and are involved in allergic diseases. Most helminths are too large to be phagocytosed, and they have thick integuments that make them resistant to many of the microbicidal substances produced by neutrophils and macrophages. The humoral immune response to helminths is dominated by IgE antibodies. The IgE antibody may bind to the worms, and could promote the attachment of eosinophils via the high-affinity Fc receptor for IgE, called FcεRI, that is expressed on eosinophils (and mast cells). In humans the eosinophil FcεRI appears incapable of transducing activating signals, and these cells are likely activated by cytokines such as IL-5 that are secreted by T cells in the vicinity of the parasites. Upon activation, the eosinophils release their granule contents, which include proteins that can kill helminths. Bound IgE antibodies may also activate mast cells, which secrete cytokines, including chemokines, that attract more leukocytes that function to destroy the helminths. This IgE-mediated reaction illustrates how Ig isotype switching is designed for optimal host defense: B cells respond to helminths by switching to IgE, which is useful against helminths, but B cells respond to most bacteria and viruses by switching to IgG antibodies that promote phagocytosis via FcγRI. As we discussed in Chapters 5 and 7, these patterns of isotype switching are determined by the cytokines produced by helper T cells responding to the different types of microbes.

IgE antibodies also are involved in allergic diseases, which are discussed in Chapter 11.

Activation of the Complement System

The complement system is a collection of circulating and cell membrane proteins that play important roles in host defense against microbes and in anti-

body-mediated tissue injury. The term *complement* refers to the ability of these proteins to assist, or complement, the antimicrobial activity of antibodies. The complement system may be activated by microbes in the absence of antibody, as part of the innate immune response to infection, and by antibodies attached to microbes, as part of adaptive immunity (see Fig. 2-12, Chapter 2). There are several features of the complement system that are important for its functions. The activation of complement proteins involves sequential proteolytic cleavage of these proteins and leads to the generation of effector molecules that participate in eliminating microbes in different ways. This cascade of complement protein activation, like all enzymatic cascades, is capable of achieving tremendous amplification, because of which an initially small number of activated complement molecules produced early in the cascade may generate a large number of effector molecules. Activated complement proteins become covalently attached to the cell surfaces where the activation occurs, ensuring that activation is limited to the correct sites. The complement system is tightly regulated by molecules present on normal host cells, and this regulation prevents uncontrolled and potentially harmful complement activation.

In the following section we describe the activation, functions, and regulation of the complement system.

PATHWAYS OF COMPLEMENT ACTIVATION

There are three major pathways of complement activation, two initiated by microbes in the absence of antibody, called the alternative and lectin pathways, and the third initiated by certain isotypes of antibodies attached to antigens, called the classical pathway (Fig. 8-5). There are several proteins in each

FIGURE 8-5 **The early steps of complement activation. A,** The steps in the activation of the alternative, classical, and lectin pathways are shown. Note that the sequence of events is similar in all three pathways, although they differ in their requirement for antibody and in the proteins used.

(B) Protein	Serum conc. (ug/mL)	Function
C3	1000-1200	C3b binds to the surface of a microbe where it functions as an opsonin and as a component of C3 and C5 convertases C3a stimulates inflammation
Factor B	200	Bb is a serine protease and the active enzyme of C3 and C5 convertases
Factor D	1-2	Plasma serine protease which cleaves Factor B when it is bound to C3b
Properdin	25	Stabilizes the C3 convertase (C3bBb) on microbial surfaces

(C) Protein	Serum conc. (ug/mL)	Function
C1 (C1qr$_2$s$_2$)		Initiates the classical pathway; C1q binds to Fc portion of antibody; C1r and C1s are proteases that lead to C4 and C2 activation
C4	300-600	C4b covalently binds to surface of microbe or cell where antibody is bound and complement is activated C4b binds to C2 for cleavage by C1s C4a stimulates inflammation
C2	20	C2a is a serine protease functioning as an active enzyme of C3 and C5 convertases
Mannose binding lectin (MBL)	0.8-1	Initiates the lectin pathway; MBL binds to terminal mannose residues of microbial carbohydrates. A MBL-associated protease activates C4 and C2, as in the classical pathway.

FIGURE 8-5, cont'd   **B,** The important properties of the proteins involved in the early steps of the alternative pathway of complement activation are summarized. **C,** The important properties of the proteins involved in the early steps of the classical and lectin pathways are summarized. Note that C3, which is listed among the alternative pathway proteins (**B**), also is the central component of the classical and lectin pathways.

pathway that interact in a precise sequence. The most abundant complement protein in the plasma, called C3, plays a central role in all three pathways. C3 is spontaneously hydrolyzed in plasma at a low level, but its products are unstable and they are rapidly broken down and lost. The **alternative pathway** is triggered when a breakdown product of C3 hydrolysis, called C3b, is deposited on the surface of a microbe. Here, the C3b forms stable covalent bonds with microbial proteins or polysaccharides and is thus protected from further degradation. (As will be described later, C3b is prevented from binding stably to normal host cells by several regulatory proteins that are present on host cells but absent from microbes.) The microbe-bound C3b becomes a substrate for the binding of another protein called factor B, which is broken down by a plasma protease to generate the Bb fragment. This fragment remains attached to the C3b, and the C3bBb complex enzymatically breaks down more C3, functioning as the "alternative pathway C3 convertase." As a result of this convertase activity, many more C3b and C3bBb molecules are produced and become attached to the microbe. Some of the C3bBb molecules bind additional C3b, and the C3bBb3b complex functions as a C5 convertase, to break down the complement protein C5 and initiate the late steps of complement activation.

The **classical pathway** is triggered when IgM or certain subclasses of IgG (IgG1 and IgG3 in humans) bind to antigens (e.g., on a microbial cell surface). As a result of this binding, the Fc regions of the antibodies become accessible to complement proteins and two or more Fc regions come close together. When this happens, the C1 complement protein binds to two adjacent Fc regions. The attached C1 becomes enzymatically active, thus resulting in the binding and cleavage of two other proteins, C4 and C2. The resultant C4b2a complex becomes covalently attached to the antibody and to the microbial surface where the antibody is bound. This complex is the "classical pathway C3 convertase," which functions to break down C3, and the C3b that is generated again becomes attached to the microbe. Some of the C3b binds to the C4b2a complex, and the resultant C4b2a3b complex functions as a C5 convertase.

The **lectin pathway** is initiated in the absence of antibody by the attachment of plasma mannose-binding lectin (MBL) to microbes. MBL is structurally similar to a component of C1 of the classical pathway and serves to activate C4. The subsequent steps are essentially the same as in the classical pathway.

The net result of these early steps of complement activation is that microbes acquire a coat of covalently attached C3b. Note that the alternative and lectin pathways are effector mechanisms of innate immunity whereas the classical pathway is a mechanism of adaptive humoral immunity. These pathways differ in how they are initiated, but once they are triggered, their late steps are the same.

The late steps of complement activation (Fig. 8-6) are initiated by the binding of C5 to the C5 convertase, and the subsequent proteolysis of C5, generating C5b. The remaining components, C6, C7, C8, and C9, bind sequentially. The final protein in the pathway, C9, polymerizes to form a pore in the cell membrane through which water and ions can enter, causing death of the cell. This poly-C9 is called the **membrane attack complex,** and its formation is the end result of complement activation.

FUNCTIONS OF THE COMPLEMENT SYSTEM

The complement system plays an important role in the elimination of microbes during innate and adaptive immune responses. The main effector functions of the complement system are illustrated in Figure 8-7.

Microbes coated with C3b are phagocytosed by virtue of the C3b's being recognized by the type 1 complement receptor (CR1 or CD35), expressed on phagocytes. Thus, C3b functions as an opsonin. Opsonization is probably the most important function of complement in defense against microbes. The membrane attack complex can induce osmotic lysis of cells, including microbes. MAC-induced lysis is effective only against microbes that have thin cell walls and little or no glycocalyx, such as bacteria of the *Neisseria* species. Small peptide fragments of C3, C4, and C5, which are produced by proteolysis, are chemotactic for neutrophils, stimulate the release of inflammatory mediators from various leukocytes, and act on endothelial cells to enhance movement of leukocytes and plasma proteins into tissues. In this way, complement fragments induce inflammatory reactions that also serve to eliminate microbes.

In addition to its antimicrobial effector functions, the complement system provides stimuli for the development of humoral immune responses. When C3 is activated by a microbe, one of its breakdown products, C3d, is recognized by the CR2 receptor on B lymphocytes. Signals delivered by this receptor stimulate B cell responses against the microbe. This process is described in Chapter 7 (see Fig. 7-5) and is an example of an innate immune response to a microbe (complement activation) stimulating an adaptive immune response to the same microbe (B cell activa-

Protein	Serum conc. (μg/mL)	Function
C5	80	C5b initiates assembly of the MAC C5a stimulates inflammation
C6	45	Component of the MAC: binds to C5b and accepts C7
C7	90	Component of the MAC: binds C5b, 6 and inserts into lipid membranes
C8	60	Component of the MAC: binds C5b, 6, 7 and initiates binding and polymerization of C9
C9	60	Component of the MAC: binds C5b, 6, 7, 8 and polymerizes to form membrane pores

FIGURE 8-6   The late steps of complement activation. A, The late steps of complement activation start after the formation of the C5 convertase and are identical in the alternative and classical pathways. Products generated in the late steps induce inflammation (C5a) and cell lysis (the membrane attack complex [MAC]). **B,** The properties of the proteins of the late steps of complement activation are listed.

tion and antibody production). Complement proteins bound to antigen-antibody complexes are recognized by follicular dendritic cells in germinal centers, allowing the antigens to be displayed for further B cell activation and selection of high-affinity B cells. This complement-dependent antigen display is another way in which the complement system promotes antibody production.

Inherited deficiencies of complement proteins are the cause of human diseases. Deficiency of C3 results in profound susceptibility to infections and usually is fatal in early life. Somewhat surprisingly, deficiencies of the early proteins of the classical pathway, C2 and C4, do not cause immune deficiencies. C2 and C4 deficiencies are associated with an increased incidence of immune complex diseases

(A) Opsonization and phagocytosis

C3b

Microbe

Binding of C3b
(or C4b) to microbe
(opsonization)

CR1

Microbe

Recognition of bound
C3b by phagocyte
C3b receptor

Phagocytosis
and killing
of microbe

(B) Complement-mediated cytolysis

C3b

Microbe

Binding of C3b to microbe,
activation of late components
of complement

MAC

Microbe

Formation of the
membrane attack
complex (MAC)

Osmotic lysis
of microbe

(C) Stimulation of inflammatory reactions

C3b

C3a
(C4a, C5a)

Microbe

Proteolysis of
C3, C4, and C5
to release C3a,
C4a, and C5a

Recruitment and
activation of
leukocytes by
C5a, C3a, C4a

Microbe

Destruction
of microbes
by leukocytes

FIGURE 8-7   The functions of complement. A, C3b opsonizes microbes and is recognized by the type 1 complement receptor (CR1) of phagocytes, resulting in ingestion and intracellular killing of the opsonized microbes. Thus, C3b is an opsonin. CR1 also recognizes C4b, which may serve the same function. Other complement products, such as the inactivated form of C3b (iC3b), also bind to microbes and are recognized by other receptors on phagocytes (e.g., the type 3 complement receptor, a member of the integrin family of proteins). **B,** The membrane attack complex creates pores in cell membranes and induces osmotic lysis of the cells. **C,** Small peptides released during complement activation bind to receptors on neutrophils and stimulate inflammatory reactions. The peptides that serve this function are C5a, C3a, and C4a (in decreasing order of potency).

resembling systemic lupus erythematosus, perhaps because the classical pathway functions to eliminate immune complexes from the circulation. Deficiencies of C9 and membrane attack complex formation result in increased susceptibility to *Neisseria* infections. Some individuals inherit polymorphisms in the gene encoding mannose-binding lectin, leading to production of a protein that is functionally defective;

such defects are associated with increased susceptibility to infections.

REGULATION OF COMPLEMENT ACTIVATION

Mammalian cells express regulatory proteins that inhibit complement activation, thus preventing complement-mediated damage to host cells (Fig.

8-8). Many such regulatory proteins have been described. Decay-accelerating factor (DAF) is a membrane protein that disrupts the binding of factor B to C3b or the binding of C4b2a to C3b, thus terminating complement activation by both the alternative and the classical pathways. Membrane cofactor protein (MCP) serves as a cofactor for the proteolysis of C3b into inactive fragments, a process that is mediated by a plasma enzyme called factor I. The type 1 complement receptor (CR1) may serve both functions. A regulatory protein called C1 inhibitor (C1 INH) stops complement activation early, at the stage of C1 activation. Still other proteins regulate complement activation at the late steps, such as the formation of the membrane attack complex. The presence of these

regulatory proteins is an adaptation of mammals. Microbes lack the regulatory proteins and are therefore susceptible to complement. Even in mammalian cells, the regulation can be overwhelmed by more and more complement activation. Therefore, mammalian cells can become targets of complement if they are coated with large amounts of antibodies, as in some hypersensitivity diseases (see Chapter 11).

Inherited deficiencies of regulatory proteins cause uncontrolled and pathologic complement activation. Deficiency of C1 INH is the cause of a disease called **hereditary angioneurotic edema,** in which excessive C1 activation and the production of vasoactive protein fragments lead to leakage of fluid (edema) in the larynx and many other tissues. A disease called **par-**

FIGURE 8-8 Regulation of complement activation. A, The cell surface proteins decay-accelerating factor (DAF) and the type 1 complement receptor (CR1) interfere with the formation of the C3 convertase by removing Bb (in the alternative pathway) or C4b (in the classical pathway, *not shown*). Membrane cofactor protein (MCP) and CR1 serve as cofactors for cleavage of C3b by a plasma enzyme called factor I, thus destroying any C3b that may be formed. **B,** C1 inhibitor (C1 INH) prevents the assembly of the C1 complex, which consists of C1q, C1r, and C1s proteins, thereby blocking complement activation by the classical pathway.

Ⓒ Plasma proteins

Protein	Distribution	Function
C1 inhibitor (C1 INH)	Plasma; conc. 200 µg/mL	Inhibits C1r and C1s serine protease activity
Factor I	Plasma; conc. 35 µg/mL	Proteolytically cleaves C3b and C4b
Factor H	Plasma; conc. 480 µg/mL	Causes dissociation of alternative pathway C3 convertase subunits Co-factor for Factor I-mediated cleavage of C3b
C4-binding protein (C4BP)	Plasma; conc. 300 µg/mL	Causes dissociation of classical pathway C3 convertase subunits Co-factor for factor I–mediated cleavage of C4b

Membrane proteins

Protein	Distribution	Function
Membrane cofactor protein (MCP, CD46)	Leukocytes, epithelial cells, endothelial cells	Co-factor for factor I–mediated cleavage of C3b and C4b
Decay-accelerating factor (DAF)	Blood cells, endothelial cells, epithelial cells	Causes dissociation of C3 convertase subunits
CD59	Blood cells, endothelial cells, epithelial cells	Blocks C9 binding and prevents formation of the MAC
Type 1 complement receptor (CR1, CD35)	Mononuclear phagocytes, neutrophils, B and T cells, erythrocytes, eosinophils, FDCs	Causes dissociation of C3 convertase subunits Co-factor for factor I–mediated cleavage of C3b and C4b

FIGURE 8-8, cont'd   C, The major regulatory proteins of the complement system and their functions are listed. FDCs, follicular dendritic cells; MAC, membrane attack complex.

oxysmal nocturnal hemoglobinuria results from deficiency of an enzyme that synthesizes the glycolipid anchor for several membrane proteins, including the complement regulatory proteins DAF and MCP. Unregulated complement activation occurs on the erythrocytes of these patients, leading to lysis of the erythrocytes.

Functions of Antibodies at Special Anatomic Sites

The effector mechanisms of humoral immunity that have been described so far may be active at any site in the body to which antibodies gain access. As has been mentioned previously, antibodies are produced in peripheral lymphoid organs and readily enter the blood, from where they may go virtually anywhere. Antibodies also serve protective functions at two special anatomic sites, the mucosal organs and the fetus. There are special mechanisms for transporting antibodies across epithelia and across the placenta, and antibodies play vital roles in defense in these locations.

MUCOSAL IMMUNITY

IgA antibody is produced in mucosal lymphoid tissues, actively transported across epithelia, and binds to and neutralizes microbes in the lumens of the mucosal organs (Fig. 8-9). Microbes often are inhaled or ingested, and antibodies that are secreted into the lumens of the respiratory or gastrointestinal tract bind to the microbes and prevent them from colonizing the host. This type of immunity is called mucosal immunity (or secretory immunity). The principal class of antibody produced in mucosal tissues is IgA. In fact, because of the vast surface area of the intestines, IgA accounts for 60% to 70% of the approximately 3 g of antibody produced daily by a healthy adult. The propensity of mucosal lymphoid tissues to produce IgA is, at least in part, because the cytokines that induce switching to this isotype, including transforming growth factor-β, are produced at high levels in these tissues. Also, some of the IgA may be pro-duced by a subset of B cells, called B-1 cells, that migrate to mucosal tissues and secrete IgA in response to nonprotein antigens without T cell help.

The mucosal lymphoid tissues are located in the lamina propria, and IgA is produced in this region. This IgA has to be transported from the lamina propria into the lumen. Transport through the epithelium is carried out by a special Fc receptor, called the **poly-Ig receptor,** which is expressed on the basal surface of the epithelial cells. This receptor binds IgA, endocytoses it into vesicles, and transports it to the luminal surface. Here the receptor is cleaved by a protease, and the IgA is released into the lumen still carrying a portion of the bound poly-Ig receptor. The antibody can then recognize microbes in the lumen and block their binding to and entry through the epithelium. Mucosal immunity is the mechanism of protective immunity against poliovirus infection that is induced by oral immunization with the attenuated virus.

NEONATAL IMMUNITY

Maternal antibodies are actively transported across the placenta to the fetus and across the gut epithelium of neonates, protecting the newborn from infections. Newborn mammals have incompletely developed immune systems and are unable to mount

FIGURE 8-9 **Transport of IgA through epithelium.** In the mucosa of the gastrointestinal and respiratory tracts, IgA is produced by plasma cells in the lamina propria and is actively transported through epithelial cells by an IgA-specific Fc receptor (called the poly-Ig receptor because it recognizes IgM as well). On the luminal surface, the IgA with a portion of the bound receptor is released. Here the antibody recognizes ingested or inhaled microbes and blocks their entry through the epithelium. Ig, immunoglobulin.

effective immune responses against many microbes. During their early life, they are protected from infections by antibodies acquired from their mothers. This is an excellent example of passive immunity. Neonates acquire maternal antibodies via two routes, both of which rely on the neonatal Fc receptor (FcRn). During pregnancy, some classes of maternal IgG bind to the neonatal Fc receptor expressed in the placenta, and the IgG is actively transported into the fetal circulation. After birth, neonates ingest maternal antibodies in their mothers' milk. The neonate's intestinal epithelial cells also express the Fc receptor, which binds the ingested antibody and carries it across the epithelium. Thus, neonates acquire the IgG antibody profiles of their mothers and are protected from infectious microbes to which the mothers were exposed or vaccinated.

Evasion of Humoral Immunity by Microbes

Microbes have evolved numerous mechanisms to evade humoral immunity (Fig. 8-10). Many bacteria and viruses mutate their antigenic surface molecules so that they can no longer be recognized by antibodies produced in response to previous infections. Antigenic variation commonly is seen in viruses, such as influenza virus, human immunodeficiency virus (HIV), and rhinovirus. There are so many variants of the major antigenic surface glycoprotein of HIV, called gp120, that antibodies against one HIV isolate may not protect against other HIV isolates. This is one reason why gp120 vaccines are not effective for protecting people from HIV infection. Bacteria such as *Escherichia coli* vary the antigens contained in their pili and thus evade antibody-mediated defense. The trypanosome parasite expresses new surface glycoproteins whenever it encounters antibodies against the original glycoprotein. As a result, infection with this protozoal parasite is characterized by waves of parasitemia, each wave consisting of an antigenically new parasite that is not recognized by antibodies produced against the parasites in the preceding wave. Other microbes inhibit complement activation or resist phagocytosis.

Mechanism of immune evasion	Example(s)	
Antigenic variation	Many viruses, e.g., influenza, HIV *Neisseria gonorrhoeae, E. coli, Salmonella typhimurium*	
Inhibition of complement activation	Many bacteria	
Resistance to phagocytosis	Pneumococcus	

FIGURE 8-10   Evasion of humoral immunity by microbes. The principal mechanisms by which microbes evade humoral immunity are listed, with illustrative examples. HIV, human immunodeficiency virus.

Type of vaccine	Examples	Form of protection
Live attenuated, or killed, bacteria	BCG, cholera	Antibody response
Live attenuated viruses	Polio, rabies	Antibody response; cell-mediated immune response
Subunit (antigen) vaccines	Tetanus toxoid, diphtheria toxoid	Antibody response
Conjugate vaccines	*Haemophilus influenzae infection*	Helper T cell–dependent antibody response
Synthetic vaccines	Hepatitis (recombinant proteins)	Antibody response
Viral vectors	Clinical trials of HIV antigens in canary pox vector	Cell-mediated and humoral immune responses
DNA vaccines	Clinical trials ongoing for several infections	Cell mediated and humoral immune responses

FIGURE 8-11 Vaccination strategies. Examples of different types of vaccines are provided, and the nature of the protective immune responses induced by these vaccines is summarized. BCG, bacille Calmette-Guérin; HIV, human immunodeficiency virus.

Vaccination

Vaccination is the process of stimulating protective adaptive immune responses against microbes by exposure to nonpathogenic forms or components of the microbes. The development of vaccines against infections has been one of the great successes of immunology. The only human disease to be intentionally eradicated from the earth is smallpox, and this was achieved by a worldwide program of vaccination. Polio is likely to be the second such disease, and as mentioned in Chapter 1, many other diseases have been largely controlled by vaccination (Fig. 1-2, Chapter 1). Several types of vaccines are in use and are being developed (Fig. 8-11). Some of the most effective vaccines are composed of attenuated microbes, which are treated to abolish their infectivity and pathogenicity while retaining their antigenicity. Immunization with these attenuated microbes stimulates the production of neutralizing antibodies against microbial antigens that protect vaccinated individuals from subsequent infections. For some infections, such as polio, as mentioned earlier, the vaccines are given orally, to stimulate mucosal IgA responses that protect individuals from natural infection, which occurs by the oral route. Vaccines composed of microbial proteins and polysaccharides, called subunit vaccines, work in the same way. Some microbial polysaccharide antigens (which cannot stimulate T cell help) are chemically coupled to proteins, so that helper T cells are activated and high-affinity antibodies are produced against the polysaccharides. These are called conjugate vaccines, and they are excellent examples of the practical application of our knowledge of helper T cell–B cell interactions. Immunization with inactivated microbial toxins and with microbial proteins synthesized in the laboratory stimulate antibodies that bind to and neutralize the native toxins and the microbes, respectively.

One of the continuing challenges in vaccination is to develop vaccines that stimulate cell-mediated immunity against intracellular microbes. Injected or fed microbial antigens are extracellular antigens, and they induce mainly antibody responses. To elicit T cell–mediated immune responses, it may be necessary to deliver the antigens to the interior of antigen-presenting cells, particularly dendritic cells. Attenuated viruses can achieve this goal, but only a few viruses have been successfully treated such that they remain able to infect cells, retain immunogenicity, and are safe. Many newer approaches are being tried to stimulate cell-mediated immunity by vaccination. These approaches include incorporating microbial antigens into viral "vectors," which will infect host cells and produce the antigens inside the cells. A new technique is to immunize individuals with DNA encoding a microbial antigen in a bacterial plasmid. The plasmid is ingested by host antigen-presenting cells, and the antigen is produced inside the cells. Intracellular antigens induce cell-mediated immunity (see Chapters 5 and 6), which may be effective against infections by intracellular microbes. Many of these strategies are now undergoing clinical trials for different infections.

SUMMARY

■ Humoral immunity is the type of adaptive immunity that is mediated by antibodies. Antibodies prevent infections by blocking the ability of microbes to invade host cells, and they eliminate microbes by activating several effector mechanisms.

■ In antibody molecules, the antigen-binding (Fab) regions are spatially separate from the effector (Fc) regions. The ability of antibodies to neutralize microbes and toxins is entirely a function of the antigen-binding regions. Even Fc-dependent effector functions are activated after antibodies bind antigens.

■ Antibodies are produced in lymphoid tissues and bone marrow, but they enter the circulation and are able to reach any site of infection. Heavy chain isotype switching and affinity maturation enhance the protective functions of antibodies.

■ Antibodies neutralize the infectivity of microbes and the pathogenicity of microbial toxins by binding to and interfering with the ability of these microbes and toxins to attach to host cells.

■ Antibodies coat (opsonize) microbes and promote their phagocytosis by binding to Fc receptors on phagocytes. The binding of antibody Fc regions to Fc receptors also stimulates the microbicidal activities of phagocytes.

■ The complement system is a collection of circulating and cell surface proteins that play important roles in host defense. The complement system may be activated on microbial surfaces without antibodies (called the alternative and lectin pathways, components of innate immunity) and after the binding of antibodies to antigens (the classical pathway, a component of adaptive humoral immunity). Complement proteins are sequentially cleaved, and active components, mainly C3b, become covalently attached to the surfaces on which complement is activated. The late steps of complement activation lead to the formation of the cytolytic membrane attack complex. Different products of complement activation promote phagocytosis of microbes, induce cell lysis, and stimulate inflammation. Mammals express cell surface and circulating regulatory proteins that prevent inappropriate complement activation on host cells.

■ IgA antibody is produced in the lamina propria of mucosal organs and is actively transported by a special Fc receptor through the epithelium into the lumen, where it blocks the ability of microbes to invade the epithelium.

■ Neonates acquire IgG antibodies from their mothers through the placenta and from the milk through gut epithelium, using a neonatal Fc receptor to capture and transport the maternal antibodies.

■ Microbes have developed strategies to resist or evade humoral immunity, such as varying their antigens and becoming resistant to complement and phagocytosis.

■ Most vaccines in current use work by stimulating the production of neutralizing antibodies. Many approaches are being tested to develop vaccines that can stimulate protective cell-mediated immune responses.

REVIEW QUESTIONS

1 *What regions of antibody molecules are involved in the functions of antibodies?*

2 *How do heavy chain isotype (class) switching and affinity maturation improve the abilities of antibodies to combat infectious pathogens?*

3 *In what situations does the ability of antibodies to neutralize microbes protect the host from infections?*

4 *How do antibodies assist in the elimination of microbes by phagocytes?*

5 *How is the complement system activated, and why is it effective against microbes but does not react against host cells and tissues?*

6 *What are the functions of the complement system, and what components of complement mediate these functions?*

7 *How do antibodies prevent infections by ingested and inhaled microbes?*

8 *How do neonatal animals develop the capacity to protect themselves from infections even before their immune systems have reached maturity?*

Chapter 9

IMMUNOLOGICAL TOLERANCE AND AUTOIMMUNITY

Self-Nonself Discrimination in the Immune System and Its Failure

One of the remarkable characteristics of the normal immune system is that it is capable of reacting to an enormous variety of microbes, but it does not react against each individual's own (self) antigens. This unresponsiveness to self antigens, also called **immunological tolerance,** is maintained despite the fact that the mechanisms by which lymphocyte receptors are expressed are not inherently biased to produce receptors for nonself antigens. In other words, lymphocytes with the ability to recognize self antigens are constantly being generated during the normal process of lymphocyte maturation. Furthermore, many self antigens have ready access to the immune system, so that unresponsiveness to these antigens cannot be maintained simply by concealing them from lymphocytes. It follows that there must exist mechanisms that prevent immune responses to self antigens. These mechanisms are responsible for one of the cardinal features of the immune system, namely, its ability to discriminate between self and nonself (usually microbial) antigens. If these mechanisms fail, the immune system may attack the individual's own cells and tissues. Such reactions are called **autoimmunity,** and the diseases they cause are called autoimmune diseases.

In this chapter we will address the following questions.

- How does the immune system maintain its unresponsiveness to self antigens?

• What are the factors that may contribute to the development of autoimmunity?

This chapter begins with a discussion of the important principles and features of self-tolerance. Then we discuss the different mechanisms that maintain tolerance to self antigens, including how each mechanism may fail, resulting in autoimmunity.

Immunological Tolerance: Significance and Mechanisms

Immunological tolerance is a lack of response to antigens that is induced by exposure of lymphocytes to these antigens. When lymphocytes with receptors for a particular antigen are exposed to this antigen, any of several outcomes is possible. The lymphocytes may be activated to proliferate and to differentiate into effector cells, leading to a productive immune response; antigens that elicit such a response are said to be immunogenic. The lymphocytes may be functionally inactivated or killed, resulting in tolerance; antigens that induce tolerance are said to be tolerogenic. In some situations, the antigen-specific lymphocytes may not react in any way; this phenomenon has been called immunological ignorance, implying that the lymphocytes simply ignore the presence of the antigen. Normally, microbes are immunogenic and self antigens are tolerogenic. The choice between lymphocyte activation and tolerance is determined by the nature of the antigen-specific lymphocytes and by the nature of the antigen and how it is displayed to the immune system. In fact, the same antigen may be administered in different ways to induce an immune response or tolerance. This experimental observation has been exploited to analyze what factors determine whether activation or tolerance develops as a consequence of encounter with an antigen.

The phenomenon of immunological tolerance is important for several reasons. First, as we stated at the outset, self antigens normally induce tolerance. Second, if we learn how to induce tolerance in lymphocytes specific for a particular antigen, we may be able to use this knowledge to prevent or control unwanted immune reactions. Strategies for inducing tolerance are being tested to treat allergic and autoimmune diseases and to prevent the rejection of organ transplants. The same strategies may be valuable in gene therapy, to prevent immune responses against the products of newly expressed genes or vectors, and even for stem cell transplantation if the stem cell donor is genetically different from the recipient.

Immunological tolerance to different self antigens may be induced when developing lymphocytes encounter these antigens in the generative (central) lymphoid organs, called central tolerance, or when mature lymphocytes encounter self antigens in peripheral tissues, called peripheral tolerance (Fig. 9-1). Central tolerance is a mechanism of tolerance only to self antigens that are present in the generative lymphoid organs, namely, the bone marrow and thymus. Tolerance to self antigens that are not present in these organs must be induced and maintained by peripheral mechanisms. We have only limited knowledge of how many and which self antigens induce central or peripheral tolerance or are ignored by the immune system.

With this brief background, we proceed to a discussion of the mechanisms of immunological tolerance and how the failure of each mechanism may result in autoimmunity. Tolerance in CD4+ helper T lymphocytes is described first, because more is known about the process involving this cell type than about any other. Recall that CD4+ helper T cells control virtually all immune responses to protein antigens. Therefore, if helper T cells are made unresponsive to self protein antigens, this may be enough to prevent both cell-mediated and humoral immune responses against these antigens. Conversely, failure of tolerance in helper T cells may result in autoimmunity manifested by T cell–mediated attack against self antigens or by the production of autoantibodies against self proteins.

Central T Lymphocyte Tolerance

The principal mechanisms of central tolerance in T cells are cell death and, for CD4+ cells, the generation of regulatory T cells (Fig. 9-2). The lymphocytes that develop in the thymus consist of cells with receptors capable of recognizing many antigens, both self and foreign. If an immature lymphocyte strongly interacts with a self antigen, displayed as a peptide bound to a self major histocompatibility complex (MHC) molecule, that lymphocyte receives signals that trigger apoptosis, and the cell dies before it can complete its maturation. This process also is termed

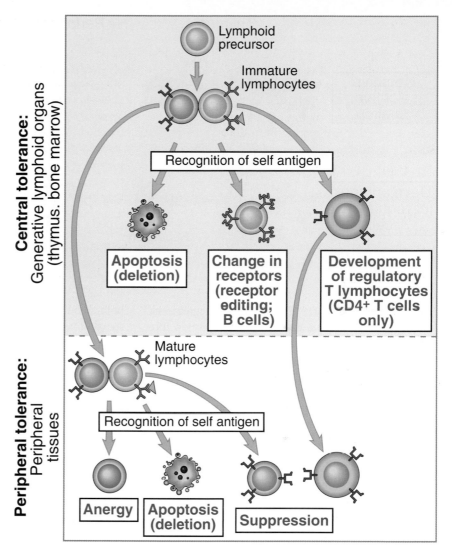

FIGURE 9-1 **Central and periph-eral tolerance to self antigens.** *Central tolerance*: Immature lympho-cytes specific for self antigens may encounter these antigens in the gen-erative lymphoid organs and are deleted; B lymphocytes change their specificity (receptor editing), and some T lymphocytes develop into regulatory T cells. Some self-reactive lymphocytes may complete their mat-uration and enter peripheral tissues. *Peripheral tolerance*: Mature self-reactive lymphocytes may be inacti-vated or deleted by encounter with self antigens in peripheral tissues. B lym-phocytes are shown in this illustra-tion, but the general principles apply to T lymphocytes as well.

negative selection (see Chapter 4), and it is a major mechanism of central tolerance. Immature lympho-cytes may interact strongly with an antigen if the antigen is present at high concentrations in the thymus and if the lymphocytes express receptors that recog-nize the antigen with high affinity. Antigens that induce negative selection may include proteins that are abun-dant throughout the body, such as plasma proteins and common cellular proteins. Surprisingly, many self pro-teins that are thought to be expressed mainly or exclu-sively in peripheral tissues are actually also expressed in some of the epithelial cells of the thymus. A protein called AIRE (*a*utoimmune *r*egulator) is responsible for thymic expression of many of these otherwise periph-eral tissue–restricted protein antigens. Mutations in the *AIRE* gene are the cause of a rare autoimmune dis-order called autoimmune polyendocrine syndrome. The process of negative selection affects self-reactive CD4+ T cells and CD8+ T cells, which recognize self peptides displayed by class II MHC and class I MHC molecules, respectively. It is not known what signals induce apoptosis in immature lymphocytes that recog-nize antigens with high affinity in the thymus. Defec-tive negative selection is postulated to be a reason why some autoimmunity-prone inbred strains of mice contain abnormally large numbers of mature T cells specific for various self antigens. Why deletion may fail in these mice also is not known.

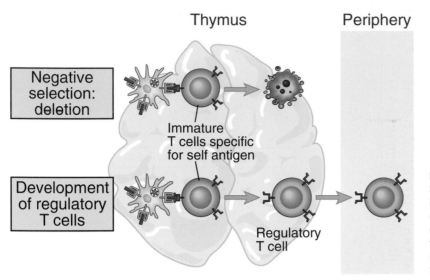

Thymus   Periphery

Negative selection: deletion

Immature T cells specific for self antigen

Development of regulatory T cells

Regulatory T cell

FIGURE 9-2   Central T cell tolerance. Strong recognition of self antigens by immature T cells in the thymus may lead to death of the cells (negative selection, or deletion). Self antigen recognition in the thymus also may lead to the development of regulatory T cells that enter peripheral tissues.

Some immature CD4+ T cells that recognize self antigens in the thymus do not die but develop into regulatory T cells and enter peripheral tissues (see Fig. 9-2). The functions of regulatory T cells are described later in the chapter. What determines whether a thymic T cell that recognizes a self antigen will die or become a regulatory T cell is not known.

Peripheral T Lymphocyte Tolerance

Peripheral tolerance is induced when mature T cells recognize self antigens in peripheral tissues, leading to functional inactivation (anergy) or death, or when the self-reactive lymphocytes are suppressed by regulatory T cells. Each of these mechanisms of peripheral T cell tolerance is described in this section. Peripheral tolerance is clearly important for preventing T cell responses to self antigens that are present mainly in peripheral tissues and not in the thymus. Peripheral tolerance also may provide "back-up" mechanisms for preventing autoimmunity in situations where central tolerance is incomplete.

ANERGY

Anergy is the functional inactivation of T lymphocytes that occurs when these cells recognize antigens without adequate levels of the costimulators (second signals) that are needed for full T cell activation (Fig. 9-3). In previous chapters we have

pointed out that naive T lymphocytes need at least two signals for their proliferation and differentiation into effector cells: Signal 1 is always antigen, and signal 2 is provided by costimulators that are expressed on antigen-presenting cells (APCs) in response to microbes. It is believed that, normally, APCs in tissues and peripheral lymphoid organs, including dendritic cells, are in a resting state, in which they express little or no costimulators such as B7 proteins (see Chapter 5). These APCs are constantly processing and displaying the self antigens that are present in the tissues. T lymphocytes with receptors for the self antigens are able to recognize the antigens and thus receive prolonged signals from their antigen receptors (signal 1), but the T cells do not receive strong costimulation because there is no accompanying innate immune response. Under these conditions, the T cell antigen receptors (TCRs) may lose their ability to transmit activating signals, or the T cells may preferentially engage one of the inhibitory receptors of the CD28 family, CTLA-4 (cytotoxic T lymphocyte–associated antigen-4 or CD152) or PD-1 (programmed [cell] death protein-1) (see Chapter 5). The net result is long-lasting T cell anergy (see Fig. 9-3). It is intriguing that CTLA-4, which is involved in shutting off T cell responses, recognizes the same B7 costimulators that bind to CD28 and initiate T cell activation. How T cells choose to use CD28 or CTLA-4, with these very different outcomes, is not understood.

FIGURE 9-3 T cell anergy. An antigen presented by costimulator-expressing antigen-presenting cells (APCs) induces a normal T cell response. If the T cell recognizes antigen without strong costimulation or innate immunity, the T cell receptors may lose their ability to deliver activating signals, or the T cell may engage inhibitory receptors, such as CTLA-4 (cytotoxic T lymphocyte–associated protein-4), that block activation.

Several experimental animal models support the importance of T cell anergy in the maintenance of self-tolerance. Forced expression of high levels of B7 costimulators in a tissue in a mouse, by transgenic technology, results in autoimmune reactions against antigens in that tissue. Thus, artificially providing second signals "breaks" anergy and activates autoreactive T cells. If CTLA-4 molecules are blocked (by treatment with antibodies) or deleted (by gene knockout) in a mouse, that mouse develops widespread autoimmune reactions against its own tissues. These results suggest that the inhibitory receptors are constantly functioning to keep autoreactive T cells in

check. Polymorphisms in the *CTLA4* gene have been associated with some autoimmune diseases in humans. Although anergy is well documented by experimental mouse models, it is still not known which types of self antigens induce anergy by which mechanism, or even if anergic T cells are present in normal humans.

IMMUNE SUPPRESSION BY REGULATORY T CELLS

Regulatory T cells develop in the thymus or peripheral tissues on recognition of self antigens

FIGURE 9-4 **T cell–mediated suppression of immune responses.** CD4+ T cells that recognize self antigens may differentiate into regulatory cells in the thymus or peripheral tissues, in a process that is dependent on the transcription factor Foxp3 and requires interleukin-2 (IL-2). (The *larger arrow* from the thymus, compared to the one from peripheral tissues, indicates that most of these cells probably arise in the thymus.) These regulatory cells inhibit the activation of naive T cells and their differentiation into effector T cells, by contact-dependent mechanisms or by secreting cytokines that inhibit T cell responses. APC, antigen-presenting cell.

and block the activation of potentially harmful lymphocytes specific for these self antigens (Fig. 9-4). A majority of self-reactive regulatory T cells probably develop in the thymus (see Fig. 9-2), but they also may arise in peripheral lymphoid organs. Most regulatory T cells are CD4+ and express high levels of CD25, the α chain of the interleukin-2 (IL-2) receptor. The development and function of these cells are dependent on a transcription factor called Foxp3. Mutations of Foxp3 in humans or knockout of the gene in mice causes a systemic, multiorgan autoimmune disease, demonstrating the importance of regulatory T cells for the maintenance of self-tolerance. The survival and function of regulatory T cells are dependent on the cytokine IL-2, and this role of IL-2 accounts for the severe autoimmune disease that develops in mice in which the gene encoding IL-2 or the α or β chain of the IL-2 receptor is deleted. The cytokine transforming growth factor-β (TGF-β) also plays a role in the generation of regulatory T cells, perhaps by stimulating expression of the Foxp3 transcription

factor. The source of TGF-β for inducing these cells in the thymus or peripheral tissues is not defined. We know little about the mechanisms by which regulatory T cells inhibit immune responses in vivo. Some regulatory cells produce cytokines, such as IL-10 and TGF-β, that block the activation of lymphocytes and macrophages. Regulatory cells also may directly interact with and suppress other lymphocytes or APCs, by undefined mechanisms that require cell–cell contact. It is worth pointing out that there may be regulatory populations in addition to the CD25+Foxp3+ cells that have been the focus of most current investigations.

It has been suggested that an underlying abnormality in some autoimmune diseases in humans is defective regulatory T cell function or resistance of pathogenic T cells to regulation. However, convincing evidence for these hypotheses is lacking, mainly because it has proved difficult to define the maintenance, heterogeneity, and functions of regulatory T cells in humans.

FIGURE 9-5 Activation-induced death of T lymphocytes. T cells respond to antigen presented by normal antigen-presenting cells (APCs) by secreting interleukin-2 (IL-2), expressing anti-apoptotic proteins, and undergoing proliferation and differentiation. Self antigen recognition by T cells without costimulation or innate immunity may lead to excess of intracellular pro-apoptotic proteins that cause cell death. Alternatively, self antigen recognition may lead to expression of death receptors and their ligands, such as Fas and Fas ligand (FasL), on lymphocytes, and engagement of the death receptor leads to apoptotic death of the cells.

DELETION: ACTIVATION-INDUCED CELL DEATH

Recognition of self antigens may trigger pathways of apoptosis that result in elimination (deletion) of the self-reactive lymphocytes (Fig. 9-5). This process has been called activation-induced cell death because it is the consequence of antigen recognition (i.e., activation). There are two likely mechanisms of death of mature T lymphocytes induced by self antigens. First, antigen recognition induces the production of pro-apoptotic proteins in T cells that induce cell death by the "mitochondrial pathway," in which various mito-

chondrial proteins leak out and activate caspases, cytosolic enzymes that induce apoptosis. In immune responses to microbes, the activity of these pro-apoptotic proteins is counteracted by anti-apoptotic proteins that are induced by costimulation and by growth factors produced during immune responses. But self antigens, which are recognized without strong costimulation, do not stimulate production of anti-apoptotic proteins, resulting in death of the cells that recognize these antigens. Second, recognition of self antigens may lead to the coexpression of death receptors and their ligands. This ligand–receptor interaction generates signals through the death receptor that culminate in the activation of caspases and apoptosis by what is called the "death receptor pathway." The best-defined death receptor: ligand pair involved in self-tolerance is a protein called Fas (CD95), which is expressed on many cell types, and Fas ligand (FasL), which is expressed mainly on activated T cells. Binding of FasL to Fas has been shown to induce death of both T and B cells exposed to self antigens and to mimics of self antigens in experimental animals. Whether the Fas death receptor has functions in addition to triggering apoptosis is not established.

Evidence supporting the role of apoptosis in self-tolerance has come from genetic studies. Blocking the mitochondrial pathway of apoptosis in mice results in a failure of deletion of self-reactive T cells in the thymus and also in peripheral tissues. Mice with mutations in the *fas* and *fasL* genes and children with mutations in *FAS* all develop autoimmune diseases with lymphocyte accumulation. The human disease, called the autoimmune lymphoproliferative syndrome, is rare and the only known example of a defect in

apoptosis causing a complex autoimmune phenotype in humans.

From this discussion of the mechanisms of T cell tolerance, it should be clear that self antigens differ from foreign microbial antigens in several ways, which contribute to the choice between tolerance induced by the former and activation by the latter (Fig. 9-6). Self antigens are present in the thymus, where they induce deletion and generate regulatory T cells; by contrast, microbial antigens are actively transported to and concentrated in peripheral lymphoid organs. Self antigens are displayed by resting APCs in the absence of innate immunity and second signals, thus favoring the induction of T cell anergy or death. By contrast, microbes elicit innate immune reactions, leading to the expression of costimulators and cytokines that function as second signals and promote T cell proliferation and differentiation into effector cells. Self antigens are present throughout life and may therefore cause prolonged or repeated TCR engagement, again promoting anergy and apoptosis. It is apparent that much of our

Feature of antigen	Tolerogenic self antigens	Immunogenic foreign antigens
	Tissue	Microbe
Presence in generative organs	Yes (some self antigens): high concentrations induce negative selection and regulatory T cells (central tolerance)	No: microbial antigens are concentrated in peripheral lymphoid organs
Presentation with second signals (costimulation, innate immunity)	No: deficiency of second signals may lead to T cell anergy or apoptosis	Yes: typically seen with microbes; second signals promote lymphocyte survival and activation
Persistence of antigen	Long-lived (throughout life); prolonged TCR engagement may induce anergy and apoptosis	Usually short lived; immune response eliminates antigen

FIGURE 9-6 Features of protein antigens that influence the choice between T cell tolerance and activation. This table summarizes some of the characteristics of self and foreign (e.g., microbial) protein antigens that determine why the self antigens induce tolerance and microbial antigens stimulate T cell–mediated immune responses. TCR, T cell receptor.

understanding of the mechanisms of T cell tolerance, and their roles in preventing autoimmunity, is based on studies with experimental animal models. Extending these studies to humans remains an important challenge.

B Lymphocyte Tolerance

Self polysaccharides, lipids, and nucleic acids are T-independent antigens that are not recognized by T cells. These antigens must induce tolerance in B lymphocytes to prevent autoantibody production. As we mentioned earlier, self protein antigens may fail to elicit autoantibody responses because of tolerance in helper T cells. However, there is experimental evidence that protein antigens can also induce tolerance in B cells. It is suspected that diseases associated with autoantibody production, such as systemic lupus erythematosus, are caused by defective tolerance in both B lymphocytes and helper T cells.

CENTRAL B CELL TOLERANCE

When immature B lymphocytes interact strongly with self antigens in the bone marrow, the B cells either change their receptor specificity (receptor editing) or are killed (negative selection) (Fig. 9-7).

Some immature B cells that recognize self antigens in the bone marrow may reactivate their immunoglobulin (Ig) gene recombination machinery and begin to express a new Ig light chain (see Chapter 4). This new light chain associates with the previously expressed Ig heavy chain to produce a new antigen receptor that is no longer specific for the self antigen. This process of changing receptor specificity, called **receptor editing**, reduces the likelihood that potentially harmful self-reactive B cells will leave the marrow. It is estimated that 25% to 50% of mature B cells in a normal individual may have undergone receptor editing during their maturation. (There is no evidence that developing T cells can undergo receptor editing.) If editing fails, immature B cells that recognize self antigens with high affinity receive death signals and die by apoptosis. This process of deletion is similar to negative selection of immature T lymphocytes. As in the T cell compartment, negative selection of B cells eliminates lymphocytes with high-affinity receptors for abundant, and usually widely expressed, cell membrane or soluble self antigens. Although central tolerance in developing B cells is a well-established phenomenon, there are no known examples of autoimmune diseases that can be attributed to loss of central B cell tolerance.

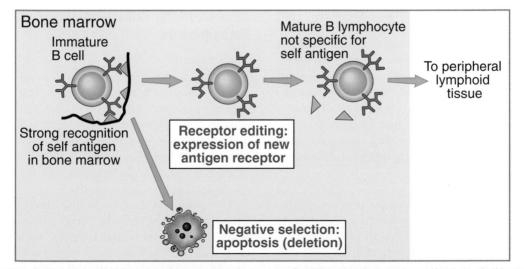

FIGURE 9-7   Central tolerance in immature B lymphocytes. An immature B cell that strongly recognizes self antigens (in this case, a multivalent self antigen with several epitopes) in the bone marrow either changes its antigen receptor (receptor editing) or dies by apoptosis (negative selection, or deletion).

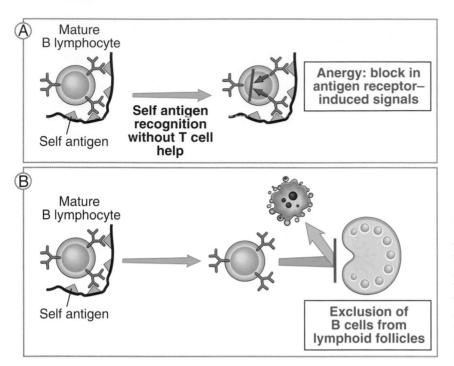

FIGURE 9-8 **Peripheral tolerance in B lymphocytes. A,** A mature B cell that recognizes a self antigen without T cell help is functionally inactivated and becomes incapable of responding to that antigen. **B,** B cells that are partially activated by recognition of self antigens without T cell help may be excluded from lymphoid follicles and may die by apoptosis because they are deprived of survival stimuli.

PERIPHERAL B CELL TOLERANCE

Mature B lymphocytes that encounter high concentrations of self antigens in peripheral lymphoid tissues become anergic and cannot again respond to that self antigen (Fig. 9-8). According to one hypothesis, if B cells recognize an antigen and do not receive T cell help (because helper T cells are absent or tolerant), the B cells become anergic. Presumably, T-independent antigens activate B lymphocytes without T cell help only when such antigens trigger strong signals in the B cells (see Chapter 7). Anergic B cells may leave lymphoid follicles and are subsequently excluded from the follicles. These excluded B cells may die because they do not receive necessary survival stimuli.

Now that we have discussed the principal mechanisms of self-tolerance, we can turn to a consideration of the consequences of failure of self-tolerance—namely, the development of autoimmunity. We start with general principles and then proceed to a discussion of the major known factors involved in the pathogenesis of autoimmune diseases. The mechanisms of

tissue injury in these diseases, and therapeutic strategies for autoimmune disorders, are described in Chapter 11.

Autoimmunity: Principles and Pathogenesis

Autoimmunity is defined as an immune response against self (autologous) antigens. It is an important cause of disease, estimated to affect at least 1% to 2% of persons in developed countries, and with an apparently increasing prevalence. It is worth adding a cautionary note that in many cases, diseases associated with uncontrolled immune responses are called autoimmune without formal evidence that the responses are directed against self antigens.

The principal factors in the development of autoimmunity are the inheritance of susceptibility genes and environmental triggers, such as infections (Fig. 9-9). Autoimmunity may result in the production of antibodies against self antigens or the activation of T cells reactive with self antigens. Much has been learned from experimental animal models

Genetic susceptibility

Environmental stimuli

Susceptibility genes

Tissue

Infection, tissue injury, inflammation

Failure of self-tolerance

Activation of tissue APCs

Self-reactive lymphocytes

Influx of self-reactive lymphocytes into tissues

Activation of self-reactive lymphocytes

Tissue injury: autoimmune disease

FIGURE 9-9 Postulated mechanisms of autoimmunity. In this proposed model of an organ-specific T cell–mediated autoimmune disease, various genetic loci may confer susceptibility to autoimmunity, probably by influencing the maintenance of self-tolerance. Environmental triggers, such as infections and other inflammatory stimuli, promote the influx of lymphocytes into tissues and the activation of self-reactive T cells, resulting in tissue injury. APCs, antigen-presenting cells.

about how self-tolerance may fail and how self-reactive lymphocytes may become pathogenic. Susceptibility genes may interfere with pathways of self-tolerance and lead to the persistence of self-reactive T and B lymphocytes. Environmental stimuli and tissue injury may result in the activation of these self-reactive lymphocytes. Nevertheless, despite our growing knowledge of the immunologic abnormalities that may result in autoimmunity, we still do not know

the etiology of any human autoimmune disease. This lack of understanding is due mainly to the following three factors: autoimmune diseases in humans usually are heterogeneous and multifactorial; the self antigens that are the inducers and targets of the autoimmune reactions often are unknown; and the diseases may manifest clinically long after the autoimmune reactions have been initiated. Recent advances, including the identification of disease-associated genes, better techniques for studying antigen-specific immune responses in humans, and the analysis of animal models that can be extrapolated to clinical situations, hold great promise for providing answers to the enigma of autoimmunity.

Genetic Factors in Autoimmunity

Most autoimmune diseases are polygenic and are associated with multiple gene loci, the most important of which are the MHC genes. The genetic predisposition to autoimmunity was appreciated when it was noted that if an autoimmune disease develops in one of two twins, the same disease is more likely to develop in the other twin than in an unrelated member of the general population. Furthermore, this increased incidence is greater among monozygotic (identical) twins than among dizygotic twins. Genome-wide association analyses, as well as breeding studies in animals, are revealing some of the genes that may contribute to different autoimmune diseases.

Many autoimmune diseases in humans and inbred animals are linked to particular MHC alleles (Fig. 9-10). The association between HLA alleles and autoimmune diseases in humans was recognized many years ago and was one of the first indications that T cells played an important role in these disorders (because the only known function of MHC molecules is to present peptide antigens to T cells). The incidence of a particular autoimmune disease often is greater among individuals who inherit a particular HLA allele(s) than in the general population. This increased incidence is called the "relative risk" of an HLA-disease association. It is important to point out that an HLA allele may increase the risk of developing a particular autoimmune disease, but the HLA allele is not, by itself, the cause of the disease. In fact, in the vast majority of people who inherit an HLA allele that frequently is disease associated, that disease never develops. Particular MHC alleles may contribute to the development of autoimmunity because they are inefficient at displaying self antigens, leading to defective negative selection of T cells, or because peptide anti-

Evidence	Examples		
	Disease	MHC allele	Relative risk
"Relative risk" of developing an autoimmune disease in individuals who inherit particular HLA allele(s) compared with individuals lacking these alleles	Ankylosing spondylitis	HLA-B27	90
	Rheumatoid arthritis	HLA-DR4	4
	Type 1 diabetes mellitus	HLA-DR3/DR4	25
	Pemphigus vulgaris	HLA-DR4	14
Animal models: breeding studies establish association of disease with particular MHC alleles	Type 1 diabetes mellitus (nonobese diabetic mouse strain)	I-A^{g7}	

FIGURE 9-10   Association of autoimmune diseases with alleles of the major histocompatibility complex (MHC) locus. Several lines of evidence support the association of certain MHC alleles with certain autoimmune diseases. Family and linkage studies show a greater likelihood of developing certain autoimmune diseases in persons who inherit particular human leukocyte antigen (HLA) alleles than in persons who lack these alleles ("relative risk"). Selected examples of HLA disease associations are listed. For instance, in people who have the HLA-B27 allele, the risk of development of the disease ankylosing spondylitis is 90 to 100 times higher than in B27-negative people; other diseases show various degrees of association with other HLA alleles. Breeding studies in animals have shown that the incidence of some autoimmune diseases correlates strongly with the inheritance of particular MHC alleles (e.g., type 1 diabetes mellitus with the mouse class II allele called I-A^{g7}).

Gene(s)	Disease association	Mechanism
AIRE	Autoimmune polyendocrine syndrome	Defective expression of tissue antigens and elimination of self-reactive T cells in the thymus
Complement proteins (C2, C4)	Lupus-like disease	Defective clearance of immune complexes? Defects in B cell tolerance?
Fas, FasL	Lpr, gld mouse strains; human ALPS	Defective elimination of self-reactive lymphocytes
FcγRIIb	Lupus-like diseases	Defective feedback inhibition of B cell activation
Foxp3	X-linked polyendocrinopathy and enteropathy (IPEX)	Deficiency of regulatory T cells
IL-2; IL-2Rα/β	Several autoimmune diseases (increased risk with polymorphisms)	Deficiency of regulatory T cells
NOD-2	Crohn's disease (inflammatory bowel disease)	Defective resistance or abnormal responses to intestinal microbes?
PTPN22	Several autoimmune diseases	Abnormal tyrosine phosphatase regulation of lymphocyte activation?

FIGURE 9-11 The roles of some non–major histocompatibility complex (MHC) genes in autoimmunity. Shown here are examples of some genes (listed alphabetically) other than MHC genes that may contribute to the development of autoimmune diseases. The roles of many of these individual genes have been inferred from the autoimmune diseases that develop in humans with mutations or in mouse gene knockouts. Note, however, that autoimmune diseases caused by single gene abnormalities are rare, and most human autoimmune diseases are complex, multigenic traits. Lpr and gld are, respectively, the mouse mutations "lymphoproliferation" and "generalized lymphoproliferative disease." AICD, activation-induced cell death; AIRE, autoimmune regulator; ALPS, autoimmune lymphoproliferative syndrome; IL, interleukin; IPEX, immunodysregulation–polyendocrinopathy–enteropathy X-linked syndrome; NOD-2, nucleotide-binding oligomerization domain–containing protein-2; PTPN22, protein tyrosine phosphatase N22.

gens presented by these MHC alleles may fail to stimulate regulatory T cells.

Numerous non-HLA genes also are associated with various autoimmune diseases. Some of these associated genes are known (Fig. 9-11), and their roles in the development of autoimmunity have been the focus of many hypotheses. More recent linkage analyses and genome-wide association studies have enormously expanded the number and diversity of genetic loci thought to be associated with various autoimmune diseases. Two genes that recently have been associated with autoimmune diseases in humans encode the tyrosine phosphatase PTPN22 (protein tyrosine phosphatase N22), which may regulate T cell activation and is associated with numerous autoimmune diseases, and the cytoplasmic microbial sensor NOD-2 (nucleotide-binding oligomerization domain–

containing protein-2), which may lower resistance to intestinal microbes. Other polymorphisms that are associated with multiple autoimmune diseases include genes encoding the IL-2 receptor α chain CD25, believed to influence the balance of effector and regulatory T cells, and the receptor for the cytokine IL-23, which promotes the development of pro-inflammatory T_H17 cells. It is hoped that elucidation of these genetic associations will reveal pathogenic mechanisms or provide new ideas for better prediction and treatment.

Role of Infections in Autoimmunity

Infections may activate self-reactive lymphocytes, thereby triggering the development of autoimmune diseases. Clinicians have recognized for many years

FIGURE 9-12 **Mechanisms by which microbes may promote autoimmunity. A,** Normally, encounter of mature T cells with self antigens presented by resting tissue antigen-presenting cells (APCs) results in peripheral tolerance by anergy or deletion. **B,** Microbes may activate the APCs to express costimulators, and when these APCs present self antigens, the specific T cells are activated, rather than being rendered tolerant. **C,** Some microbial antigens may cross-react with self antigens (mimicry). Therefore, immune responses initiated by the microbes may become directed at self cells and tissues. This figure illustrates concepts as they apply to T cells; molecular mimicry also may apply to self-reactive B lymphocytes.

that the clinical manifestations of autoimmunity often are preceded by infectious prodromes. This association between infections and autoimmune tissue injury has been formally established in animal models. Infections may contribute to autoimmunity in several ways (Fig. 9-12). An infection of a tissue may induce a local innate immune response, and this may lead to increased production of costimulators and cytokines by tissue APCs. These activated tissue APCs may be able to stimulate self-reactive T cells that encounter self antigens in the tissue. In other words, infection may "break" T cell anergy and promote the activation of self-reactive lymphocytes. Some infectious microbes may produce peptide antigens that are similar to, and

cross-react with, self antigens. Immune responses to these microbial peptides may result in an immune attack against self antigens. Such cross-reactions between microbial and self antigens are termed **molecular mimicry.** Although the contribution of molecular mimicry to autoimmunity has fascinated immunologists, its actual significance in the development of most autoimmune diseases remains unknown. There are some rare disorders in which antibodies produced against a microbial protein bind to self proteins. One example is rheumatic fever, in which antibodies against streptococci cross-react with a myocardial antigen and cause heart disease. Infections also may injure tissues and release antigens that normally are sequestered from the immune system. For instance, some sequestered antigens (e.g., in the testis and eye) normally are not "seen" by the immune system and are ignored. Release of these antigens (e.g., by trauma or infection) may initiate an autoimmune reaction against the tissue.

Paradoxically, some infections appear to confer protection from autoimmune diseases. This conclusion is based on epidemiologic data and limited experimental studies. The basis of this effect of infections is unknown.

SUMMARY

■ Immunological tolerance is specific unresponsiveness to an antigen induced by exposure of lymphocytes to that antigen. All individuals are tolerant of (unresponsive to) their own (self) antigens. Tolerance against antigens may be induced by administering that antigen in particular ways, and this strategy may be useful for treating immunological diseases and for preventing the rejection of transplants.

■ Central tolerance is induced by the death of or other changes in immature lymphocytes that encounter antigens in the generative lymphoid organs. Peripheral tolerance results from the recognition of antigens by mature lymphocytes in peripheral tissues.

■ Central tolerance of T cells is the result of high-affinity recognition of antigens in the thymus. Some of these self-reactive T cells die (negative selection), thus eliminating the potentially most dangerous T cells, which express high-affinity receptors for self antigens. Other T cells of the CD4 lineage develop into regulatory T cells that suppress self reactivity in the periphery.

■ Peripheral tolerance in T cells is induced by multiple mechanisms. Anergy (functional inactivation) results from the recognition of antigens without innate immunity and costimulators (second signals). The mechanisms of anergy include a block in TCR signaling and engagement of inhibitory receptors such as CTLA-4 and PD-1. Self-reactive regulatory T cells suppress potentially pathogenic T cells. Deletion (death by apoptosis) may occur when T cells encounter self antigens.

■ In B lymphocytes, central tolerance occurs when immature cells recognize self antigens in the bone marrow. Some of the cells change their receptors (receptor editing) and others die by apoptosis (negative selection, or deletion). Peripheral tolerance is induced when mature B cells recognize self antigens without T cell help, and this results in anergy and death of the B cells.

■ Autoimmune diseases result from a failure of self-tolerance. Multiple factors contribute to autoimmunity, including the inheritance of susceptibility genes and environmental triggers such as infections.

■ Many genes contribute to the development of autoimmunity. The strongest associations are between HLA genes and various T cell–mediated autoimmune diseases.

■ Infections predispose to autoimmunity, by causing inflammation and stimulating the expression of costimulators, or because of cross-reactions between microbial and self antigens.

REVIEW QUESTIONS

1 *What is immunological tolerance? Why is it important?*

2 *How is central tolerance induced in T lymphocytes and B lymphocytes?*

3 *How is functional anergy induced in T cells? How may anergy be "broken" to give rise to autoimmune disorders?*

4 *What are some of the genes that contribute to autoimmunity? How may MHC genes play a role in the development of autoimmune diseases?*

5 *What are some possible mechanisms by which infections promote the development of autoimmunity?*

Chapter 10

IMMUNE RESPONSES AGAINST TUMORS AND TRANSPLANTS

Immunity to Noninfectious Transformed and Foreign Cells

Cancer and organ transplantation represent two clinical situations in which the role of the immune system has received a great deal of attention. In cancer, it is widely believed that enhancing immunity against the tumors holds much promise for treatment. In organ transplantation, of course, the situation is precisely the reverse: Immune responses against the transplants are a barrier to successful transplantation, and learning how to suppress these responses is a major goal of transplant immunologists. Because of the importance of the immune system in host responses to tumors and transplants, tumor immunology and transplantation immunology have become subspecialties in which researchers and clinicians come together to address both fundamental and clinical questions.

Immune responses against tumors and transplants share several characteristics. These are situations in which the immune system is not responding to microbes, as it usually does, but to noninfectious cells that are perceived as foreign. The antigens that mark tumors and transplants as foreign may be expressed in virtually any cell type that is the target of malignant transformation or is grafted from one individual to another. Therefore, there have to be special mechanisms for inducing immune responses against diverse cell types. Also, an important, and perhaps major, mechanism by which tumor cells and the cells of tissue transplants are destroyed involves cytotoxic T lymphocytes (CTLs). For all of these reasons, immunity to tumors and transplants is discussed in one chapter, focusing on the following questions:

- What are the antigens in tumors and tissue transplants that are recognized as foreign by the immune system?
- How does the immune system recognize and react to tumors and transplants?
- How can the immune responses to tumors and grafts be manipulated to enhance tumor rejection and inhibit graft rejection?

We discuss tumor immunity first, and then transplantation, with an emphasis on the principles that are common to both.

Immune Responses against Tumors

Since the 1950s it has been thought that a physiologic function of the adaptive immune system is to prevent the outgrowth of transformed cells or to destroy these cells before they become harmful tumors. This phenomenon is called **immune surveillance.** Several lines of evidence support the idea that immune surveillance against tumors is important for preventing tumor growth (Fig. 10-1). However, the fact that common malignant tumors develop in immunocompetent individuals indicates that tumor immunity

often is weak compared with antimicrobial immunity, and is easily overwhelmed by rapidly growing tumors. Immunologists have been interested in defining the kinds of tumor antigens against which the immune system reacts and how antitumor immunity may be maximally enhanced.

TUMOR ANTIGENS

Malignant tumors express various types of molecules that may be recognized by the immune system as foreign antigens (Fig. 10-2). If the immune system of an individual is able to react against a tumor in that individual, it follows that the tumor must express antigens that are seen as nonself by that individual's immune system. In experimental tumors induced by chemical carcinogens or radiation, the tumor antigens may be mutants of normal cellular proteins. Virtually any gene may be mutagenized randomly in different tumors, and most of the mutated genes play no role in tumorigenesis. Such mutants of diverse cellular proteins are much less common in spontaneous human tumors than in experimentally induced tumors. Some tumor antigens are products of mutated or translocated oncogenes or tumor suppressor genes that presumably are involved in the process of malignant transformation. Surprisingly, in several human

Evidence	Conclusion
Histopathologic and clinical observations: lymphocytic infiltrates around some tumors and enlargement of draining lymph nodes correlate with better prognosis	Immune responses against tumors inhibit tumor growth
Experimental: transplants of a tumor are rejected by animals previously exposed to that tumor; immunity to tumor transplants can be transferred by lymphocytes from a tumor-bearing animal	Tumor rejection shows features of adaptive immunity (specificity, memory) and is mediated by lymphocytes
Clinical and experimental: immunodeficient individuals have an increased incidence of some types of tumors	The immune system protects against the growth of tumors (the concept of "immune surveillance")

FIGURE 10-1   **Evidence supporting the concept that the immune system reacts against tumors.** Several lines of clinical and experimental evidence indicate that defense against tumors is mediated by reactions of the adaptive immune system.

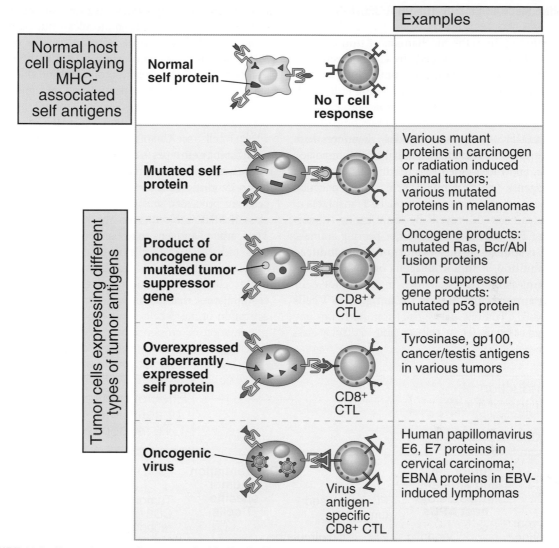

	Examples
Normal host cell displaying MHC-associated self antigens — Normal self protein / No T cell response	
Mutated self protein	Various mutant proteins in carcinogen or radiation induced animal tumors; various mutated proteins in melanomas
Product of oncogene or mutated tumor suppressor gene — CD8+ CTL	Oncogene products: mutated Ras, Bcr/Abl fusion proteins; Tumor suppressor gene products: mutated p53 protein
Overexpressed or aberrantly expressed self protein — CD8+ CTL	Tyrosinase, gp100, cancer/testis antigens in various tumors
Oncogenic virus — Virus antigen-specific CD8+ CTL	Human papillomavirus E6, E7 proteins in cervical carcinoma; EBNA proteins in EBV-induced lymphomas

Tumor cells expressing different types of tumor antigens

FIGURE 10-2   Types of tumor antigens recognized by T cells. Tumor antigens that are recognized by tumor-specific CD8+ T cells may be mutated forms of normal self proteins, products of oncogenes or tumor suppressor genes, overexpressed or aberrantly expressed self proteins, or products of oncogenic viruses. Tumor antigens also may be recognized by CD4+ T cells, but less is known about the role that CD4+ T cells play in tumor immunity. CTL, cytotoxic T lymphocyte; EBNA, Epstein-Barr virus nuclear antigen; EBV, Epstein-Barr virus; gp100, glycoprotein of 100 KD; MHC, major histocompatibility complex.

tumors, the antigens that elicit immune responses appear to be normal proteins that are over-expressed, or whose expression normally is limited to particular tissues or stages of development but is dysregulated in the tumors. These normal self antigens would not be expected to elicit immune responses, but their aberrant expression may be enough to elicit such responses. For example, self proteins that are expressed only in embryonic tissues may not induce tolerance in adults, so that the same proteins expressed in tumors may be recognized as foreign by the immune system. In tumors caused by oncogenic viruses, tumor antigens may be products of the viruses.

IMMUNE MECHANISMS OF TUMOR REJECTION

The principal immune mechanism of tumor eradication is killing of tumor cells by CTLs specific for tumor antigens. A majority of tumor antigens that elicit immune responses in tumor-bearing individuals are endogenously synthesized cytosolic proteins that are displayed as class I major histocompatibility complex (MHC)–associated peptides. Therefore, these antigens are recognized by class I MHC–restricted CD8+ CTLs, whose function is to kill cells producing the antigens. The role of CTLs in tumor rejection has been established in animal models: Transplants of tumors can be destroyed by transferring tumor-reactive CD8+ T cells into the tumor-bearing animals.

CTL responses against tumors often are induced by recognition of tumor antigens on host antigen-presenting cells (APCs), which ingest tumor cells or their antigens and present the antigens to T cells (Fig. 10-3). Tumors may arise from virtually any nucleated cell type. These cells are able to display class I MHC–associated peptides (because all nucleated cells express class I MHC molecules), but often the tumor cells do not express costimulators or class II MHC molecules. We know, however, that the activation of naive CD8+ T cells to proliferate and differentiate into active CTLs requires not only recognition of antigen (class I MHC–associated peptide) but also costimulation and/or help from class II MHC–restricted CD4+ T cells (see Chapter 5). How, then, can tumors of different cell types stimulate CTL responses? The likely answer is that tumor cells are ingested by the host's dendritic cells, and the antigens of the tumor cells are processed and displayed by the class I and class II MHC molecules on the host dendritic cells. Thus, tumor antigens may be recognized by CD8+ T cells and by CD4+ T cells in much the same manner as for any other protein antigens displayed by dendritic cells. At the same time, these APCs express costimulators that provide "second signals" for the activation of the T cells. This process is called cross-presentation or cross-priming, because one cell type

FIGURE 10-3 Induction of CD8+ T cell responses against tumors. CD8+ T cell responses to tumors may be induced by cross-priming (also called cross-presentation), in which the tumor cells or tumor antigens (or both) are taken up by dendritic cells, processed, and presented to T cells. In some cases, B7 costimulators expressed by these antigen-presenting cells (APCs) provide the second signals for the differentiation of the CD8+ T cells. The APCs may also stimulate CD4+ helper T cells, which may provide signals for CTL development (see Chapter 5, Fig. 5-7). Differentiated CTLs kill tumor cells without a requirement for costimulation or T cell help. CTL, cytotoxic T lymphocyte.

(the dendritic cell) presents antigens of another cell (the tumor cell) and activates (or primes) T lymphocytes specific for the second cell type. (Cross-presentation was discussed in Chapter 3, as the mechanism by which CTL responses are initiated to viruses that do not directly infect dendritic cells.) The concept of cross-presentation has been exploited to develop methods for vaccinating against tumors, as is discussed later in this chapter. Once naive CD8+ T cells have differentiated into effector CTLs, they are able to kill tumor cells expressing the relevant antigens without a requirement for costimulation or T cell help. Thus, CTL differentiation may be induced by cross-presentation of tumor antigens by host APCs, but the CTLs are effective against the tumor itself.

Several other immune mechanisms may play a role in tumor rejection. Antitumor CD4+ T cell responses and antibodies have been detected in patients, but there is little convincing evidence that these responses actually protect individuals against tumor growth. Experimental studies have shown that activated macrophages and natural killer (NK) cells are capable of killing tumor cells in vitro, but again the protective role of these effector mechanisms in tumor-bearing individuals is unclear.

EVASION OF IMMUNE RESPONSES BY TUMORS

Immune responses often fail to check tumor growth, because these responses are ineffective or because tumors evolve to evade immune attack. The immune system faces a daunting challenge if it is to be effective against malignant tumors, because immune responses must kill all tumor cells and tumors grow rapidly. Often, the growth of the tumor simply outstrips immune defenses. Immune responses against tumors may be weak because many tumor antigens are weakly immunogenic, perhaps because they differ only slightly from self antigens.

Growing tumors also develop mechanisms for evading immune responses (Fig. 10-4). Some tumors stop expressing the antigens that are the targets of immune attack. These tumors are called "antigen loss variants." If the lost antigen is not involved in maintaining the malignant properties of the tumor, the variant tumor cells continue to grow and spread. Other tumors stop expressing class I MHC molecules,

FIGURE 10-4 How tumors evade immune responses. Antitumor immunity develops when T cells recognize tumor antigens and are activated. Tumor cells may evade immune responses by losing expression of antigens or major histocompatibility complex (MHC) molecules or by producing immunosuppressive cytokines.

so they cannot display antigens to CD8+ T cells. NK cells recognize molecules expressed on tumor cells, but not on normal cells, and are activated when their target cells lack class I MHC molecules. Therefore, NK cells may provide a mechanism for killing class I MHC–negative tumors. Still other tumors may secrete cytokines, such as transforming growth factor-β, that suppress immune responses. Some tumors engage normal T cell inhibitory pathways, such as those mediated by CTLA-4 or PD-1 (Chapter 9), and thus suppress anti-tumor immune responses.

IMMUNOLOGICAL APPROACHES FOR CANCER THERAPY

The main strategies for cancer immunotherapy aim to provide antitumor effectors (antibodies and T cells) to patients, actively immunize patients against their tumors, and stimulate the patients' own antitumor immune responses. At present, the treatment of disseminated cancers (which cannot be surgically resected) relies on chemotherapy and irradiation, both of which have devastating effects on normal nontumor tissues. Because the immune response is highly specific, it has long been hoped that tumor-specific immunity may be used to selectively eradicate tumors without injuring the patient. Immunotherapy remains a major goal of tumor immunologists, and many approaches to therapy have been tried in experimental animals and in humans.

One of the earliest strategies for tumor immunotherapy relied on various forms of passive immunization, in which immune effectors are injected into cancer patients. Monoclonal antibodies against various tumor antigens, often coupled to potent toxins, have been tried in many cancers. The antibodies bind to tumor antigens and either activate host effector mechanisms, such as phagocytes or the complement system, or deliver the toxins to the tumor cells. Antibodies specific for CD20, which is expressed on B cells, are used to treat B cell tumors, usually in combination with chemotherapy. Because CD20 is not expressed by hematopoietic stem cells, normal B cells are replenished after the antibody treatment is stopped. Other monoclonal antibodies that are used in cancer therapy may work by blocking growth factor signaling (e.g., anti-Her2/Neu for breast cancer) or by inhibiting angiogenesis (e.g., antibody against the vascular endothelial growth factor for colon cancer and other tumors). T lymphocytes may be isolated from the blood or tumor infiltrates of a patient, expanded by culture with growth factors, and injected back into the same patient. The T cells presumably contain tumor-specific CTLs, which find the tumor and destroy it. This approach, called "adoptive cellular immunotherapy," has been tried as a therapy for several types of metastatic cancers, but results have been variable among different patients and tumors.

Many new strategies for cancer immunotherapy rely on boosting the host's own immune responses against tumors (Fig. 10-5). One way of stimulating immune responses against tumors is to vaccinate patients with their own tumor cells or with antigens from these cells. An important reason for defining tumor antigens is to produce and use these antigens to vaccinate individuals against their own tumors. Vaccines may be administered as recombinant proteins with adjuvants. More recently, there has been great interest in growing dendritic cells from individuals (by isolating precursors from the blood and expanding them by culture with growth factors), exposing the dendritic cells to tumor cells or tumor antigens, and using these "tumor-pulsed" dendritic cells as vaccines. It is hoped that the dendritic cells bearing tumor antigens will mimic the normal pathway of cross-presentation and will generate CTLs against the tumor cells. Another approach to vaccination uses a plasmid containing a complementary DNA (cDNA) encoding a tumor antigen. Injection of the plasmid results in expression of the cDNA in host cells, including APCs, that take up the plasmid. The APCs produce the tumor antigen, thus inducing specific T cell responses. Tumors caused by oncogenic viruses can be prevented by vaccinating against these viruses. Two such vaccines that are proving to be remarkably effective are against hepatitis B virus (the cause of many liver cancers) and human papillomavirus (the cause of cervical cancer).

Problems in identifying immunogenic tumor antigens and in developing effective vaccines have convinced some tumor immunologists that the best therapeutic strategy may be to let patients generate their own tumor-specific immune responses and to design therapies to optimize these responses. One approach for achieving this goal is to treat patients with cytokines that stimulate immune responses. The first cytokine to be used in this way was interleukin-2 (IL-2), but its applications are limited by serious toxic effects at the high doses that are needed to stimulate anti-tumor T cell responses. Many other cytokines

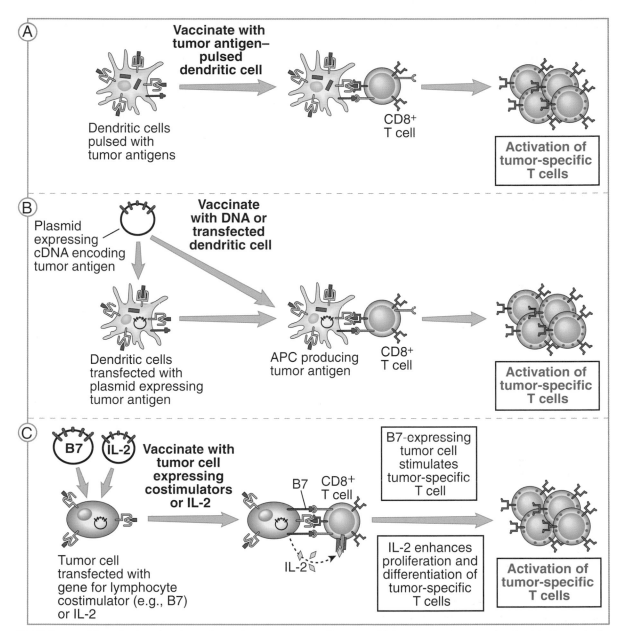

FIGURE 10-5 Strategies for enhancing antitumor immune responses. Tumor-specific immune responses may be stimulated by vaccinating with host dendritic cells that have been pulsed (incubated) with tumor antigens (**A**), or with plasmids containing complementary DNAs encoding tumor antigens that are injected directly into patients or used to transfect dendritic cells (**B**), or by vaccinating with tumor cells transfected with genes encoding B7 costimulators or the T cell growth factor interleukin-2 (IL-2) (**C**). APC, antigen-presenting cell; cDNA, complementary DNA.

have been tried for systemic therapy or local administration at sites of tumors. In a variation of this approach, a cytokine gene may be expressed in tumor cells and used to immunize the patient (see Fig. 10-5). In this way, it is hoped that T cell responses against tumor antigens become enhanced. The same principle underlies experimental studies in which the costimulator B7 is expressed in tumor cells, and the B7-expressing tumor cells are used as tumor vaccines. An interesting recent variation on the idea of boosting host immune responses against tumors is to eliminate normal inhibitory signals for lymphocytes. In some animal models, blocking the inhibitory receptor CTLA-4 has led to strong immune responses against transplanted tumors. Clinical trials of these approaches are currently underway.

Immune Responses against Transplants

From the advent of tissue transplantation, it was realized that individuals reject grafts from other individuals in a normal, outbred population. Rejection results from inflammatory reactions that damage the transplanted tissues. Studies in the 1940s and 1950s established that graft rejection is mediated by the adaptive immune system, because it shows specificity and memory and is dependent on lymphocytes (Fig. 10-6). Much of the knowledge about the immunology of transplantation came from studies with inbred strains of rodents, particularly mice. All members of an inbred strain are identical to each other and different from the members of other strains. Transplants exchanged between animals of the same and other inbred strains showed that grafts among members of an inbred strain are accepted and grafts among different strains are rejected. It was soon established that graft rejection is determined by inherited genes whose products are expressed in all tissues. The language of transplantation immunology evolved from these studies. The individual that provides the graft is called the **donor,** and the individual in which the graft is placed is the **recipient** or **host.** Animals that are identical to one another (and grafts exchanged among these animals) are said to be **syngeneic;** animals (and grafts) of one species that differ from other animals of the same species are said to be **allogeneic;** and animals (and grafts) of different species are **xenogeneic.** Allogeneic and xenogeneic grafts, also called **allografts** and **xenografts,** are always rejected. The antigens that serve as the targets of rejection are called alloantigens and xenoantigens, and the antibodies and T cells that react against these antigens are said to be alloreactive and xenoreactive, respectively. In the clinical situation, transplants usually are exchanged between allogeneic individuals, who are members of an outbred species who differ from one another (except, of course, for identical twins). Most of the following discussion focuses on immune responses to allografts.

Evidence	Conclusion
Prior exposure to donor MHC molecules leads to accelerated graft rejection	Graft rejection shows memory and specificity, two cardinal features of adaptive immunity
The ability to reject a graft rapidly can be transferred to a naive individual by lymphocytes from a sensitized individual	Graft rejection is mediated by lymphocytes
Depletion or inactivation of T lymphocytes by drugs or antibodies results in reduced graft rejection	Graft rejection can be mediated by T lymphocytes

FIGURE 10-6   Evidence indicating that the rejection of tissue transplants is an immune reaction. Clinical and experimental evidence indicates that rejection of grafts is a reaction of the adaptive immune system. MHC, major histocompatibility complex.

TRANSPLANTATION ANTIGENS

The antigens of allografts that serve as the principal targets of rejection are proteins encoded in the MHC. As we mentioned in Chapter 3, the MHC was discovered (and named) on the basis of its role in the rejection of grafts exchanged between mice of different inbred strains. Homologous MHC genes and molecules are present in all mammals; the human MHC is the human leukocyte antigen (HLA) complex. It took more than 20 years after the discovery of the MHC to show that the physiologic function of MHC molecules is to display peptide antigens for recognition by T lymphocytes (see Chapter 3). Recall that every human being expresses six class I MHC alleles (one allele of HLA-A, -B, and -C from each parent) and at least six class II MHC alleles (one allele of HLA-DQ and -DP and one or two of -DR from each parent, and some combinations of these). MHC genes are highly polymorphic; it is estimated that in the population there are at least 350 alleles of HLA-A genes, 620 alleles of HLA-B genes, 400 alleles of DR genes, and 90 alleles of DQ genes. Because these alleles can be inherited and expressed in many different combinations, every individual is likely to express some MHC proteins that appear foreign to another individual's immune system, except in the case of identical twins. All of the MHC molecules may be targets of rejection, although HLA-C and HLA-DP have limited polymorphism and probably are of minor significance.

The recognition of the MHC antigens on another individual's cells is one of the strongest immune responses known. The reason why individuals react against MHC molecules of other individuals is now understood quite well. T cell antigen receptors (TCRs) have evolved to recognize MHC molecules, which is essential for surveillance of cells harboring infectious microbes. In each individual, all CD4+ T cells and CD8+ T cells are selected during their maturation to recognize peptides displayed by that individual's (self) MHC molecules. This selection is the basis for the "self MHC restriction" of T lymphocytes, a fundamental property of T cells. If all mature T cells are selected to recognize only peptides displayed by self MHC molecules, why should T cells from one individual recognize the MHC molecules of another (allogeneic) individual as foreign? Recall that as a result of positive selection in the thymus, mature T cells that have some

affinity for self MHC molecules survive, and many of these will have high affinity for self MHC displaying foreign peptides. Allogeneic MHC molecules, containing peptides derived from the allogeneic cells, may look like self MHC molecules plus bound foreign peptides (Fig. 10-7). Therefore, recognition of allogeneic MHC molecules in allografts is an example of an immunologic cross-reaction. The process of negative selection in the thymus eliminates cells that strongly recognize self MHC, but there is no opportunity to selectively eliminate T cells whose TCRs have a high affinity for allogeneic MHC molecules, which are never present in the thymus. Many clones of T cells specific for different foreign peptides bound to the same self MHC molecule may cross-react with any one allogeneic MHC molecule, so long as the allogeneic MHC molecule resembles complexes of self MHC plus foreign peptides. As a result, many self MHC–restricted T cells specific for different peptide antigens may recognize any one allogeneic MHC molecule. Furthermore, a single allogeneic graft cell will express thousands of MHC molecules, every one of which may be recognized as foreign by a graft recipient's T cells. By contrast, in the case of an infected cell, only a small fraction of the self MHC molecules on the cell surface will carry a foreign microbial peptide recognized by the host's T cells. These are the main reasons why allogeneic cells evoke very strong T cell reactions.

Although MHC proteins are the major antigens that stimulate graft rejection, other polymorphic proteins also may play a role in rejection. Non-MHC antigens that induce graft rejection are called minor histocompatibility antigens, and most of them are allelic forms of normal cellular proteins that happen to differ between donor and recipient. The rejection reactions that minor histocompatibility antigens elicit usually are not as strong as reactions against foreign MHC proteins. Two clinical situations in which minor antigens are important targets of rejection are blood transfusion and bone marrow transplantation; these are discussed later in the chapter.

INDUCTION OF IMMUNE RESPONSES AGAINST TRANSPLANTS

The induction of T cell–mediated immune responses against tissue transplants has to overcome the same

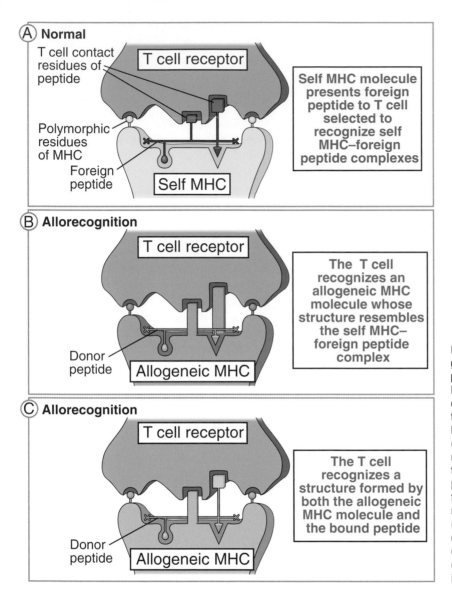

FIGURE 10-7 **Recognition of allogeneic major histocompatibility complex (MHC) molecules by T lymphocytes.** Recognition of allogeneic MHC molecules may be thought of as a cross-reaction in which a T cell specific for a self MHC molecule–foreign peptide complex (**A**) also recognizes an allogeneic MHC molecule whose structure resembles that of a self MHC molecule–foreign peptide complex (**B, C**). Peptides derived from the graft (labeled "donor peptides") may not contribute to allorecognition (**B**), or they may form part of the complex that the T cell "sees" (**C**). As discussed later in the chapter, the type of T cell recognition depicted in **B** and **C** is called direct allorecognition.

problem as in responses against tumors: Because a graft may contain many cell types, often including epithelial and connective tissue cells, how can the immune system recognize and react against all these cells? The answer is that T cells in the recipient may recognize donor alloantigens in the graft in different ways, depending on what cells in the graft are displaying these alloantigens.

T cells may recognize allogeneic MHC molecules in the graft displayed by dendritic cells in the graft, or graft alloantigens may be processed and presented by the host's dendritic cells (Fig. 10-8). Many tissues contain dendritic cells, and these APCs are carried into the recipients with grafts of these tissues. When T cells in the recipient recognize donor allogeneic MHC molecules on graft dendritic cells, the T cells are activated; this process is called **direct recognition** (or direct presentation of alloantigens). Direct recognition stimulates the development of alloreactive T cells (e.g., CTLs) that recognize and attack

FIGURE 10-8 *Direct and indirect recognition of alloantigens.* **A,** *Direct* alloantigen recognition occurs when T cells bind directly to intact allogeneic major histocompatibility complex (MHC) molecules on professional antigen-presenting cells (APCs) in a graft, as illustrated in Figure 10-7. **B,** *Indirect* alloantigen recognition occurs when allogeneic MHC molecules from graft cells are taken up and processed by recipient APCs, and peptide fragments of the allogeneic MHC molecules are presented by recipient (self) MHC molecules. Recipient APCs also may process and present graft proteins other than allogeneic MHC molecules.

the cells of the graft. Alloantigens can be recognized by the recipient by a second pathway, which is much like that for recognition of any foreign antigen. If graft cells (or alloantigens) are ingested by dendritic cells in the recipient, donor alloantigens are processed and presented by the self MHC molecules on recipient APCs. This process is called **indirect recognition** (or indirect presentation) and is similar to the cross-presentation of tumor antigens discussed earlier. The dendritic cells that present alloantigens by the direct or indirect pathway also provide costimulators and can stimulate helper T cells as well as alloreactive CTLs. However, if alloreactive CTLs are induced by the indirect pathway, these CTLs are specific for alloantigens displayed by self MHC molecules on host APCs, and they cannot recognize and kill cells in the

graft. It is likely that when graft alloantigens are recognized by the indirect pathway, the subsequent rejection of the graft is mediated mainly by alloreactive CD4+ T cells. These T cells may enter the graft together with host APCs, recognize graft antigens displayed by the APCs, and secrete cytokines that injure the graft by a delayed-type hypersensitivity (DTH) reaction. We do not know the relative importance of the direct and indirect pathways of allorecognition in the rejection of allografts. It has been suggested that the direct pathway is most important for CTL-mediated acute rejection and that the indirect pathway plays a greater role in chronic rejection.

The **mixed lymphocyte reaction** (MLR) is an in vitro model of T cell recognition of alloantigens. In this model, T cells from one individual are cultured with leukocytes of another individual, and the responses of the T cells are assayed. The magnitude of this response is proportional to the extent of the MHC differences between these individuals and is a rough predictor of the outcomes of grafts exchanged between these individuals.

Although much of the emphasis on allograft rejection has been on the role of T cells, it also is clear that alloantibodies contribute to rejection. Most of these antibodies are helper T cell–dependent high-affinity antibodies. In order to produce alloantibodies, recipient B cells recognize donor alloantigens and then process and present peptides derived from these antigens to helper T cells, thus initiating the process of antibody production. This is a good example of indirect presentation of alloantigens, in this case by B lymphocytes.

IMMUNE MECHANISMS OF GRAFT REJECTION

Graft rejection is classified into hyperacute, acute, and chronic, on the basis of clinical and pathologic features (Fig. 10-9). This historical classification was devised by clinicians and has stood the test of time remarkably well. It also has become apparent that each type of rejection is mediated by a particular type of immune response.

Hyperacute rejection occurs within minutes of transplantation and is characterized by thrombosis of graft vessels and ischemic necrosis of the graft. Hyperacute rejection is mediated by circulating antibodies, specific for antigens on graft endothelial cells, that are present before transplantation. These preformed antibodies may be natural IgM antibodies specific for blood group antigens (discussed later), or they may be antibodies specific for allogeneic MHC molecules that are present because of exposure to allogeneic cells due to blood transfusions, pregnancy, or prior organ transplantation. These antibodies bind to antigens in the graft vascular endothelium and activate the complement and clotting systems, leading to injury to the endothelium and thrombus formation. Hyperacute rejection is not a common problem in clinical transplantation, because every recipient is tested for blood type and for antibodies against the cells of the potential donor. (The test for antibodies is called a cross-match.) However, hyperacute rejection is the

major barrier to xenotransplantation, as discussed later.

Acute rejection occurs within days or weeks after transplantation and is the principal cause of early graft failure. Acute rejection is mediated mainly by T cells, which react against alloantigens in the graft. These T cells may be CTLs that directly destroy graft cells, or the T cells may react against cells in graft vessels, leading to vascular damage. Antibodies also contribute to acute rejection, especially the vascular component of this reaction, when injury to graft vessels is caused mainly by complement activation by the classical pathway. Current immunosuppressive therapy is designed mainly to prevent and reduce acute rejection by blocking the activation of alloreactive T cells, as is discussed later.

Chronic rejection is an indolent form of graft damage that occurs over months or years, leading to progressive loss of graft function. Chronic rejection may be manifested as fibrosis of the graft and by gradual narrowing of graft blood vessels, called graft arteriosclerosis. In both lesions, the culprits are believed to be T cells that react against graft alloantigens and secrete cytokines, which stimulate the proliferation and activities of fibroblasts and vascular smooth muscle cells in the graft. As treatment for acute rejection has improved, chronic rejection is becoming the principal cause of graft failure.

PREVENTION AND TREATMENT OF GRAFT REJECTION

The mainstay of preventing and treating the rejection of organ transplants is immunosuppression, designed mainly to inhibit T cell activation and effector functions (Fig. 10-10). The most useful immunosuppressive drug in clinical transplantation is cyclosporine, which functions by blocking the T cell phosphatase (called calcineurin) that is required to activate the transcription factor NFAT (nuclear factor of activated T cells) and thus inhibits transcription of cytokine genes in the T cells. The advent of cyclosporine as a clinically useful drug opened up a new era in transplantation medicine and has allowed the transplantation of heart, liver, and lung. Many other immunosuppressive agents are now used as adjuncts to or instead of cyclosporine (see Fig. 10-10). All of these immunosuppressive drugs carry the problem of

FIGURE 10-9 Mechanisms of graft rejection. A, In *hyperacute rejection,* preformed antibodies react with alloantigens on the vascular endothelium of the graft, activate complement, and trigger rapid intravascular thrombosis and necrosis of the vessel wall. **B,** In *acute cellular rejection,* CD8+ T lymphocytes reactive with alloantigens on graft endothelial cells and parenchymal cells cause damage to these cell types. Inflammation of the endothelium sometimes is called "endotheliitis." Alloreactive antibodies also may contribute to vascular injury. **C,** In *chronic rejection* with graft arteriosclerosis, T cells reactive with graft alloantigens may produce cytokines that induce proliferation of endothelial cells and intimal smooth muscle cells, leading to luminal occlusion. This type of rejection probably is a chronic delayed-type hypersensitivity (DTH) reaction to alloantigens in the vessel wall.

Drug	Mechanism of action
Cyclosporine and FK506	Blocks T cell cytokine production by inhibiting the phosphatase calcineurin and thus blocking activation of the NFAT transcription factor
Mycophenolate mofetil	Blocks lymphocyte proliferation by inhibiting guanine nucleotide synthesis in lymphocytes
Rapamycin	Blocks lymphocyte proliferation by inhibiting IL-2 signaling
Corticosteroids	Reduce inflammation by inhibiting macrophage cytokine secretion
Anti-CD3 monoclonal antibody	Depletes T cells by binding to CD3 and promoting phagocytosis or complement-mediated lysis (used to treat acute rejection)
Anti–IL-2 receptor antibody	Inhibits T cell proliferation by blocking IL-2 binding; may also opsonize and help eliminate activated IL-2R–expressing T cells
CTLA4-Ig	Inhibits T cell activation by blocking B7 costimulator binding to T cell CD28 (clinical trials)

FIGURE 10-10   Treatments for graft rejection. Agents that commonly are used to treat the rejection of organ grafts, and the mechanisms of action of these agents, are listed. Like cyclosporine, FK506 is a calcineurin inhibitor, but it is not as widely used. CTLA4-Ig, cytotoxic T lymphocyte–associated protein-4–immunoglobulin (fusion protein); IL, interleukin; NFAT, nuclear factor of activated T cells.

nonspecific immunosuppression (i.e., the drugs inhibit responses to more than the graft). Therefore, patients receiving these drugs as part of their posttransplantation regimen become susceptible to infections, particularly infections by intracellular microbes, and demonstrate an increased incidence of cancers, especially tumors caused by oncogenic viruses.

The matching of donor and recipient HLA alleles by tissue typing had an important role in minimizing graft rejection in the days before cyclosporine became available for clinical use. Now, however, immunosuppression is so effective that HLA matching is not considered necessary for many types of organ transplants, especially because recipients often are too sick to wait for the closest match.

The long-term goal of transplant immunologists is to induce immunological tolerance specifically for the graft alloantigens. If this is achieved, it will allow graft acceptance without shutting off any other immune responses in the host. Attempts to induce graft-specific tolerance are ongoing in experimental models (e.g., by stimulating alloreactive T cells to become regulatory cells).

A major problem in transplantation is the shortage of suitable donor organs. **Xenotransplantation** is a possible solution for this problem. Experimental studies with xenotransplants have shown that hyperacute rejection is a frequent cause of the loss of these grafts. The reason for the high incidence of hyperacute rejection of xenografts is that individuals often contain antibodies that react with cells from other species. These antibodies, like antibodies against blood group antigens discussed subsequently, are called "natural antibodies" because their production does not require prior exposure to the xenoantigens. It is thought that these antibodies are produced against bacteria that normally inhabit the gut and that the antibodies cross-react with cells of other species. Xenografts also are subject to acute rejection, much like allografts. Attempts are ongoing to genetically modify xenogeneic tissues in ways that prevent their rejection by recipients of other species.

TRANSPLANTATION OF BLOOD CELLS AND BONE MARROW CELLS

Transplantation of blood cells, called **transfusion,** is the oldest form of transplantation in clinical medicine. The major barrier to transfusion is the presence of foreign **blood group antigens,** the prototypes of which are the ABO antigens. These antigens are expressed on red blood cells, endothelial cells, and many other cell types. ABO molecules are glycosphingolipids containing a core glycan with sphingolipids attached.

The names A and B refer to the terminal sugars (*N*-acetylgalactosamine and galactose, respectively); AB means that both are present; and O means that neither is present. Individuals expressing one blood group antigen are tolerant to that antigen but contain antibodies against the other. It is believed that these antibodies are produced against similar antigens that are expressed by intestinal microbes and cross-react with the ABO blood group antigens. The preformed antibodies react against transfused blood cells expressing the target antigens, and the result may be a severe **transfusion reaction.** This problem is avoided by matching blood donors and recipients, a standard practice in medicine. Because the blood group antigens are sugars, they do not elicit T cell responses. Blood group antigens other than the ABO antigens also are involved in transfusion reactions, and these usually are less severe.

Hematopoietic stem cell transplantation is being used increasingly to correct hematopoietic defects or to restore bone marrow cells that have been damaged by irradiation and chemotherapy for cancer. Either whole bone marrow cells or enriched populations of hematopoietic stem cells derived from a donor's blood or bone marrow are injected into the circulation of a recipient, and the cells home to the marrow. The transplantation of bone marrow cells poses many special problems. Before transplantation, some of the bone marrow of the recipient has to be destroyed to create "space" to receive the transplanted marrow cells, and this depletion of the recipient's marrow inevitably causes deficiency of blood cells, including immune cells. The immune system reacts very strongly against allogeneic bone marrow cells, so that successful transplantation requires careful HLA matching of donor and recipient. If mature allogeneic T cells are transplanted with the marrow cells, these mature T cells can attack the recipient's tissues, resulting in a serious clinical reaction called **graft-versus-host disease.** Even if the graft is successful, recipients often are severely immunodeficient while their immune systems are being reconstituted. Despite these problems, there is great interest in hematopoietic stem cell transplantation as a therapy for a wide variety of diseases affecting the hematopoietic and lymphoid systems.

SUMMARY

- A physiologic function of the immune system is to eradicate tumors and prevent the growth of tumors.

- Tumor antigens may be products of oncogenes or tumor suppressor genes, mutated cellular proteins, overexpressed or aberrantly expressed molecules, or products of oncogenic viruses.

- Tumor rejection is mediated mainly by CTLs recognizing peptides derived from tumor antigens. The induction of CTL responses against tumor antigens often involves ingestion of tumor cells or their antigens by dendritic cells and presentation of the antigens to T cells.

- Tumors may evade immune responses by losing expression of their antigens, shutting off expression of MHC molecules or molecules involved in antigen processing, and secreting cytokines that suppress immune responses.

- Immunotherapy for cancer aims to enhance antitumor immunity by passively providing immune effectors to patients or by actively boosting the host's own effectors. Approaches for active boosting include vaccination with tumor antigens or with tumor cells engineered to express costimulators and cytokines.

- Tissue transplants are rejected by the immune system, and the major antigen targets of rejection are MHC molecules.

- The antigens of allografts that are recognized by T cells are allogeneic MHC molecules that resemble peptide-loaded self MHC molecules that the T cells are selected to recognize. Graft antigens either are directly presented to recipient T cells or are picked up and presented by host APCs.

- Grafts may be rejected by different mechanisms. Hyperacute rejection is mediated by preformed antibodies that cause endothelial injury and thrombosis of blood vessels in the graft. Acute rejection is mediated by T cells, which injure graft cells and endothelium, and by antibodies that bind to the endothelium. Chronic rejection is caused by T cells that produce cytokines that stimulate growth of vascular smooth muscle cells and tissue fibroblasts.

■ Treatment for graft rejection is designed to suppress T cell responses and inflammation. The mainstay of treatment has been the immunosuppressive drug cyclosporine; many other agents are in clinical use now.

■ Bone marrow transplants elicit strong rejection reactions, carry the risk of graft-versus-host disease, and often lead to temporary immunodeficiency in recipients.

REVIEW QUESTIONS

1   *What are the types of tumor antigens that the immune system reacts against? What is the evidence that tumor rejection is an immunologic phenomenon?*

2   *How do CD8+ T cells recognize tumor antigens, and how are these cells activated to differentiate into effector CTLs?*

3   *What are some of the mechanisms by which tumors may evade the immune response?*

4   *What are some strategies for enhancing host immune responses to tumor antigens?*

5   *Why do normal T cells, which recognize foreign peptide antigens bound to self MHC molecules, react strongly against the allogeneic MHC molecules of a graft?*

6   *What are the principal mechanisms of rejection of allografts?*

7   *What is the mixed leukocyte reaction, and what is its importance?*

8   *What are some of the problems associated with the transplantation of bone marrow cells?*

Chapter 11

HYPERSENSITIVITY

Disorders Caused by Immune Responses

The concept that the immune system is required for defending the host against infections has been emphasized throughout this book. However, immune responses are themselves capable of causing tissue injury and disease. Injurious, or pathologic, immune reactions are called **hypersensitivity reactions.** This term is derived from the idea that an immune response to an antigen may result in sensitivity to challenge with that antigen and, therefore, hypersensitivity is a reflection of excessive or aberrant immune responses. Hypersensitivity reactions may occur in two situations. First, responses to foreign antigens may be dysregulated or uncontrolled, resulting in tissue injury. Second, the immune responses may be directed against self (autologous) antigens, as a result of the failure of self-tolerance (see Chapter 9). Responses against self antigens are termed **autoimmunity,** and disorders caused by such responses are called **autoimmune diseases.**

This chapter describes the important features of hypersensitivity reactions and the diseases they cause, focusing on their pathogenesis. Details of the clinical and pathologic features of these diseases may be found in many other textbooks and are summarized only briefly in this chapter. The following questions are addressed:

- What are the mechanisms of different types of hypersensitivity reactions?
- What are the major clincal and pathologic features of diseases caused by these reactions, and what principles underlie treatment of such diseases?

Types of Hypersensitivity Reactions

Hypersensitivity reactions commonly are classified on the basis of the principal immunologic mechanism that is responsible for tissue injury and disease (Fig. 11-1). We prefer the more informative descriptive designations, rather than the numerical ones, so these descriptors are used throughout this chapter. Immediate hypersensitivity, or type I hypersensitivity, is a type of pathologic reaction that is caused by the release of mediators from mast cells. This reaction most commonly is triggered by the production of IgE antibody against environmental antigens and the binding of IgE to mast cells in various tissues. Antibodies other than IgE may cause diseases in two ways: Antibodies directed against cell or tissue antigens can damage these cells or tissues or impair their functions. These diseases are said to be antibody-mediated and represent type II hypersensitivity. Sometimes, antibodies against soluble antigens may form complexes with the antigens, and the immune complexes may deposit in blood vessels in various tissues, causing inflammation and tissue injury. Such diseases are called immune complex diseases and represent type III hypersensitivity. Finally, some diseases result from the reactions of T lymphocytes, often against self antigens in tissues. These T cell–mediated diseases represent type IV hypersensitivity.

In the remainder of this chapter, we describe the important features of each type of hypersensitivity disease.

Immediate Hypersensitivity

Immediate hypersensitivity is a rapid, IgE antibody– and mast cell–mediated vascular and smooth muscle reaction, often followed by inflammation, that occurs in some individuals on encounter with certain foreign antigens to which they have been exposed previously. Immediate hypersensitivity reactions are also called **allergy**, or **atopy**, and individuals with a strong propensity to develop these reactions are said to be "atopic." Such reactions may affect various tissues and may be of varying severity in different individuals. Common types of immediate hypersensitivity reactions include hay fever, food allergies, bronchial asthma, and anaphylaxis. The clinical features of these reactions are discussed later in the chapter. Allergies are the most frequent disorders of the immune system, estimated to affect about 20% of the population.

The sequence of events in the development of immediate hypersensitivity reactions consists of the production of IgE antibodies in response to an antigen, binding of IgE to Fc receptors of mast cells, cross-linking of the bound IgE by the antigen, and release of mast cell mediators (Fig. 11-2). Some mast cell mediators cause a rapid increase in vascular permeability and smooth muscle contraction, resulting in many of the symptoms of these reactions. This vascular and smooth muscle reaction may occur within minutes of reintroduction of antigen into a previously sensitized individual—hence the name immediate hypersensitivity. Other mast cell mediators are cytokines that recruit neutrophils and eosinophils to the site of the reaction over several hours. This inflammatory component is called the **late phase reaction**, and it is mainly responsible for the tissue injury that results from repeated bouts of immediate hypersensitivity.

With this background, we proceed to a discussion of the steps in immediate hypersensitivity reactions.

PRODUCTION OF IgE ANTIBODY

In individuals who are prone to allergies, encounter with some antigens results in the activation of T_H2 cells and the production of IgE antibody (see Fig. 11-2). Normal individuals do not mount strong T_H2 responses to most foreign antigens. For unknown reasons, when some individuals encounter antigens such as proteins in pollen, certain foods, insect venoms, or animal dander, or if they are exposed to certain drugs such as penicillin, the dominant T cell response is the development of T_H2 cells. Any atopic individual may be allergic to one or more of these antigens. Immediate hypersensitivity develops as a consequence of the activation of T_H2 cells in response to protein antigens or chemicals that bind to proteins.

Type of hypersensitivity	Pathologic immune mechanisms	Mechanisms of tissue injury and disease
Immediate hypersensitivity (Type I)	T_H2 cells, IgE antibody, mast cells, eosinophils	Mast cell-derived mediators (vasoactive amines, lipid mediators, cytokines) Cytokine-mediated inflammation (eosinophils, neutrophils)
Antibody-mediated diseases (Type II)	IgM, IgG antibodies against cell surface or extracellular matrix antigens	Complement and Fc receptor-mediated recruitment and activation of leukocytes (neutrophils, macrophages) Opsonization and phagocytosis of cells Abnormalities in cellular function, e.g. hormone receptor signaling
Immune complex-mediated diseases (Type III)	Immune complexes of circulating antigens and IgM or IgG antibodies deposited in vascular basement membrane	Complement and Fc receptor-mediated recruitment and activation of leukocytes
T cell-mediated diseases (Type IV)	1. CD4+ T cells (delayed type hypersensitivity) 2. CD8+ CTLs (T cell-mediated cytolysis)	1. Macrophage activation, cytokine-mediated inflammation 2. Direct target cell lysis, cytokine-mediated inflammation

FIGURE 11-1 Types of hypersensitivity reactions. In the four major types of hypersensitivity reactions, different immune effector mechanisms cause tissue injury and disease. CTLs, cytotoxic T lymphocytes; Ig, immunoglobulin.

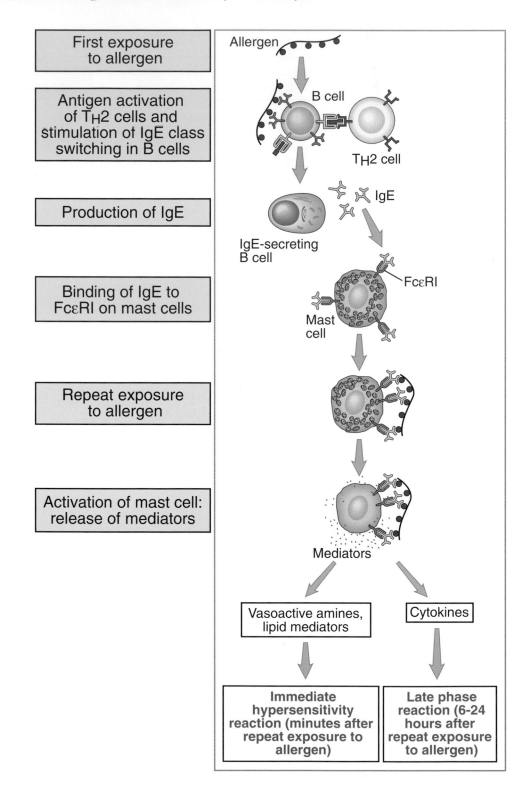

First exposure to allergen

Antigen activation of T$_H$2 cells and stimulation of IgE class switching in B cells

Production of IgE

Binding of IgE to FcεRI on mast cells

Repeat exposure to allergen

Activation of mast cell: release of mediators

Allergen

B cell

T$_H$2 cell

IgE

IgE-secreting B cell

FcεRI

Mast cell

Mediators

Vasoactive amines, lipid mediators

Cytokines

Immediate hypersensitivity reaction (minutes after repeat exposure to allergen)

Late phase reaction (6-24 hours after repeat exposure to allergen)

FIGURE 11-2   The sequence of events in immediate hypersensitivity. Immediate hypersensitivity diseases are initiated by the introduction of an allergen, which stimulates T_H2 reactions and immunoglobulin E (IgE) production. IgE binds to Fc receptors (FcεRI) on mast cells, and subsequent exposure to the allergen activates the mast cells to secrete the mediators that are responsible for the pathologic reactions of immediate hypersensitivity.

Antigens that elicit immediate hypersensitivity (allergic) reactions often are called allergens.

Two of the cytokines secreted by T_H2 cells, interleukin (IL)-4 and IL-13, stimulate B lymphocytes specific for the foreign antigens to switch to IgE-producing plasma cells. Therefore, atopic persons produce large amounts of IgE antibody in response to antigens that do not elicit IgE responses in most people. We know that the propensity toward T_H2 development, IgE production, and immediate hypersensitivity has a strong genetic basis, with many different genes playing contributory roles.

ACTIVATION OF MAST CELLS AND SECRETION OF MEDIATORS

IgE antibody produced in response to an allergen binds to high-affinity Fc receptors specific for the ε heavy chain expressed on mast cells (Fig. 11-3). Thus, in an atopic individual, mast cells are coated with IgE antibody specific for the antigen(s) to which the individual is allergic. This process of coating mast cells with IgE is called "sensitization," because coating with IgE specific for an antigen makes the mast cells sensitive to activation by subsequent encounter with that antigen. In normal individuals, by contrast, mast cells may carry IgE molecules of many different specificities, because many antigens may elicit small IgE responses, not enough to cause immediate hypersensitivity reactions. Mast cells are present in all connective tissues, and which of the body's mast cells are activated by cross-linking of allergen-specific IgE often depends on the route of entry of the allergen. For instance, inhaled allergens activate mast cells in the submucosal tissues of the bronchus, whereas ingested allergens activate mast cells in the wall of the intestine.

The high-affinity Fcε receptor, called FcεRI, consists of three chains, one of which binds the Fc portion of the ε heavy chain very strongly, with a K_d of approximately 10^{-11} M. (The concentration of IgE in the plasma is approximately 10^{-9} M, so that even in normal individuals, mast cells are always coated with IgE bound to FcεRI.) The other two chains of the receptor are signaling proteins. The same FcεRI also is present on basophils, the circulating counterpart of mast cells, but the role of basophils in immediate hypersensitivity is not as well established as the role of mast cells.

When mast cells sensitized by IgE are exposed to the allergen, the cells are activated to secrete their mediators (see Fig. 11-3). Thus, immediate hypersensitivity reactions occur after initial exposure to an allergen elicits specific IgE production and repeat exposure activates sensitized mast cells. Mast cell activation results from binding of the allergen to two or more IgE antibodies on the mast cell. When this happens, the IgE and the FcεRI molecules that are carrying the IgE are cross-linked, triggering biochemical signals from the signal-transducing chains of FcεRI. The signals lead to three types of responses in the mast cell: rapid release of granule contents (degranulation), synthesis and secretion of lipid mediators, and synthesis and secretion of cytokines.

The most important mediators produced by mast cells are vasoactive amines and proteases that are released from granules, products of arachidonic acid metabolism, and cytokines (Fig. 11-4). These mediators have different actions. The major amine, histamine, causes the dilation of small blood vessels, increases vascular permeability, and stimulates the transient contraction of smooth muscles. Proteases may cause damage to local tissues. Arachidonic acid metabolites include prostaglandins, which cause vascular dilation, and leukotrienes, which stimulate prolonged smooth muscle contraction. Cytokines induce local inflammation (the late phase reaction, described next). Thus, mast cell mediators are responsible for acute vascular and smooth muscle reactions and inflammation, the hallmarks of immediate hypersensitivity.

IgE-coated resting mast cell

Antigen-activated mast cell

Mast cell activation; degranulation

FIGURE 11-3   The activation of mast cells. Mast cells are sensitized by the binding of immunoglobulin E (IgE) to FcεRI receptors (**A**), and binding of the allergen to the IgE cross-links the Fcε receptors and activates the mast cells (**B**). Mast cell activation leads to degranulation, as seen in the light micrographs, in which the granules are stained with a red dye (**C, D**) and in the electron micrographs of a resting and an activated mast cell (**E, F**). (Courtesy of Dr. Daniel Friend, Department of Pathology, Harvard Medical School, Boston.)

Cytokines produced by mast cells stimulate the recruitment of leukocytes, which cause the late phase reaction. The principal leukocytes involved in this reaction are eosinophils, neutrophils, and T$_H$2 cells. Mast cell–derived tumor necrosis factor (TNF) and IL-4 promote neutrophil- and eosinophil-rich inflammation. Chemokines produced by mast cells and by epithelial cells in the tissues also contribute to leukocyte recruitment. Eosinophils and neutrophils liberate proteases, which cause tissue damage, and

T$_H$2 cells may exacerbate the reaction by producing more cytokines. Eosinophils are prominent components of many allergic reactions and are an important cause of tissue injury in these reactions. These cells are activated by the cytokine IL-5, which is produced by T$_H$2 cells and mast cells. Cytokines have effects in addition to leukocyte recruitment in immediate hypersensitivity reactions. For instance, the T$_H$2 cytokine IL-13 acts on airway epithelial cells to stimulate the secretion of mucus.

FIGURE 11-4 Biochemical events in mast cell activation. Cross-linking of immunoglobulin E (IgE) on a mast cell by an allergen stimulates phosphorylation of immunoreceptor tyrosine–based activation motifs (ITAMs) in the signaling chains of the IgE Fc receptor (FcεRI), which then initiates multiple signaling pathways. These signaling pathways stimulate the release of mast cell granule contents (amines, proteases), the synthesis of arachidonic acid metabolites (prostaglandins, leukotrienes), and the synthesis of various cytokines. These mast cell mediators stimulate the various reactions of immediate hypersensitivity. TNF, tumor necrosis factor.

CLINICAL SYNDROMES AND THERAPY

Immediate hypersensitivity reactions have diverse clinical and pathologic features, all of which are attributable to mediators produced by mast cells in different amounts and in different tissues (Fig. 11-5). Some mild reactions, such as allergic rhinitis and sinusitis, which commonly are seen in hay fever, are reactions to inhaled allergens, such as the ragweed protein of pollen. Mast cells in the nasal mucosa produce histamine, and T_H2 cells produce IL-13, and these two mediators cause increased production of mucus. Late phase reactions may lead to more prolonged inflammation. In food allergies, ingested allergens trigger mast cell degranulation, and the released histamine causes increased peristalsis. Bronchial asthma is a form of respiratory allergy in which inhaled allergens (often undefined) stimulate bronchial mast cells to release mediators, including leukotrienes, which cause repeated bouts of bronchial constriction and airway obstruction. In chronic asthma, there are large numbers of eosinophils in the bronchial mucosa and excessive secretion of mucus in the airways, and the bronchial smooth muscle becomes hyperreactive to various stimuli. Some cases of asthma are not associated with IgE production, although all are caused by mast cell activation. In some affected persons, asthma may be triggered by cold or exercise; how either of these causes mast cell activation is unknown. The most severe form of immediate hypersensitivity is **anaphylaxis,** a systemic reaction characterized by edema in many tissues, including the larynx, accompanied by a fall in blood pressure. This reaction is caused by widespread mast cell degranulation in response to a systemic antigen, and it is life-threatening because of the sudden fall in blood pressure and airway obstruction.

The therapy for immediate hypersensitivity reactions is aimed at inhibiting mast cell degranulation, antagonizing the effects of mast cell mediators, and reducing inflammation (Fig. 11-6). Commonly used drugs include antihistamines for hay fever, drugs that relax bronchial smooth muscles in asthma, and epinephrine in anaphylaxis. In diseases in which inflammation is an important component of the pathology, such as asthma, corticosteroids are used to inhibit inflammation. Many patients benefit from repeated administration of small doses of allergens, called desensitization. This treatment may work by changing the T cell response away from T_H2 dominance or by inducing tolerance (anergy) in allergen-specific T cells.

Before concluding the discussion of immediate hypersensitivity, it is important to address the question of why evolution has preserved an IgE antibody– and mast cell–mediated immune response whose major effects are pathologic. There is no good answer to this puzzle. It is known that IgE antibody and eosinophils are important mechanisms of defense against helminthic infections, and mast cells play a role in innate immunity against some bacteria. But it is not understood why common environmental antigens elicit reactions of T_H2 cells and mast cells that are capable of causing considerable damage.

Clinical syndrome	Clinical and pathologic manifestations
Allergic rhinitis, sinusitis (hay fever)	Increased mucus secretion; inflammation of upper airways, sinuses
Food allergies	Increased peristalsis due to contraction of intestinal muscles
Bronchial asthma	Bronchial hyperresponsiveness caused by smooth muscle contraction; inflammation and tissue injury caused by late phase reaction
Anaphylaxis (may be caused by drugs, bee sting, food)	Fall in blood pressure (shock) caused by vascular dilation; airway obstruction due to laryngeal edema

FIGURE 11-5 Clinical manifestations of immediate hypersensitivity reactions. The manifestations of some common immediate hypersensitivity reactions are listed. Immediate hypersensitivity may be manifested in many other ways, as in development of skin lesions such as urticaria and eczema.

Syndrome	Therapy	Mechanism of action
Anaphylaxis	Epinephrine	Causes vascular smooth muscle contraction; increases cardiac output (to counter shock); inhibits further mast cell degranulation
Bronchial asthma	Corticosteroids	Reduce inflammation
	Phosphodiesterase inhibitors	Relax bronchial smooth muscles
Various allergic diseases	"Desensitization" (repeated administration of low doses of allergens)	Unknown; may inhibit IgE production and increase production of other Ig isotypes; may induce T cell tolerance.
	Anti-IgE antibody (in clinical trials)	Neutralizes and eliminates IgE
	Antihistamines	Block actions of histamine on vessels and smooth muscles
	Cromolyn	Inhibits mast cell degranulation

FIGURE 11-6 **Treatment of immediate hypersensitivity reactions.** Various drugs are used to treat immediate hypersensitivity reactions. The principal mechanisms of action of these drugs are summarized. Ig, immunoglobulin.

Diseases Caused by Antibodies and Antigen-Antibody Complexes

Antibodies, other than IgE, may cause disease by binding to their target antigens in cells and tissues or by forming immune complexes that deposit in blood vessels (Fig. 11-7). Antibody-mediated hypersensitivity reactions were recognized many years ago and are common to many chronic immunologic diseases in humans. Antibodies against cells or extracellular matrix components may deposit in any tissue that expresses the relevant target antigen. Diseases caused by such antibodies usually are specific for a particular tissue. Immune complexes tend to deposit in blood vessels at sites of turbulence (branches of vessels) or high pressure (kidney glomeruli and synovium). Therefore, immune complex diseases tend to be systemic and often manifest as widespread vasculitis, arthritis, and nephritis.

ETIOLOGY OF ANTIBODY-MEDIATED DISEASES

The antibodies that cause disease most often are autoantibodies against self antigens and less commonly are specific for foreign (e.g., microbial) antigens. The production of autoantibodies results from a failure of self-tolerance. In Chapter 9 we discussed the mechanisms by which self-tolerance may fail, but, as has been pointed out, it is still not understood why this happens in any human autoimmune disease. Autoantibodies may bind to self antigens in tissues, or they may form immune complexes with circulating self antigens.

There are several examples of diseases caused by antibodies that are produced against microbial antigens. Two of the best described are rare, late sequelae of streptococcal infections. After such infections, some individuals produce antistreptococcal antibodies that cross-react with an antigen in heart muscle. Deposition of these antibodies in the heart triggers an inflammatory disease called rheumatic fever. Other individuals make antistreptococcal antibodies that deposit in kidney glomeruli, causing poststreptococcal glomerulonephritis. Some immune complex diseases are caused by the formation of complexes of antibodies against microbial antigens with the antigens. This may occur in patients with chronic infections with certain viruses (e.g., Epstein-Barr virus) or parasites (malaria).

FIGURE 11-7 Types of antibody-mediated diseases. Antibodies (other than immunoglobulin E [IgE]) may cause tissue injury and disease by binding directly to their target antigens in cells and extracellular matrix (**A**, type II hypersensitivity) or by forming immune complexes that deposit mainly in blood vessels (**B**, type III hypersensitivity).

MECHANISMS OF TISSUE INJURY AND DISEASE

Antibodies specific for cell and tissue antigens may deposit in tissues and cause injury by inducing local inflammation, or they may interfere with normal cellular functions (Fig. 11-8). Antibodies against tissue antigens and immune complexes deposited in vessels induce inflammation by attracting and activating leukocytes. IgG antibodies of the IgG1 and IgG3 subclasses bind to neutrophil and macrophage Fc receptors and activate these leukocytes, resulting in inflammation. The same antibodies, as well as IgM, activate the complement system by the classical pathway, resulting in the production of complement byproducts that recruit leukocytes and induce inflammation. When leukocytes are activated at sites of antibody deposition, these cells release substances such as reactive oxygen species and lysosomal enzymes that damage the adjacent tissues. If antibodies bind to cells, such as erythrocytes and platelets, the cells are opsonized and may be ingested and destroyed by host phagocytes. Some antibodies may cause disease without directly inducing tissue injury. For instance, antibodies against hormone receptors may inhibit receptor function; in some cases of myasthenia gravis, antibodies against the acetylcholine receptor inhibit

FIGURE 11-8 Effector mechanisms of antibody-mediated diseases. Antibodies may cause disease by inducing inflammation at the site of deposition (**A**), by opsonizing cells for phagocytosis (**B**), and by interfering with normal cellular functions, such as hormone receptor signaling (**C**). All three mechanisms are seen with antibodies that bind directly to their target antigens, but immune complexes cause disease mainly by inducing inflammation (**A**). TSH, thyroid-stimulating hormone.

neuromuscular transmission, causing paralysis. Other antibodies may directly activate receptors, mimicking their physiologic ligands; in a form of hyperthyroidism called Graves' disease, antibodies against the receptor for thyroid-stimulating hormone stimulate thyroid cells even in the absence of the hormone.

CLINICAL SYNDROMES AND THERAPY

Many chronic hypersensitivity disorders in humans are known to be caused by, or are associated with, anti-tissue antibodies (Fig. 11-9) and immune complexes (Fig. 11-10). Two experimental models of

Antibody-mediated disease	Target antigen	Mechanisms of disease	Clinicopathologic manifestations
Autoimmune hemolytic anemia	Erythrocyte membrane proteins (Rh blood group antigens, I antigen)	Opsonization and phagocytosis of erythrocytes	Hemolysis, anemia
Autoimmune (idiopathic) thrombocytopenic purpura	Platelet membrane proteins (gpIIb/IIIa integrin)	Opsonization and phagocytosis of platelets	Bleeding
Pemphigus vulgaris	Proteins in intercellular junctions of epidermal cells (epidermal cadherin)	Antibody-mediated activation of proteases, disruption of intercellular adhesions	Skin vesicles (bullae)
Goodpasture's syndrome	Noncollagenous protein in basement membranes of kidney glomeruli and lung alveoli	Complement and Fc receptor–mediated inflammation	Nephritis, lung hemorrhages
Acute rheumatic fever	Streptococcal cell wall antigen; antibody cross-reacts with myocardial antigen	Inflammation, macrophage activation	Myocarditis, arthritis
Myasthenia gravis	Acetylcholine receptor	Antibody inhibits acetycholine binding, down-modulates receptors	Muscle weakness, paralysis
Graves' disease (hyperthyroidism)	Thyroid-stimulating hormone (TSH) receptor	Antibody-mediated stimulation of TSH receptors	Hyperthyroidism
Pernicious anemia	Intrinsic factor of gastric parietal cells	Neutralization of intrinsic factor, decreased absorption of vitamin B_{12}	Abnormal erythropoiesis, anemia

FIGURE 11-9   Human antibody-mediated diseases. Examples of human diseases that are caused by antibodies are listed. In most of these diseases, the role of antibodies is inferred from the detection of antibodies in the blood or the lesions, and in some cases by similarities with experimental models in which the involvement of antibodies can be formally established by transfer studies.

Immune complex disease	Antibody specificity	Clinicopathologic manifestations
Systemic lupus erythematosus	DNA, nucleoproteins, others	Nephritis, arthritis, vasculitis
Polyarteritis nodosa	Hepatitis B virus surface antigen	Vasculitis
Poststreptococcal glomerulonephritis	Streptococcal cell wall antigen(s)	Nephritis
Serum sickness (clinical and experimental)	Various protein antigens	Systemic vasculitis, nephritis, arthritis
Arthus reaction (experimental)	Various protein antigens	Cutaneous vasculitis

FIGURE 11-10 Immune complex diseases. Examples of human diseases that are caused by the deposition of immune complexes, and two experimental models, are listed. In these diseases, immune complexes are detected in the blood or in the tissues that are the sites of injury. In all of the disorders, injury is caused by complement- and Fc receptor–mediated inflammation.

immune complex diseases have provided valuable information about pathogenic mechanisms. **Serum sickness** is induced by systemic administration of a protein antigen, which elicits an antibody response and leads to the formation of circulating immune complexes. (Human serum sickness can occur after a person receives injections of serum from other individuals or animals, which sometimes is used for the treatment of snakebite or exposure to rabies virus.) The **Arthus reaction** is induced by subcutaneous administration of a protein antigen to a previously immunized animal; it results in the formation of immune complexes at the site of antigen injection, and a local vasculitis.

Therapy for these diseases is intended mainly to limit inflammation and its injurious consequences, with drugs such as corticosteroids. In severe cases, plasmapheresis is used to reduce levels of circulating antibodies or immune complexes. Treatment of patients with an antibody specific for CD20, a surface protein of mature B cells, results in depletion of the B cells, and is useful for treating antibody and immune complex–mediated diseases. There is great interest in trying novel approaches for inhibiting the production of autoantibodies (e.g., by treating patients with antagonists that block CD40 ligand and thus inhibit helper T cell–dependent B cell activation). There is also great interest in inducing tolerance in cases in which the

autoantigens are known. These newer therapies are at the stage of preclinical testing and early clinical trials.

Diseases Caused by T Lymphocytes

The role of T lymphocytes in human immunological diseases has been increasingly recognized as methods for identifying and isolating these cells from lesions have improved and animal models of human diseases have been developed in which a pathogenic role of T cells can be established by experiments. In fact, much of the recent interest in the pathogenesis and treatment of human autoimmune diseases is focused on disorders in which tissue injury is caused mainly by T lymphocytes.

ETIOLOGY OF T CELL–MEDIATED DISEASES

T cell–mediated hypersensitivity reactions are caused by autoimmunity and by responses to environmental antigens. The autoimmune reactions usually are directed against cellular antigens with restricted tissue distribution. Therefore, T cell–mediated autoimmune diseases tend to be limited to a few organs and usually are not systemic. Contact sensitivity to chemicals (e.g., those found in poison ivy) is a T cell-mediated reaction. Tissue injury also may accompany T cell responses to microbes. For instance, in tuberculosis, a T cell–mediated immune response is raised against *Mycobacterium tuberculosis*, and the response becomes chronic because the infection is difficult to eradicate. The resultant granulomatous inflammation causes injury to normal tissues at the site of infection. In hepatitis virus infection, the virus itself may not be highly cytopathic, but the cytotoxic T lymphocyte (CTL) response to infected hepatocytes may cause liver injury.

Excessive polyclonal T cell activation by certain microbial toxins produced by some bacteria and viruses can lead to production of large amounts of inflammatory cytokines, causing a syndrome similar to septic shock. These toxins are called **superantigens** because they stimulate large numbers of T cells. Superantigens bind to invariant parts of T cell receptors on many different clones of T cells, regardless of antigen specificity, thereby activating these cells.

MECHANISMS OF TISSUE INJURY

In different T cell–mediated diseases, tissue injury is caused by a delayed-type hypersensitivity reaction mediated by CD4+ T cells or by killing of host cells by CD8+ CTLs (Fig. 11-11). The mechanisms of tissue injury are the same as the mechanisms used by T cells to eliminate cell-associated microbes. CD4+ T cells may react against cell or tissue antigens and secrete cytokines that induce local inflammation and activate macrophages. Different diseases may be associated with activation of T_H1 and T_H17 cells. T_H1 cells are the source of IFN-γ, the principal macrophage-activating cytokine, and T_H17 cells are thought to be responsible for recruitment of leukocytes, including neutrophils. The actual tissue injury in these

FIGURE 11-11 Mechanisms of T cell–mediated tissue injury. T cells may cause tissue injury and disease by two mechanisms: (1) delayed-type hypersensitivity reactions (**A**), which may be triggered by CD4+ and CD8+ T cells and in which tissue injury is caused by activated macrophages and inflammatory cells, and (2) direct killing of target cells (**B**), which is mediated by CD8+ CTLs. APC, antigen-presenting cell; CTLs, cytotoxic T lymphocytes.

Disease	Specificity of pathogenic T cells	Genetic associations	Clinicopathologic manifestations
Type 1 (insulin-dependent) diabetes mellitus	Pancreatic islet antigens	Insulin, PTPN22	Impaired glucose metabolism, vascular disease
Rheumatoid arthritis	Unknown antigens in joint	PTPN22	Inflammation of synovium and erosion of cartilage and bone in joints
Multiple sclerosis	Myelin proteins	CD25	Demyelination of neurons in the central nervous system, sensory and motor dysfunction
Inflammatory bowel disease	Unknown, ? role of intestinal microbes	NOD2	Inflammation of the bowel wall; adbominal pain, diarrhea, hemorrhage
Contact sensitivity (e.g. poison ivy reaction)	Modified skin proteins		DTH reaction in skin, rash
Chronic infections (e.g. tuberculosis)	Microbial proteins		Chronic (e.g. granulomatous) inflammation
Viral hepatitis (HBV, HCV)	Virally encoded proteins (e.g. EBNA)		CTL-mediated hepatocyte death, liver dysfunction; fibrosis
Superantigen mediated diseases (toxic shock syndrome)	Polyclonal (microbial superantigens activate many T cells of different specificities)		Fever, shock related to systemic inflammatory cytokine release

Abbreviations: DTH, delayed-type hypersensitivity; NOD2, nucleotide-binding oligomerization domain containing 2; PTPN22, protein tyrosine phosphatase N22

FIGURE 11-12 **T cell–mediated diseases.** Listed here are diseases in which T cells play a dominant role in causing tissue injury; antibodies and immune complexes may also contribute. Note that type 1 diabetes, rheumatoid arthritis, and multiple sclerosis are autoimmune disorders; inflammatory bowel disease has components of autoimmunity and reactions against microbes in the intestine; and the other diseases listed are caused by reactions against foreign (microbial or environmental) antigens. In most of these diseases, the role of T cells is inferred from the detection and isolation of T cells reactive with various antigens from the blood or lesions, and from the similarity with experimental models in which the involvement of T cells has been established by transfer studies. The specificity of pathogenic T cells has been defined in animal models and in some of the lesions in humans. The genetic associations in the autoimmune diseases listed are based on a variety of linkage studies; we referred to some of these associations in Chapter 9, when we discussed the genetic basis of autoimmunity. CTL, cytotoxic T lymphocyte; DTH, delayed-type hypersensitivity; EBNA, Epstein-Barr (virus) nuclear antigen; HBV, HCV, hepatitis B virus, hepatitis C virus; IL-2, interleukin-2; NOD-2, nucleotide-binding oligomerization domain–containing protein-2; PTPN22, protein tyrosine phosphatase N22.

diseases is caused by the macrophages and neutrophils. CD8$^+$ T cells specific for antigens on host cells may directly kill these cells. In many T cell–mediated autoimmune diseases, both CD4$^+$ T cells and CD8$^+$ T cells specific for self antigens are present, and both contribute to tissue injury.

CLINICAL SYNDROMES AND THERAPY

Many organ-specific autoimmune diseases in humans are believed to be caused by T cells, based on the identification of these cells in lesions and similarities with animal models in which the diseases are known to be T cell mediated (Fig. 11-12). These disorders typically are chronic and progressive, in part because T cell–macrophage interactions tend to amplify the reaction. Also, tissue injury with release and alteration of self proteins may result in reactions against these proteins, a phenomenon that has been called "epitope spreading" to indicate that the initial immune response against one or a few self antigen epitopes may expand to include responses against many more self antigens. Chronic inflammatory diseases that are initiated by immune reactions are called **immune-mediated inflammatory diseases.**

The therapy for T cell–mediated hypersensitivity disorders is designed to reduce inflammation, using corticosteroids and antagonists against cytokines such as TNF, and to inhibit T cell responses with immunosuppressive drugs such as cyclosporine. Antagonists of TNF have proved to be beneficial in patients with rheumatoid arthritis and inflammatory bowel disease. Many newer agents are being developed to inhibit T cell responses. These include agents that block costimulators such as B7 and antagonists against receptors for cytokines such as IL-2. There also is great hope for inducing tolerance in pathogenic T cells, but no successful clinical trials have been reported yet.

SUMMARY

■ Immune responses that cause tissue injury are called hypersensitivity reactions, and the diseases caused by these reactions are called hypersensitivity diseases or immune-mediated inflammatory diseases.

■ Hypersensitivity reactions may arise from uncontrolled or abnormal responses to foreign antigens or autoimmune responses against self antigens.

■ Hypersensitivity reactions are classified according to the mechanism of tissue injury.

■ Immediate hypersensitivity (type I, commonly called allergy) is caused by the production of IgE antibody against environmental antigens or drugs (allergens), sensitization of mast cells by the IgE, and degranulation of these mast cells on subsequent encounter with the allergen.

■ The clinical and pathologic manifestations of immediate hypersensitivity are due to the actions of mediators secreted by the mast cells. These include amines, which dilate vessels and contract smooth muscles; arachidonic acid metabolites, which also contract muscles; and cytokines, which induce inflammation, the hallmark of the late phase reaction. Treatment of allergies is designed to inhibit the production of and antagonize the actions of mediators and to counteract their effects on end organs.

■ Antibodies against cell and tissue antigens may cause tissue injury and disease (type II hypersensitivity). IgM and IgG antibodies promote the phagocytosis of cells to which they bind, induce inflammation by complement- and Fc receptor–mediated leukocyte recruitment, and may interfere with the functions of cells by binding to essential molecules and receptors.

■ Antibodies may bind to circulating antigens to form immune complexes, which deposit in vessels and cause tissue injury (type III hypersensitivity). Injury is due mainly to leukocyte recruitment and inflammation.

■ T cell–mediated diseases (type IV hypersensitivity) are caused by T_H1-mediated delayed-type hypersensitivity reactions or T_H17-mediated inflammatory reactions, or by killing of host cells by CD8$^+$ CTLs.

REVIEW QUESTIONS

1 *What types of antigens may induce immune responses that cause hypersensitivity reactions?*

2 *What is the sequence of events in a typical immediate hypersensitivity reaction? What is the late phase reaction, and what is it caused by?*

3 *What are some examples of immediate hypersensitivity disorders, what is their pathogenesis, and how are they treated?*

4 *How do antibodies cause tissue injury and disease? What are some of the differences in the manifestations of diseases caused by antibodies against extracellular matrix proteins and by immune complexes that deposit in tissues?*

5 *What are some examples of diseases caused by IgG or IgM antibodies or immune complexes, what is their pathogenesis, and what are their principal clinical and pathologic manifestations?*

6 *What are some examples of diseases caused by T cells, what is their pathogenesis, and what are their principal clinical and pathologic manifestations?*

Chapter 12

CONGENITAL AND ACQUIRED IMMUNODEFICIENCIES

Diseases Caused by Defective Immune Responses

Defects in the development and functions of the immune system result in increased susceptibility to infections; reactivation of latent infections (such as cytomegalovirus, Epstein-Barr virus, and tuberculosis) in which the normal immune response keeps the infection in check but does not eradicate it; and increased incidence of certain cancers. These consequences of defective immunity are predictable because, as emphasized throughout this book, the normal function of the immune system is to defend individuals against infections and some cancers. Disorders caused by defective immunity are called **immunodeficiency diseases.** Some of these diseases may result from genetic abnormalities in one or more components of the immune system; these are called **congenital** (or **primary**) **immunodeficiencies.** Other defects in the immune system may result from infections, nutritional abnormalities, or medical treatments that cause loss or inadequate function of various components of the immune system; these are called **acquired** (or **secondary**) **immunodeficiencies.** In this chapter we describe the causes and pathogenesis of congenital and acquired immunodeficiencies. Among the acquired diseases, we emphasize the acquired immunodeficiency syndrome (AIDS), the disease that results from infection by the human immunodeficiency virus (HIV) and is one of the most devastating health problems worldwide. We will address the following questions:

- What are the mechanisms of immune compromise in the common immunodeficiency diseases?

(Information about the clinical features of these disorders may be found in textbooks of pediatrics and medicine.)

- How does HIV cause the clinical and pathologic abnormalities of AIDS?
- What approaches are being used to treat immunodeficiency diseases?

Congenital (Primary) Immunodeficiencies

Congenital immunodeficiencies are caused by genetic defects that lead to blocks in the maturation or functions of different components of the immune system. It is estimated that as many as 1 in 500 individuals in the United States and Europe suffer from congenital immune deficiencies of varying severity. Congenital immunodeficiencies share several features, the most common being infectious complications (Fig. 12-1). Different congenital immunodeficiency diseases, however, may differ considerably in clinical and pathologic manifestations. Some of these disorders result in greatly increased susceptibility to infections that may be manifested early after birth and may

be fatal unless the immunologic defects are corrected. Other congenital immunodeficiencies lead to mild infections and may be detected in adult life. In the following discussion, the pathogenesis of selected immunodeficiencies is summarized, several of which were mentioned in earlier chapters to illustrate the physiologic importance of various components of the immune system. Congenital deficiencies in molecules involved in self tolerance are manifested as autoimmune disease, as discussed in Chapter 11.

DEFECTS IN LYMPHOCYTE MATURATION

Many congenital immunodeficiencies are the result of genetic abnormalities that cause blocks in the maturation of B lymphocytes, T lymphocytes, or both (Figs. 12-2 and 12-3). Disorders manifesting as defects in both the B cell and T cell arms of the adaptive immune system are classified as **severe combined immunodeficiency (SCID).**

Several different genetic abnormalities cause severe combined immunodeficiencies. About half of these cases are X-linked, affecting only male children. About 50% of the cases of **X-linked SCID** are caused by mutations in a signaling subunit of a receptor for

Type of immunodeficiency	Histopathologic and laboratory abnormalities	Common infectious consequences
B cell deficiencies	Absent or reduced follicles and germinal centers in lymphoid organs Reduced serum Ig levels	Pyogenic bacterial infections
T cell deficiencies	May be reduced T cell zones in lymphoid organs Reduced DTH reactions to common antigens Defective T cell proliferative responses to mitogens *in vitro*	Viral and other intracellular microbial infections (e.g., *Pneumocystis jiroveci*, atypical mycobacteria, fungi) Virus-associated malignancies (e.g., EBV-associated lymphomas)
Innate immune deficiencies	Variable, depending on which component of innate immunity is defective	Variable; pyogenic bacterial infections

FIGURE 12-1 Features of immunodeficiency diseases. The important diagnostic features and clinical manifestations of immune deficiencies affecting different components of the immune system are summarized. Within each group, different diseases, and even different patients with the same disease, may show considerable variation. Reduced numbers of circulating B or T cells often are detected in some of these diseases. DTH, delayed-type hypersensitivity; EBV, Epstein-Barr virus; Ig, immunoglobulin.

FIGURE 12-2 Congenital immunodeficiencies caused by defects in lymphocyte maturation. Immunodeficiencies caused by genetic defects in lymphocyte maturation are shown. Lymphocyte maturation pathways are described in more detail in Chapter 4. ADA, adenosine deaminase; PNP, purine nucleoside phosphorylase; RAG, recombination-activating gene; SCID, severe combined immunodeficiency.

cytokines. This subunit is called the common γ chain (γc), because it is a component of the receptors for numerous cytokines, including interleukin (IL)-2, IL-4, IL-7, IL-9, and IL-15. (Because the γc chain was first identified as one of the three chains of the IL-2 receptor, it often is called the IL-2Rγ chain.) When the γc chain is not functional, immature lymphocytes, especially pro-T cells, cannot proliferate in response to the major growth factor for these cells, namely, IL-7. Defective responses to IL-7 result in reduced survival and maturation of lymphocyte precursors. In humans, the defect affects mainly T cell maturation (whereas in mice, B cells also are greatly reduced). The consequence of this block is a profound decrease in the numbers of mature T cells, deficient cell-mediated

immunity, and defective humoral immunity because of absent T cell help (even though B cells may mature almost normally). Natural killer (NK) cells also are deficient, because the receptor for IL-15, the major cytokine involved in NK cell proliferation and maturation, also uses the γc chain.

About half of the cases of **autosomal SCID** are caused by mutations in an enzyme called adenosine deaminase (ADA), which is involved in the breakdown of purines. Deficiency of ADA leads to the accumulation of toxic purine metabolites in cells that are actively synthesizing DNA, namely, proliferating cells. Lymphocytes, which actively proliferate during their maturation, are injured by these accumulating toxic metabolites. ADA deficiency results in a block in T cell

Severe combined immunodeficiency (SCID)

Disease	Functional deficiencies	Mechanism of defect
X-linked SCID	Markedly decreased T cells; normal or increased B cells; reduced serum Ig	Cytokine receptor common γ chain gene mutations, defective T cell maturation due to lack of IL-7 signals
Autosomal recessive SCID due to ADA, PNP deficiency	Progressive decrease in T and B cells (mostly T); reduced serum Ig in ADA deficiency, normal B cells and serum Ig in PNP deficiency	ADA or PNP deficiency leads to accumulation of toxic metabolites in lymphocytes
Autosomal recessive SCID due to other causes	Decreased T and B cells; reduced serum Ig	Defective maturation of T and B cells; genetic basis unknown in most cases; may be mutations in *RAG* genes

B cell immunodeficiencies

Disease	Functional deficiencies	Mechanism of defect
X-linked agammaglobulinemia	Decrease in all serum Ig isotypes; reduced B cell numbers	Block in maturation beyond pre-B cells, because of mutation in B cell tyrosine kinase
Ig heavy chain deletions	IgG1, IgG2, or IgG4 absent; sometimes associated with absent IgA or IgE	Chromosomal deletion at 14q32 (Ig heavy chain locus)

T cell immunodeficiencies

Disease	Functional deficiencies	Mechanism of defect
DiGeorge syndrome	Decreased T cells; normal B cells; normal or decreased serum Ig	Anomalous development of 3rd and 4th branchial pouches, leading to thymic hypoplasia

FIGURE 12-3   **Features of congenital immunodeficiencies caused by defects in lymphocyte maturation.** The most common congenital immunodeficiencies in which the genetic blocks are known, and their principal features, are summarized. ADA, adenosine deaminase; Ig, immunoglobulin; IL-7, interleukin-7; PNP, purine nucleoside phosphorylase; RAG, recombination-activating gene; SCID, severe combined immunodeficiency.

maturation more than in B cell maturation; defective humoral immunity is largely a consequence of the lack of T cell helper function. Another important cause of autosomal SCID is mutations in a kinase that is involved in signaling by the γc cytokine receptor chain. Such mutations result in the same abnormalities as in X-linked SCID due to γc mutations, described previously. Rare cases of autosomal SCID are caused by mutations in the *RAG1* or *RAG2* gene, which encode the lymphocyte specific components of the VDJ recombinase, which is required for immunoglobulin (Ig) and T cell receptor gene recombinations and lymphocyte maturation (see Chapter 4). The cause of about 50% of both X-linked and autosomal cases of SCID is not known.

The most common clinical syndrome caused by a block in B cell maturation is **X-linked agammaglobulinemia** (first described as "Bruton's agammaglobulinemia"). In this disorder, B cells in the bone marrow fail to mature beyond the pre-B cell stage, resulting in a marked decrease or absence of mature B lymphocytes and serum immunoglobulins. The disease is caused by mutations in the gene encoding a kinase called the B cell tyrosine kinase or Bruton tyrosine kinase (Btk), resulting in defective production or function of the enzyme. The enzyme is activated by the pre-B cell receptor expressed in pre-B cells, and it delivers biochemical signals that promote maturation of these cells. The gene for this enzyme is located on the X chromosome. Therefore, women who carry a mutant allele of the *BTK* gene on one of their X chromosomes are carriers of the disease, and male offspring who inherit the abnormal X chromosome are affected. Paradoxically, in about a fourth of patients with X-linked agammaglobulinemia, autoimmune diseases, notably arthritis, develop as well. Why an immune deficiency affecting B cells should lead to a reaction typical of excessive or uncontrolled immune responses is not known.

Selective defects in T cell maturation are quite rare. The most frequent of these is the **DiGeorge syndrome,** which results from incomplete development of the thymus (and the parathyroid glands) and a failure of T cell maturation. Patients with this disease tend to improve with age, probably because the small amount of thymic tissue that does develop is able to support some T cell maturation.

Treatment of primary immunodeficiencies that affect lymphocyte maturation varies with the disease. SCID is fatal in early life unless the patient's immune system is reconstituted. The most widely used treatment is bone marrow transplantation, with careful matching of donor and recipient to avoid potentially serious graft-versus-host disease. For selective B cell defects, patients may be given pooled immunoglobulin from healthy donors to provide passive immunity. Ig replacement therapy has provided enormous benefit in patients with X-linked agammaglobulinemia. The

ideal treatment for all congenital immunodeficiencies is replacement gene therapy. This treatment, however, remains a distant goal for most diseases. The most impressive results of successful gene therapy have been reported in patients with X-linked SCID whose own bone marrow cells into which a normal γc gene was introduced were used for reconstitutive therapy. In some of these patients, however, T cell leukemia has subsequently developed, apparently because the introduced gene was inserted near an oncogene and activated this oncogene. In all patients with these diseases, infections are treated with antibiotics as needed.

DEFECTS IN LYMPHOCYTE ACTIVATION AND FUNCTION

As understanding of the molecules involved in lymphocyte activation and function has improved, mutations and other abnormalities in these molecules that result in immunodeficiency disorders also have begun to be recognized. Many such disorders are now known (Fig. 12-4). The following discussion describes some of the diseases in which lymphocytes mature normally but the activation and effector functions of the cells are defective.

The **X-linked hyper-IgM syndrome** is characterized by defective B cell heavy chain isotype (class) switching, so that IgM is the major serum antibody, and by severe deficiency of cell-mediated immunity against intracellular microbes. The disease is caused by mutations in CD40 ligand (CD40L), the helper T cell protein that binds to CD40 on B cells and macrophages and thus mediates T cell–dependent activation of B cells and macrophages. Failure to express functional CD40L leads to defective T cell–dependent B cell responses, such as isotype switching in humoral immunity, and to defective T cell–dependent macrophage activation in cell-mediated immunity.

Genetic deficiencies in the production of selected Ig isotypes are quite common. IgA deficiency is believed to affect as many as 1 in 700 people, but in most of these persons it causes no clinical problems. The defect causing these deficiencies is not known in a majority of cases; rarely, the deficiencies may be caused by mutations of Ig heavy chain constant region genes. **Common variable immunodeficiency** is a

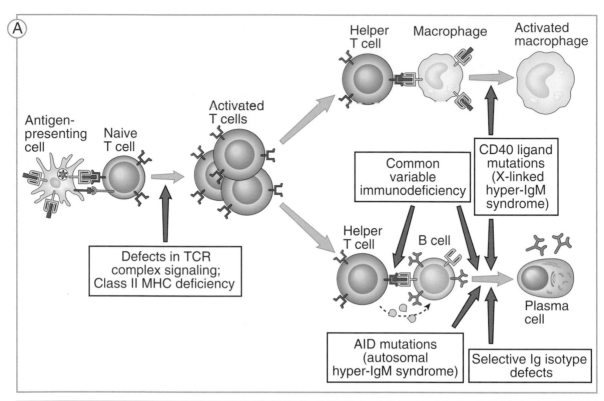

B) Disease	Functional Deficiencies	Mechanisms of Defect
X-linked hyper-IgM syndrome	Defects in helper T cell-dependent B cell and macrophage activation	Mutations in CD40 ligand
Common variable immunodeficiency	Reduced or no production of selective isotypes or subtypes of immunoglobulins; susceptibility to bacterial infections or no clinical problems	Mutations in receptor for B cell growth factors, costimulators
Defective class II MHC expression: The bare lymphocyte syndrome	Lack of class II MHC expression and impaired CD4+ T cell activation; defective cell-mediated immunity and T cell-dependent humoral immunity	Mutations in genes encoding transcription factors required for class II MHC gene expression
Defects in T cell receptor complex expression or signaling	Decreased T cells or abnormal ratios of CD4+ and CD8+ subsets; decreased cell-mediated immunity	Rare cases due to mutations or deletions in genes encoding CD3 proteins, ZAP-70

FIGURE 12-4 Congenital immunodeficiencies associated with defects in lymphocyte activation and effector functions. Congenital immunodeficiencies may be caused by genetic defects in the expression of molecules required for antigen presentation to T cells, T or B lymphocyte antigen receptor signaling, helper T cell activation of B cells and macrophages, and differentiation of antibody-producing B cells. Examples showing the sites at which immune responses may be blocked are illustrated in **A,** and the features of some of these disorders are summarized in **B.** AID, activation-induced deaminase; Ig, immunoglobulin; MHC, major histocompatibility complex; TCR, T cell receptor; ZAP-70, zeta chain–associated protein of 70 Kd.

heterogeneous group of disorders that represent a common form of primary immunodeficiency. These disorders are characterized by poor antibody responses to infections and reduced serum levels of IgG, IgA, and often IgM. The underlying causes of common variable disease are poorly understood but include defects in B cell maturation and activation. Some patients have mutations in genes encoding receptors for B cell growth factors or costimulators involved in T cell–B cell interactions. Patients suffer from recurrent infections, autoimmune disease, and lymphomas.

Defective activation of T lymphocytes may result from deficient expression of major histocompatibility complex (MHC) molecules. The **bare lymphocyte syndrome** is a disease caused by a failure to express class II MHC molecules, as a result of mutations in the transcription factors that normally induce class II MHC expression. Recall that class II MHC molecules display peptide antigens for recognition by CD4+ T cells and that this recognition is critical for maturation and activation of the T cells. The disease is manifested by a profound decrease in CD4+ T cells, because of defective maturation of these cells in the thymus and defective activation in peripheral lymphoid organs. Occasional patients have been described in whom immunodeficiency is caused by mutations in T cell signal–transducing molecules, cytokines, and various receptors. Because T cell activation defects result in impaired cell-mediated immunity and T-dependent antibody responses, these disorders are often clinically characterized as forms of SCID.

DEFECTS IN INNATE IMMUNITY

Abnormalities in two components of innate immunity, phagocytes and the complement system, are important causes of immunodeficiency (Fig. 12-5). **Chronic granulomatous disease** is caused by mutations in the enzyme phagocyte oxidase, which catalyzes the production of microbicidal reactive oxygen species in lysosomes (see Chapter 2). As a result, neutrophils and macrophages that phagocytose microbes are unable to kill the microbes. The immune system tries to compensate for this defective microbial killing by calling in more and more macrophages, and by activating T cells, which stimulate recruitment and activation of even more phagocytes. Therefore, collections of phagocytes accumulate around foci of infections by intracel-

lular microbes, but the microbes cannot be destroyed effectively. These collections resemble granulomas, giving rise to the name of this disease. **Leukocyte adhesion deficiency** is caused by mutations in genes encoding integrins or in enzymes required for the expression of ligands for selectins. Integrins and selectin ligands are involved in the adhesion of leukocytes to other cells. As a result of these mutations, blood leukocytes do not bind firmly to vascular endothelium and are not recruited normally to sites of infection.

Deficiencies of almost every complement protein, and many complement regulatory proteins, have been described, and some of these were mentioned in Chapter 8. C3 deficiency results in severe infections and usually is fatal. Deficiencies of C2 and C4, two components of the classical pathway of complement activation, result not in immunodeficiency but in immune complex–mediated diseases resembling lupus. A likely explanation for this association between complement deficiencies and lupus-like disease is that the classical complement pathway is involved in eliminating immune complexes that are constantly being formed during humoral immune responses. Failure to clear these immune complexes results in their deposition in tissues—the hallmark of immune complex disease. The observation that C2 and C4 deficiencies do not make individuals susceptible to infection suggests that the alternative pathway may be adequate for host defense. Deficiencies of complement regulatory proteins lead to excessive complement activation and not to immunodeficiencies (see Chapter 8).

The **Chédiak-Higashi syndrome** is an immunodeficiency disease in which the lysosomal granules of leukocytes do not function normally. The immune defect is thought to affect phagocytes and NK cells and is manifested by increased susceptibility to bacterial infections.

Rare patients have been described with mutations affecting Toll-like receptors (TLRs) or signaling pathways downstream of TLRs, including molecules required for activation of the NF-κB (nuclear factor-κB) transcription factor.

LYMPHOCYTE ABNORMALITIES ASSOCIATED WITH OTHER DISEASES

Some systemic diseases that involve multiple organ systems, and whose major manifestations are not

Disease	Functional Deficiencies	Mechanisms of Defect
Chronic granulomatous disease	Defective production of reactive oxygen species by phagocytes	Mutations in genes encoding components of the phagocyte oxidase enzyme, most often cytochrome b558
Leukocyte adhesion deficiency-1	Absent or deficient expression of β2 integrins causing defective leukocyte adhesion–dependent functions	Mutations in gene encoding the β chain (CD18) of β2 integrins
Leukocyte adhesion deficiency-2	Absent or deficient expression of leukocyte ligands for endothelial E- and P-selectins, causing failure of leukocyte migration into tissues	Mutations in gene encoding a protein required for synthesis of the sialyl-Lewis X component of E- and P-selectin ligands
Complement C3 deficiency	Defect in complement cascade activation	Mutations in the C3 gene
Complement C2, C4 deficiency	Deficient activation of classical pathway of complement leading to failure to clear immune complexes and development of lupus-like disease	Mutations in C2 or C4 genes
Chédiak-Higashi syndrome	Defective lysosomal function in neutrophils, macrophages, and dendritic cells, and defective granule function in natural killer cells	Mutation in a gene encoding a lysosomal trafficking regulatory protein

FIGURE 12-5 **Congenital immunodeficiencies caused by defects in innate immunity.** Immunodeficiency diseases caused by defects in various components of the innate immune system are listed.

immunologic, may have a component of immunodeficiency. The **Wiskott-Aldrich syndrome** is characterized by eczema, reduced blood platelets, and immunodeficiency. It is an X-linked disease, caused by a mutation in a gene that encodes a protein that binds to various adapter molecules and cytoskeletal components in hematopoietic cells. It is believed that because of the absence of this protein, platelets and leukocytes are small, do not develop normally, and fail to migrate normally. **Ataxia-telangiectasia** is a disease characterized by gait abnormalities (ataxia), vascular malformations (telangiectasia), and immunodeficiency. The disease is caused by mutations in a gene whose product is involved in DNA repair. Defects in this protein lead to abnormal DNA repair

(e.g., during recombination of antigen receptor gene segments), resulting in defective lymphocyte maturation.

Acquired (Secondary) Immunodeficiencies

Deficiencies of the immune system often develop because of abnormalities that are not genetic but are acquired during life (Fig. 12-6). The most serious of these abnormalities worldwide is HIV infection, which is described later in the chapter. The most frequent causes of secondary immunodeficiencies in developed countries are cancers involving the bone marrow and

Cause	Mechanism
Human immunodeficiency virus infection	Depletion of CD4$^+$ helper T cells
Irradiation and chemotherapy treatments for cancer	Decreased bone marrow precursors for all leukocytes
Involvement of bone marrow by cancers (metastases, leukemias)	Reduced site of leukocyte development
Protein-calorie malnutrition	Metabolic derangements inhibit lymphocyte maturation and function
Removal of spleen	Decreased phagocytosis of microbes

FIGURE 12-6 Acquired (secondary) immunodeficiency. The most common causes of acquired immunodeficiencies, and how they lead to defects in immune responses, are listed.

various therapies. Cancer treatment with chemotherapeutic drugs and irradiation may damage proliferating cells, including bone marrow precursors and mature lymphocytes, resulting in immunodeficiency. Treatments to prevent graft rejection and inflammatory diseases, including some of the newer therapies (such as TNF antagonists and costimulation blockade) are designed to suppress immune responses. Therefore, immunodeficiency is a frequent complication of such therapies. Protein-calorie malnutrition results in deficiencies of virtually all components of the immune system and is a common cause of immunodeficiency in developing countries.

Acquired Immunodeficiency Syndrome

A remarkable and tragic fact is that although AIDS was recognized as a distinct disease entity as recently as the 1980s, it has since become one of the most devastating afflictions in the history of mankind. AIDS is caused by infection with HIV. It is estimated that there are more than 42 million HIV-infected people in the world (of which about 70% are in Africa and 20% in Asia), more than 22 million deaths attributable to this disease, and almost 3 million deaths annually. The infection continues to spread, and in some countries in Africa, more than 30% of the population has been infected with HIV. This section describes the important features of HIV, how it infects humans, and the

disease it causes. The section concludes with a brief discussion of the current status of therapy and vaccine development.

THE HUMAN IMMUNODEFICIENCY VIRUS

HIV is a retrovirus that infects cells of the immune system, mainly CD4$^+$ T lymphocytes, and causes progressive destruction of these cells. An infectious HIV particle consists of two RNA strands within a protein core, surrounded by a lipid envelope derived from infected host cells but containing viral proteins (Fig. 12-7). The viral RNA encodes structural proteins, various enzymes, and proteins that regulate transcription of viral genes and the viral life cycle.

The life cycle of HIV consists of the following sequential steps: infection of cells, production of viral DNA and its integration into the host genome, expression of viral genes, and production of viral particles (Fig. 12-8). HIV infects cells by virtue of its major envelope glycoprotein, called gp120 (for 120-kD glycoprotein), binding to CD4 and particular chemokine receptors (CXCR4 on T cells and CCR5 on macrophages) on human cells. Therefore, the virus can efficiently infect only cells expressing CD4 and these chemokine receptors. The major cell types that may be infected by HIV are CD4$^+$ T lymphocytes, macrophages, and dendritic cells. After binding to cellular receptors, the viral membrane fuses with the

FIGURE 12-7 The structure and genes of the human immunodeficiency virus (HIV). A, An HIV-1 virion is shown next to a T cell surface. HIV-1 consists of two identical strands of RNA (the viral genome) and associated enzymes, including reverse transcriptase, integrase, and protease, packaged in a cone-shaped core composed of the p24 capsid protein with a surrounding p17 protein matrix, all surrounded by a phospholipid membrane envelope derived from the host cell. Virally encoded membrane proteins (gp41 and gp120) are bound to the envelope. CD4 and chemokine receptors on the host cell surface function as the receptors for HIV-1. MHC, major histocompatibility complex. (Adapted from front cover, The New Face of AIDS. Science 272:1841-2102, 1996. © Terese Winslow.) **B,** The HIV-1 genome consists of genes whose positions are indicated here as *differently colored blocks.* Some genes contain sequences that overlap with sequences of other genes, as shown by *overlapping blocks,* but are read differently by host cell RNA polymerase. *Similarly shaded blocks* separated by lines (*tat, rev*) indicate genes whose coding sequences are separated in the genome and require RNA splicing to produce functional messenger RNA. The major functions of the proteins encoded by different viral genes are listed. (Adapted from Greene WC: AIDS and the immune system. © 1993 by Scientific American, Inc. All rights reserved.)

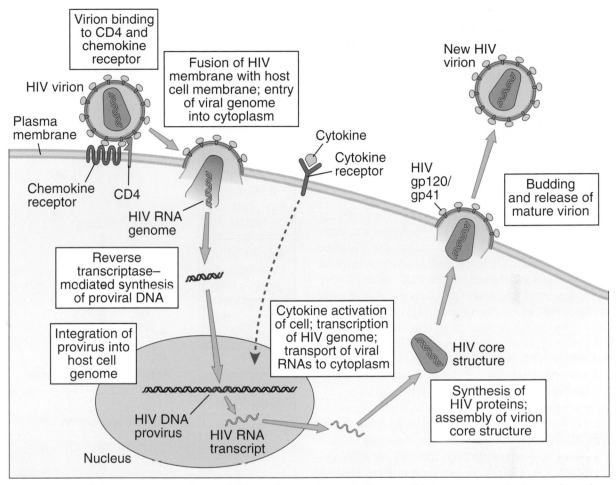

FIGURE 12-8   The life cycle of human immunodeficiency virus type 1 (HIV-1). The sequential steps in HIV reproduction are shown, from initial infection of a host cell to release of a new virus particle (virion). For the sake of clarity, the production and release of only one new virion are shown. An infected cell actually produces many virions, each capable of infecting nearby cells, leading to spread of the infection.

host cell membrane, and the virus enters the cell's cytoplasm. Here the virus is uncoated by viral protease and its RNA is released. A DNA copy of the viral RNA is synthesized by the virus's reverse transcriptase enzyme (a process that is characteristic of all retroviruses), and the DNA integrates into the host cell's DNA by the action of the integrase enzyme. The integrated viral DNA is called a provirus. If the infected T cell, macrophage, or dendritic cell is activated by some extrinsic stimulus, such as another infectious microbe, the cell responds by turning on the transcription of many of its own genes and often by producing cyto-

kines. An unfortunate consequence of this normal protective response is that the cytokines, and the process of cellular activation itself, also may activate the provirus, leading to production of viral RNAs and then proteins. The virus is now able to form a core structure, which migrates to the cell membrane, acquires a lipid envelope from the host, and is shed as an infectious viral particle, ready to infect another cell. It is possible that the integrated HIV provirus remains latent within infected cells for months or years, hidden from the patient's immune system (and even from antiviral therapies, discussed later).

Most cases of AIDS are caused by HIV-1 (i.e., HIV type 1). A related virus, HIV-2, causes some cases of the disease.

PATHOGENESIS OF AIDS

HIV establishes a latent infection in cells of the immune system and may be reactivated to produce infectious virus. This viral production leads to death of infected cells, as well as to death of uninfected lymphocytes, subsequent immune deficiencies, and clinical AIDS (Fig. 12-9). HIV infection is acquired by sexual intercourse, sharing contaminated needles used by intravenous drug users, transplacental transfer, or transfusion of infected blood or blood products. After infection there may be a brief, acute viremia, when the virus is detected in the blood, and the host may respond as in any mild viral infection. The virus infects CD4+ T cells, dendritic cells, and macrophages at sites of entry through epithelia, in lymphoid organs such as lymph nodes, and in the circulation. In mucosal tissues at the sites of entry, there may be considerable destruction of infected T cells. Because a large fraction of the body's lymphocytes, and especially of memory T cells, reside in these tissues, the result of the local destruction may be a significant functional deficit that is not reflected in the presence of infected cells in the blood or the depletion of circulating T cells. Dendritic cells may capture the virus as it enters through mucosal epithelia and transport it to peripheral lymphoid organs, where it infects T cells. Rare individuals with *CCR5* mutations that do not permit HIV entry into macrophages can remain disease-free for years after HIV infection, indicating the importance of macrophage infection in the progression toward AIDS. The integrated provirus may be activated in infected cells, as described previously, leading to production of viral particles and spread of the infection. During the course of HIV infection, the major source of infectious viral particles is activated CD4+ T cells; dendritic cells and macrophages are reservoirs of infection.

FIGURE 12-9 The pathogenesis of disease caused by human immunodeficiency virus (HIV). The stages of HIV disease correlate with a progressive spread of HIV from the initial site of infection to lymphoid tissues throughout the body. The immune response of the host temporarily controls acute infection but does not prevent establishment of chronic infection of cells in lymphoid tissues. Cytokines produced in response to HIV and other microbes serve to enhance HIV production and progression to acquired immunodeficiency syndrome (AIDS). CTLs, cytotoxic T lymphocytes.

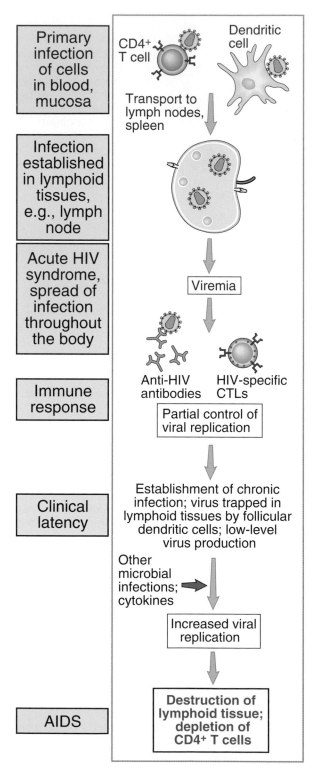

The depletion of CD4+ T cells after HIV infection is due to a cytopathic effect of the virus, resulting from production of viral particles, as well as death of uninfected cells. Active viral gene expression and protein production may interfere with the synthetic machinery of the T cells. Therefore, infected T cells in which the virus is replicating are killed during this process. The number of T cells lost during the progression to AIDS is much greater than the number of infected cells. The mechanism of this T cell loss remains poorly defined. One possibility is that T cells are chronically activated, perhaps by infections that are common in these patients, and the chronic stimulation culminates in apoptosis, by the pathway called activation-induced cell death.

Other infected cells, such as dendritic cells and macrophages, may also die, resulting in destruction of the architecture of lymphoid organs. Many studies have suggested that immune deficiency results from various functional abnormalities in T lymphocytes and other immune cells (dendritic cells and macro-phages), in addition to depletion of T cells. The significance of these functional defects has not been established, however, and loss of T cells (followed by the blood CD4+ T cell count) remains the most reliable indicator of disease progression.

CLINICAL FEATURES OF HUMAN IMMUNODEFICIENCY VIRUS INFECTION AND ACQUIRED IMMUNODEFICIENCY SYNDROME

The clinical course of HIV infection is characterized by several phases, culminating in immune deficiency (Fig. 12-10). Early after HIV infection, patients may experience a mild acute illness with fever and malaise, correlating with the initial viremia. This illness subsides within a few days, and the disease enters a period of clinical latency. During this latency, there usually is a progressive loss of CD4+ T cells in lymphoid tissues and destruction of the architecture of the lymphoid tissues. Eventually, the blood CD4+ T cell count begins to decline, and when the count falls

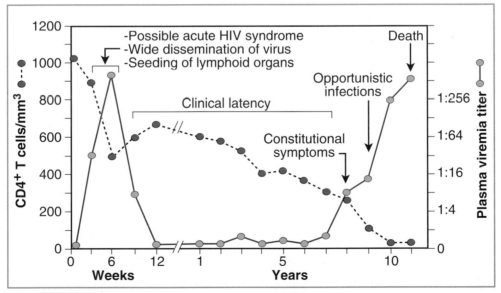

FIGURE 12-10   The clinical course of human immunodeficiency virus (HIV) disease. Blood-borne virus (plasma viremia) is detected early after infection and may be accompanied by systemic symptoms typical of acute HIV syndrome. The virus spreads to lymphoid organs, but plasma viremia falls to very low levels (detectable only by sensitive reverse transcriptase–polymerase chain reaction assays) and stays this way for many years. CD4+ T cell counts steadily decline during this clinical latency period, because of active viral replication and T cell destruction in lymphoid tissues. As the level of CD4+ T cells falls, there is increasing risk of infection and other clinical components of acquired immunodeficiency syndrome (AIDS). (Reproduced with permission from Pantaleo G, Graziosi C, Fauci A: The immunopathogenesis of human immunodeficiency virus infection. N Engl J Med 328:327-335, 1993.)

below 200 per mm³ (the normal level being about 1500 cells per mm³), patients become susceptible to infections and are said to be suffering from AIDS.

The clinical and pathologic manifestations of full-blown AIDS are primarily the result of increased susceptibility to infections and some cancers, as a consequence of immune deficiency. Patients often are infected by intracellular microbes, such as viruses, the fungal pathogen *Pneumocystis jiroveci*, and atypical mycobacteria, all of which normally are combated by T cell–mediated immunity. Many of these microbes are present in the environment, but they do not infect healthy persons with intact immune systems. Because these infections are seen in immunodeficient persons, in whom the microbes have an opportunity to establish infection, these types of infections are said to be "opportunistic." Many of the opportunistic infections are caused by viruses, such as cytomegalovirus. Patients with AIDS show defective cytotoxic T lymphocyte (CTL) responses to viruses, even though HIV does not infect CD8⁺ T cells. It is believed that the CTL responses are defective because CD4⁺ helper T cells (the main targets of HIV) are required for full CD8⁺ CTL responses against many viral antigens (see Chapters 5 and 6). Patients who have AIDS are at increased risk for infections by extracellular bacteria, probably because of impaired helper T cell–dependent antibody responses to bacterial antigens. Patients also become susceptible to cancers that are caused by oncogenic viruses. The two most common types of cancers are B cell lymphomas, caused by the Epstein-Barr virus, and a tumor of small blood vessels called Kaposi's sarcoma, caused by a herpesvirus. Patients in the advanced stages of AIDS often suffer from a wasting syndrome with a significant loss of body mass, due to altered metabolism and reduced caloric intake. The dementia that develops in some patients with AIDS is believed to be caused by infection of macrophages (microglial cells) in the brain.

The clinical course of the disease has been dramatically changed by effective antiretroviral drug therapy. With appropriate treatment, patients exhibit much slower progression of the disease, fewer opportunistic infections, and greatly reduced incidence of cancers and dementia.

The immune response to HIV is ineffective in controlling spread of the virus and its pathologic effects. Infected individuals produce antibodies and CTLs against viral antigens, and the responses help to limit the early acute HIV syndrome. But these immune responses usually do not prevent chronic progression of the disease. Antibodies against envelope glycoproteins, such as gp120, may be ineffective because the virus rapidly mutates the region of gp120 that is the target of most antibodies. CTLs often are ineffective in killing infected cells because the virus inhibits the expression of class I MHC molecules by the infected cells. Immune responses to HIV may paradoxically promote spread of the infection. Antibody-coated viral particles may bind to Fc receptors on macrophages and follicular dendritic cells in lymphoid organs, thus increasing virus entry into these cells and creating additional reservoirs of infection. If CTLs are able to kill infected cells, the dead cells may be cleared by phagocytosis, resulting in spread of the virus to macrophages. And, of course, by infecting and thereby interfering with the function of immune cells, the virus is able to prevent its own eradication.

THERAPY AND VACCINATION STRATEGIES

The current treatment for AIDS is aimed at controlling replication of HIV and the infectious complications of the disease. Cocktails of drugs that block the activity of the viral reverse transcriptase, protease, and integrase enzymes are now being administered early in the course of the infection, with considerable benefit. This therapeutic approach, called highly active antiretroviral treatment (HAART) or combination antiretroviral therapy (cART), is expensive, and its long-term efficacy is not known. The virus is capable of mutations that may render it resistant to the drugs used, and reservoirs of latent virus are not eradicated by these drugs.

The control of HIV worldwide will require the development of effective vaccines. A successful vaccine probably will have to induce an innate immune response, high titers of neutralizing antibodies, and a strong T cell response, as well as mucosal immunity. It has proven difficult to achieve all these goals with current vaccination strategies. An additional challenge is to be able to protect against all subtypes of HIV. Early efforts were focused on gp120 as an immunogen, but these were largely unsuccessful because of the high rate of mutations in gp 120. More recent attempts have involved combinations of DNA immunization and recombinant poxviruses encoding several different HIV proteins. It will take years to judge the effectiveness of new vaccines in clinical trials.

SUMMARY

■ Immunodeficiency diseases are caused by defects in various components of the immune system that result in increased susceptibility to infections and some cancers. Congenital (primary) immunodeficiency diseases are caused by genetic abnormalities, and acquired (secondary) immunodeficiencies are the result of infections, cancers, malnutrition, or treatments for other conditions that adversely affect the cells of the immune system.

■ Some congenital immunodeficiency diseases are the result of mutations that block the maturation of lymphocytes. SCID may be caused by mutations in the cytokine receptor γc chain that reduces the IL-7–driven proliferation of immature lymphocytes, by mutations in enzymes involved in purine metabolism, or by other defects in lymphocyte maturation. Selective B cell maturation defects are seen in X-linked agammaglobulinemia, caused by abnormalities in an enzyme involved in B cell maturation (Btk), and selective T cell maturation defects are seen in the DiGeorge syndrome, in which the thymus does not develop normally.

■ Some immunodeficiency diseases are caused by defects in lymphocyte activation and functions, despite their normal maturation. The X-linked hyper-IgM syndrome is caused by mutations in CD40 ligand, because of which helper T cell–dependent B cell responses (e.g., Ig heavy chain class switching) and T cell–dependent macrophage activation are defective. The bare lymphocyte syndrome is due to defective expression of class II MHC proteins, resulting in defective maturation and activation of CD4+ T cells.

■ AIDS is caused by the retrovirus HIV. HIV infects CD4+ T cells, macrophages, and dendritic cells by using an envelope protein (gp120) to bind to CD4 and chemokine receptors. The viral DNA integrates into the host genome, where it may be activated to produce infectious virus. Infected cells die during this process of virus replication, and death of cells of the immune system is the principal mechanism by which the virus causes immune deficiency.

■ The clinical course of HIV infection typically consists of an acute viremia, a period of clinical latency during which there is progressive destruction of CD4+ T cells and dissolution of lymphoid tissues, and, ultimately, AIDS, with severe immunodeficiency with opportunistic infections, some cancers, weight loss, and, occasionally, dementia. Treatment of HIV infection is designed to interfere with the life cycle of the virus. Many attempts at vaccine development are ongoing.

REVIEW QUESTIONS

1 *What are the most common clinical and pathologic manifestations of immunodeficiency diseases?*

2 *What are some of the mutations that may block the maturation of T and B lymphocytes?*

3 *What are some of the mutations that may block the activation or effector functions of CD4+ T cells, and what are the clinical and pathologic consequences of these mutations?*

4 *How does HIV infect cells and replicate inside infected cells?*

5 *What are the principal clinical manifestations of HIV infection, and what is the pathogenesis of these manifestations?*

SUGGESTED READINGS

CHAPTER 1

Burnet FM: A modification of Jerne's theory of antibody production using the concept of clonal selection. Australian Journal of Science 20:67–69, 1957.

Drayton DL, Liao S, Mounzer RW, Ruddle NH: Lymphoid organ development: From ontogeny to neogenesis. Nature Immunology 7:344–353, 2006.

Jerne NK: The natural-selection theory of antibody formation. Proceedings of the National Academy of Sciences of the United States of America 41:849–857, 1955.

Kunkel EJ, Butcher EC: Chemokines and the tissue-specific migration of lymphocytes. Immunity 16:1–4, 2002.

Luster AD, Alon R, von Andrian UH: Immune cell migration in inflammation: Present and future therapeutic targets. Nature Immunology 6:1182–1190, 2005.

Marrack P, Kappler J: Control of T cell viability. Annual Review of Immunology 22:765–787, 2004.

Mebius RE, Kraal G: Structure and function of the spleen. Nature Reviews Immunology 5:606–616, 2005.

Sallusto F, Geginat J, Lanzavecchia A: Central memory and effector memory T cell subsets: Function, generation, and maintenance. Annual Review of Immunology 22:745–763, 2004.

Von Andrian UH, Mempel TR: Homing and cellular traffic in lymph nodes. Nature Reviews Immunology 3:867–878, 2003.

CHAPTER 2

Akira S, Takeda K: Toll-like receptor signalling. Nature Reviews: Immunology 4:499–511, 2004.

Akira S, Uematsu S, Takeuchi O: Pathogen recognition and innate immunity. Cell 124:783–801, 2006.

Bottino C, Castriconi R, Moretta L, Moretta A: Cellular ligands of activating NK receptors. Trends in Immunology 26:221–226, 2005.

Bulet P, Stocklin R, Menin L: Anti-microbial peptides: From invertebrates to vertebrates. Immunological Reviews 198:169–184, 2004.

Hotchkiss RS, Karl IE: The pathophysiology and treatment of sepsis. New England Journal of Medicine 348:138–150, 2003.

Janeway C, Medzhitov R: Innate immune recognition. Annual Review of Immunology 20:197–216, 2002.

Kawai T, Akira S: Innate immune recognition of viral infection. Nature Immunology 7:131–137, 2006.

Klotman ME, Chang TL: Defensins in innate antiviral immunity. Nature Reviews Immunology 6:447–456, 2006.

Lanier LL: NK cell recognition. Annual Review of Immunology 23:225–274, 2005.

Ley K, Laudanna C, Cybulsky MI, Nourshargh S: Getting to the site of inflammation: The leukocyte adhesion cascade updated. Nature Reviews Immunology 7:678–689, 2007.

Lieberman N, Mandelboim O: The role of NK cells in innate immunity. Advances in Experimental Medicine and Biology 479:137–145, 2000.

Meylan E, Tschopp J, Karin M: Intracellular pattern recognition receptors in the host response. Nature 442:39–44, 2006.

Natarajan K, Dimasi N, Wang J, et al: Structure and function of natural killer cell receptors: Multiple molecular solutions to self, non-self. Annual Review of Immunology 20:853–885, 2002.

Pichlmair A, Reis e Sousa C: Innate recognition of viruses. Immunity 27:370–383, 2007.

Selsted ME, Ouellette AJ: Mammalian defensins in the antimicrobial immune response. Nature Immunology 6:551–557, 2005.

Strober W, Murray PJ, Kitani A, Watanabe T: Signalling pathways and molecular interactions of NOD1 and NOD2. Nature Reviews: Immunology 6:9–20, 2006.

Takeda K, Kaisho T, Akira S: Toll-like receptors. Annual Review of Immunology 21:335–376, 2003.

Trinchieri G, Sher A: Cooperation of Toll-like receptor signals in innate immune defence. Nature Reviews Immunology 7:179–190, 2007.

Underhill DM, Ozinsky A: Phagocytosis of microbes: Complexity in action. Annual Review of Immunology 20:825–852, 2002.

CHAPTER 3

Ackerman AL, Cresswell P: Cellular mechanisms governing cross-presentation of exogenous antigens. Nature Immunology 5:678–684, 2004.

Brigl M, Brenner MB: CD1: Antigen presentation and T cell function. Annual Review of Immunology 22:817–890, 2004.

Bryant PW, Lennon-Dumenil AM, Fiebiger E, et al: Proteolysis and antigen presentation by MHC class II molecules. Advances in Immunology 80:71–114, 2002.

Germain RN, Jenkins MK: In vivo antigen presentation. Current Opinion in Immunology 16:120–125, 2004.

Guermonprez P, Valladeau J, Zitvogel L, et al: Antigen presentation and T cell stimulation by dendritic cells. Annual Review of Immunology 20:621–667, 2002.

Hewitt EW: The MHC class I antigen presentation pathway: Strategies for viral immune evasion. Immunology 110:163–169, 2003.

Klein J, Sato A: The HLA system. New England Journal of Medicine 343:702–709, 782–786, 2000.

Kumánovics A, Takada T, Lindahl KF: Genomic organization of the mammalian MHC. Annual Review of Immunology 21:629–657, 2003.

The MHC Sequencing Consortium: Complete sequence and gene map of a human major histocompatibility complex. Nature 401:921–923, 1999.

Randolph GJ, Angeli V, Swartz MA: Dendritic cell trafficking to lymph nodes through lymphatic vessels. Nature Reviews Immunology 5:617–628, 2005.

Rock KL, Goldberg AL: Degradation of cell proteins and generation of MHC class I–presented peptides. Annual Review of Immunology 17:739–779, 1999.

Rock KL, York IA, Goldberg AL: Post-proteasomal antigen processing for major histocompatibility complex class I presentation. Nature Immunology 5:670–677, 2004.

Shortman K, Liu Y-J: Mouse and human dendritic cell subtypes. Nature Reviews Immunology 2:151–161, 2003.

Tortorella D, Gewurz BE, Furman MH, et al: Viral subversion of the immune system. Annual Review of Immunology 18:861–926, 2000.

Trombetta ES, Mellman I: Cell biology of antigen processing in vitro and in vivo. Annual Review of Immunology 23:975–1028, 2005.

Villadangos JA, Schnorrer P: Intrinsic and cooperative antigen-presenting functions of dendritic-cell subsets in vivo. Nature Reviews Immunology 7:543–555, 2007.

Watts C: The exogenous pathway for antigen presentation on major histocompatibility complex class II and CD1 molecules. Nature Immunology 5:685–692, 2004.

Yewdell JW, Haeryfar SM: Understanding presentation of viral antigens to CD8+ T cells in vivo: The key to rational vaccine design. Annual Review of Immunology 23:651–682, 2005.

CHAPTER 4

Bjorkman PJ: MHC restriction in three dimensions: A view of T cell receptor/ligand interactions. Cell 89:167–170, 1997.

Call ME, Wucherpfennig KW: The T cell receptor: Critical role of the membrane environment in receptor assembly and function. Annual Review of Immunology 23:101–125, 2005.

Davis SJ, Ikemizu S, Evans EJ, et al: The nature of molecular recognition by T cells. Nature Immunology 4:217–224, 2003.

Fugmann SD, Lee AI, Shockett PE, et al: The RAG proteins and V(D)J recombination: Complexes, ends, and transposition. Annual Review of Immunology 18:495–527, 2000.

Jung D, Alt FW: Unraveling V(D)J recombination: Insights into gene regulation. Cell 116:299–311, 2004.

Muljo SA, Schlissel MS: Pre-B and pre-T-cell receptors: Conservation of strategies in regulating early lymphocyte development. Immunological Reviews 175:80–93, 2000.

Nemazee D: Receptor selection in B and T lymphocytes. Annual Review of Immunology 18:19–51, 2000.

Pillai S, Cariappa A, Moran ST: Marginal zone B cells. Annual Review of Immunology 23:161–196, 2005.

Rothenberg EV: Cell lineage regulators in B and T cell development. Nature Immunology 8:441–444, 2007.

Rudolph MG, Stanfield RL, Wilson IA: How TCRs bind MHCs, peptides, and coreceptors. Annual Review of Immunology 24:419–466, 2006.

Starr TK, Jameson SC, Hogquist KA: Positive and negative selection of T cells. Annual Review of Immunology 21:139–176, 2003.

Wang JH, Reinherz EL: Structural basis of T cell recognition of peptides bound to MHC molecules. Molecular Immunology 38:1039–1049, 2002.

CHAPTER 5

Dustin ML: A dynamic view of the immunological synapse. Seminars in Immunology 17:400–410, 2005.

Gallo EM, Cante-Barrett K, Crabtree GR: Lymphocyte calcium signaling from membrane to nucleus. Nature Immunology 7:25–32, 2006.

Germain RN, Stefanova I: The dynamics of T cell receptor signaling: Complex orchestration and the key roles of tempo and cooperation. Annual Review of Immunology 19:467–522, 1999.

Greenwald RJ, Freeman GJ, Sharpe AH: The B7 family revisited. Annual Review of Immunology 23:515–548, 2005.

Jameson SC: Maintaining the norm: T cell homeostasis. Nature Reviews Immunology 2:547–556, 2002.

Kaech SM, Wherry EJ: Heterogeneity and cell-fate decisions in effector and memory CD8+ T cell differentiation during viral infection. Immunity 27:393–405, 2007.

Kaech SM, Wherry EJ, Ahmed R: Effector and memory T cell differentiation: Implications for vaccine development. Nature Reviews Immunology 2:251–262, 2002.

Krammer PH, Arnold R, Lavrik IN: Life and death in peripheral T cells. Nature Reviews Immunology 7:532–542, 2007.

Murphy KM, Reiner SL: The lineage decisions of helper T cells. Nature Reviews Immunology 2:933–944, 2002.

Pribila JT, Quale AC, Mueller KL, Shimizu Y: Integrins and T cell-mediated immunity. Annual Review of Immunology 22:157–180, 2004.

Samelson LE: Signal transduction mediated by the T cell antigen receptor: The role of adapter proteins. Annual Review of Immunology 20:371–394, 2002.

Sharpe AH, Freeman GJ: The B7-CD28 superfamily. Nature Reviews Immunology 2:116–126, 2002.

CHAPTER 6

Bettelli E, Oukka M, Kuchroo VK: T(H)-17 cells in the circle of immunity and autoimmunity. Nature Immunology 8:345–350, 2007.

Choi J, Enis DR, Koh KP, et al: T lymphocyte–endothelial cell interactions. Annual Review of Immunology 22:683–709, 2004.

Grewal IS, Flavell RA: CD40 and CD154 in cell-mediated immunity. Annual Review of Immunology 16:111–135, 1998.

Heath WR, Carbone FR: Cross-presentation in viral immunity and self-tolerance. Nature Reviews Immunology 1:126–134, 2001.

Kapsenberg ML: Dendritic-cell control of pathogen-derived T-cell polarization. Nature Reviews Immunology 3:984–993, 2003.

Lieberman J: The ABCs of granule-mediated cytotoxicity: New weapons in the arsenal. Nature Reviews Immunology 3:361–370, 2003.

Pribila JT, Quale AC, Mueller KL, Shimizu Y: Integrins and T cell-mediated immunity. Annual Review of Immunology 22:157–180, 2004.

Reiner SL: Development in motion: Helper T cells at work. Cell 129:33–36, 2007.

Reiner SL, Sallusto F, Lanzavecchia A: Division of labor with a workforce of one: Challenges in specifying effector and memory T cell fate. Science 317:622–625, 2007.

Russell JH, Ley TJ: Lymphocyte-mediated cytotoxicity. Annual Review of Immunology 20:323–370, 2002.

Sallusto F, Geginat J, Lanzavecchia A: Central memory and effector memory T cell subsets: Function, generation, and maintenance. Annual Review of Immunology 22:745–763, 2004.

Schaible UE, Collins HL, Kaufmann SHE: Confrontation between intracellular bacteria and the immune system. Advances in Immunology 71:267–377, 1999.

Von Andrian UH, Mackay CR: T-cell function and migration. New England Journal of Medicine 343:1020–1034, 2000.

Weaver CT, Harrington LE, Mangan PR, et al: T$_H$17: An effector CD4 T cell lineage with regulatory T cell ties. Immunity 24:677–688, 2006.

Wong P, Pamer EG: CD8 T cell responses to infectious pathogens. Annual Review of Immunology 21:29–70, 2003.

CHAPTER 7

Allen CD, Okada T, Cyster JG: Germinal-center organization and cellular dynamics. Immunity 27:190–202, 2007.

Carroll MC: The complement system in B cell regulation. Molecular Immunology 41:141–146, 2004.

DeFranco AL: B-cell activation 2000. Immunological Reviews 176:5–9, 2000.

Dorner T, Radbruch A: Antibodies and B cell memory in viral immunity. Immunity 27:384–392, 2007.

Dudley DD, Chaudhuri J, Bassing CH, Alt FW: Mechanism and control of V(D)J recombination versus class switch recombination: Similarities and differences. Advances in Immunology 86:43–112, 2005.

Fagarasan S, Honjo T: T-independent immune response: New aspects of B cell biology. Science 290:89–92, 2000.

Fearon DT, Carroll MC: Regulation of B lymphocyte responses to foreign and self-antigens by the CD19/CD21 complex. Annual Review of Immunology 18:393–422, 2000.

Heyman B: Regulation of antibody responses via antibodies, complement, and Fc receptors. Annual Review of Immunology 18:709–737, 2000.

Honjo T, Muramatsu M, Fagarasan S: AID: How does it aid antibody diversity? Immunity 20:659–668, 2004.

Manz RA, Hauser AE, Hiepe F, Radbruch A: Maintenance of serum antibody levels. Annual Review of Immunology 23:367–386, 2005.

McHeyzer-Williams M, McHeyzer-Williams L, Panus J, et al: Helper T-cell–regulated B-cell immunity. Microbes and Infection 5:205–212, 2003.

Mills DM, Cambier JC: B lymphocyte interactions during cognate interactions with CD4+ T lymphocytes: Molecular dynamics and immunological consequences. Seminars in Immunology 15:325–329, 2003.

Neuberger MS, Harris RS, Di Noia J, Petersen-Mahrt SK: Immunity through DNA deamination. Trends in Biochemical Sciences 28:305–312, 2003.

Pan-Hammarstrom Q, Zhao Y, Hammarstrom L: Class switch recombination: A comparison between mouse and human. Advances in Immunology 93:1–61, 2007.

Papavasiliou FN, Schatz DG: Somatic hypermutation of immunoglobulin genes: Merging mechanisms for genetic diversity. Cell 109(Suppl):S35–S44, 2002.

Radbruch A, Muehlinghaus G, Luger EO, et al: Competence and competition: The challenge of becoming a long-lived plasma cell. Nature Reviews Immunology 6:741–750, 2006.

Shapiro-Shelef M, Calame K: Regulation of plasma cell development. Nature Reviews Immunology 5:230–242, 2005.

CHAPTER 8

Carroll MC: The complement system in regulation of adaptive immunity. Nature Immunology 5:981–986, 2004.

Fargarsan S, Honjo T: Regulation of IgA synthesis at mucosal surfaces. Current Opinion in Immunology 16:277–283, 2004.

Marshall-Clarke S, Reen D, Tasker L, Hassan J: Neonatal immunity: How well has it grown up? Immunology Today 21:35–41, 2000.

Nimmerjahn F, Ravetch JV: Fc gamma receptors: Old friends and new family members. Immunity 24:19–28, 2006.

Parren PW, Burton DR: The antiviral activity of antibodies in vitro and in vivo. Advances in Immunology 77:195–262, 2001.

Roozendaal R, Carroll MC: Emerging patterns in complement-mediated pathogen recognition. Cell 125:29–32, 2006.

Walport MJ: Complement. New England Journal of Medicine 344:1058–1066, 1141–1144, 2001.

Ward ES: Acquiring maternal immunoglobulin: Different receptors, similar functions. Immunity 20:507–508, 2004.

CHAPTER 9

Baxter AG, Hodgkin PD: Activation rules: The two-signal theories of immune activation. Nature Reviews Immunology 2:439–446, 2002.

Bluestone JA, Abbas AK: Natural versus adaptive regulatory T cells. Nature Reviews Immunology 3:253–257, 2003.

Fathman CG, Lineberry NB: Molecular mechanisms of CD4+ T-cell anergy. Nature Reviews Immunology 7:599–609, 2007.

Goodnow CC: Multistep pathogenesis of autoimmune disease. Cell 130:25–35, 2007.

Goodnow CC, Sprent J, de St Groth BF, Vinuesa CG: Cellular and genetic mechanisms of self tolerance and autoimmunity. Nature 435:590–597, 2005.

Hogquist KA, Baldwin TA, Jameson SC: Central tolerance: Learning self-control in the thymus. Nature Reviews Immunology 5:772–782, 2005.

Kyewski B, Klein L: A central role for central tolerance. Annual Review of Immunology 24:571–606, 2006.

Malek TR, Bayer AL: Tolerance, not immunity, crucially depends on IL-2. Nature Reviews: Immunology 4:665–674, 2004.

Marsden VS, Strasser A: Control of apoptosis in the immune system: Bcl-2, BH3-only proteins, and more. Annual Review of Immunology 21:71–105, 2003.

Mathis D, Benoist C: Back to central tolerance. Immunity 20:509–516, 2004.

Miller SD, Turley DM, Podojil JR: Antigen-specific tolerance strategies for the prevention and treatment of autoimmune disease. Nature Reviews Immunology 7:665–677, 2007.

Nemazee D: Receptor editing in lymphocyte development and central tolerance. Nature Reviews Immunology 6:728–740, 2006.

Roncarolo MG, Battaglia M: Regulatory T-cell immunotherapy for tolerance to self antigens and alloantigens in humans. Nature Reviews Immunology 7:585–598, 2007.

Sakaguchi S, Powrie F: Emerging challenges in regulatory T cell function and biology. Science 317:627–629, 2007.

Siegel RM, Chan FK-M, Lenardo MJ: The multi-faceted role of Fas signaling in immune cell homeostasis and autoimmunity. Nature Immunology 1:469–474, 2000.

Singh NJ, Schwartz RH: Primer: Mechanisms of immunologic tolerance. Nature Clinical Practice: Rheumatology 2:44–52, 2006.

Steinman RM, Hawiger D, Nussenzweig MC: Tolerogenic dendritic cells. Annual Review of Immunology 21:685–711, 2003.

Walker LS, Abbas AK: The enemy within: Keeping self-reactive T cells at bay in the periphery. Nature Reviews Immunology 2:11–19, 2002.

Wandstrat A, Wakeland EW: The genetics of complex autoimmune diseases: Non-MHC susceptibility genes. Nature Immunology 2:802–809, 2001.

Zheng Y, Rudensky AY: Foxp3 in control of the regulatory T cell lineage. Nature Immunology 8:457–462, 2007.

CHAPTER 10

Banchereau J, Palucka AK: Dendritic cells as therapeutic vaccines against cancer. Nature Reviews Immunology 5:296–306, 2005.

Berzofsky JA, Terabe M, Oh S, et al: Progress on new vaccine strategies for the immunotherapy and prevention of cancer. Journal of Clinical Investigations 113:1515–1525, 2004.

Boon T, Coulie PG, Van den Eynde BJ, van der Bruggen P: Human T cell responses against melanoma. Annual Review of Immunology 24:175–208, 2006.

Burnet FM: The concept of immunological surveillance. Progress in Experimental Tumor Research 13:1–27, 1970.

Clarkson MR, Sayegh MH: T-cell costimulatory pathways in allograft rejection and tolerance. Transplantation 80:555–563, 2005.

Colvin RB, Smith RN: Antibody-mediated organ-allograft rejection. Nature Reviews Immunology 5:807–817, 2005.

Dranoff G: Cytokines in cancer pathogenesis and cancer therapy. Nature Reviews Cancer 4:11–22, 2004.

Dunn GP, Old LJ, Schreiber RD: The three Es of cancer immunoediting. Annual Review of Immunology 22:329–360, 2004.

Gilboa E: The promise of cancer vaccines. Nature Reviews Cancer 4:401–411, 2004.

Gilboa E: DC-based cancer vaccines. Journal of Clinical Investigation 117:1195–1203, 2007.

Gould DS, Auchincloss H Jr: Direct and indirect recognition: The role of MHC antigens in graft rejection. Immunology Today 20:77–82, 1999.

Halloran PF: Immunosuppressive drugs for kidney transplantation. New England Journal of Medicine 351:2715–2729, 2004.

Harris M: Monoclonal antibodies as therapeutic agents for cancer. Lancet Oncology 5:292–302, 2004.

June CH: Adoptive T cell therapy for cancer in the clinic. Journal of Clinical Investigation 117:1466–1476, 2007.

June CH: Principles of adoptive T cell cancer therapy. Journal of Clinical Investigation 117:1204–1212, 2007.

Pardoll D: Does the immune system see tumors as foreign or self? Annual Review of Immunology 21:807–839, 2003.

Ricordi C, Strom TB: Clinical islet transplantation: Advances and immunological challenges. Nature Reviews Immunology 4:259–268, 2004.

Swann JB, Smyth MJ: Immune surveillance of tumors. Journal of Clinical Investigation 117:1137–1146, 2007.

Vongwiwatana A, Tasanarong A, Hidalgo LG, Halloran PF: The role of B cells and alloantibody in the host response to human organ allografts. Immunological Reviews 196:197–218, 2003.

Waldmann TA: Effective cancer therapy through immunomodulation. Annual Review of Medicine 57:65–81, 2006.

Yang Y-G, Sykes M: Xenotransplantation: Current status and a perspective on the future. Nature Reviews Immunology 7:519–531, 2007.

CHAPTER 11

Bach J-F: Infections and autoimmune diseases. Journal of Autoimmunity 25(Suppl 1):74–80, 2005.

Bischoff SC: Role of mast cells in allergic and non-allergic immune responses: Comparison of human and murine data. Nature Reviews Immunology 7:93–104, 2007.

Chatenoud L: Immune therapies of autoimmune diseases: Are we approaching a real cure? Current Opinion in Immunology 18:710–717, 2006.

Cohn L, Elias JA, Chupp GL: Asthma: Mechanisms of disease persistence and progression. Annual Review of Immunology 22:789–815, 2004.

Costa JJ, Weller PF, Galli SJ: The cells of the allergic response. Journal of the American Medical Association 278:1815–1822, 1997.

Davidson A, Diamond B: Autoimmune diseases. New England Journal of Medicine 345:340–350, 2001.

Galli SJ, Kalesnikoff J, MA Grimbaldeston MA, et al: Mast cells as "tunable" effector and immunoregulatory cells: Recent advances. Annual Review of Immunology 23:749–786, 2005.

Gould HJ, Sutton BJ, Beavil AK, et al: The biology of IgE and the basis of allergic diseases. Annual Review of Immunology 21:579–628, 2003.

Kay AB: Allergy and allergic diseases. New England Journal of Medicine 344:30–37, 109–113, 2001.

Kraft S, Kinet JP: New developments in FcεRI regulation, function and inhibition. Nature Reviews Immunology 7:365–378, 2007.

Marshak-Rothstein A: Toll-like receptors in systemic autoimmune disease. Nature Reviews Immunology 6:823–835, 2006.

Nadler MJ, Matthews SA, Turner H, Kinet J-P: Signal transduction by the high affinity immunoglobulin E receptor FcεRI: Coupling form to function. Advances in Immunology 76:325–355, 2000.

Rioux JD, Abbas AK: Paths to understanding the genetic basis of autoimmune disease. Nature 435:584–589, 2005.

Robinson DS, Kay AB, Wardlaw AJ: Eosinophils. Clinical Allergy and Immunology 16:43–75, 2002.

Wills-Karp M, Ewart SL: Time to draw breath: Asthma-susceptibility genes are identified. Nature Reviews Genetics 5:376–387, 2004.

CHAPTER 12

Blankson JN, Persaud D, Siliciano RF: The challenge of viral reservoirs in HIV-1 infection. Annual Review of Medicine 53:557–593, 2002.

Bonilla FA, Geha RS: Update on primary immunodeficiency diseases. Journal of Allergy and Clinical Immunology 117(Suppl):435–441, 2006.

Brenchley JM, Price DA, Douek DC: HIV disease: Fallout from a mucosal catastrophe? Nature Immunology 7:235–239, 2006.

Buckley RH: Molecular defects in human severe combined immunodeficiency and approaches to immune reconstitution. Annual Review of Immunology 22:625–655, 2004.

Cunningham-Rundles C, Ponda PP: Molecular defects in T- and B-cell primary immunodeficiency diseases. Nature Reviews Immunology 5:880–892, 2005.

Deeks SG, Walker BD: Human immunodeficiency virus controllers: Mechanisms of durable virus control in the absence of antiretroviral therapy. Immunity 27:406–416, 2007.

Fischer A: Human primary immunodeficiency disease: A perspective. Nature Reviews Immunology 5:23–30, 2004.

Frankel AD, Young JAT: HIV-1: Fifteen proteins and an RNA. Annual Review of Biochemistry 67:1–25, 1998.

Gandhi RT, Walker BD: Immunologic control of HIV-1. Annual Review of Medicine 53:149–172, 2002.

Grossman Z, Meier-Schellersheim M, Sousa AE, et al: CD4+ T-cell depletion in HIV infection: Are we closer to understanding the cause? Nature Medicine 8:319–323, 2002.

Hazenberg MD, Harmann D, Schuitemaker H, Miedema F: T cell depletion in HIV-1 infection: CD4+ T cells go out of stock. Nature Immunology 1:285–289, 2000.

Heyworth PG, Cross AR, Curnutte JT: Chronic granulomatous disease. Current Opinion in Immunology 15:578, 2003.

Kilby JM, Eron JJ: Novel therapies based on mechanisms of HIV-1 cell entry. New England Journal of Medicine 348:2228–2238, 2004.

Leonard WJ: Cytokines and immunodeficiency diseases. Nature Reviews Immunology 1:200–208, 2001.

Letvin NL: Progress and obstacles in the development of an AIDS vaccine. Nature Reviews Immunology 6:930–939, 2006.

Lusso P: HIV and the chemokine system: 10 years later. EMBO Journal 25:447–456, 2006.

McMichael AJ, Rowland-Jones SL: Cellular immune responses to HIV. Nature 410:980–987, 2001.

Peterlin BM, Trono D: Hide, shield and strike back: How HIV-infected cells avoid immune eradication. Nature Reviews Immunology 3:97–107, 2003.

Simon V, Ho DD: HIV-1 dynamics in vivo: Implications for therapy. Nature Reviews Microbiology 1:181–190, 2003.

Simon V, Ho DD, Abdool Karim Q: HIV/AIDS epidemiology, pathogenesis, prevention, and treatment. Lancet 368:489–504, 2006.

Stebbing J, Gazzard B, Douek DC: Where does HIV live? New England Journal of Medicine 350:1872–1880, 2004.

Stevenson M: HIV-1 pathogenesis. Nature Medicine 9:853–860, 2003.

Wu L, KewalRamani VN: Dendritic-cell interactions with HIV: Infection and viral dissemination. Nature Reviews Immunology 6:859–868, 2006.

GLOSSARY

ABO blood group antigens. Glycosphingolipid antigens present on many cell types, including red blood cells and endothelial cells, which differ between different individuals depending on inherited alleles encoding the enzymes required for synthesis of the antigens. The ABO antigens act as alloantigens responsible for blood transfusion reactions and hyperacute rejection of allografts.

Accessory molecule. A lymphocyte cell surface molecule distinct from the antigen receptor complex that mediates adhesive or signaling functions important for activation or migration of the lymphocyte.

Acquired immunodeficiency. A deficiency in the immune system that is acquired after birth, because of infections, malnutrition, or therapies that deplete immune cells, and is not related to a genetic defect.

Acquired immunodeficiency syndrome (AIDS). A disease caused by human immunodeficiency virus (HIV) infection that is characterized by depletion of CD4+ T cells, leading to a profound defect in cell-mediated immunity. Clinically, AIDS includes opportunistic infections, malignancies, wasting, and encephalopathy.

Activation-induced deaminase (AID). An enzyme required for immunoglobulin (Ig) class switch recombination and somatic hypermutation of the Ig variable regions. AID deficiency causes one form of hyper-IgM syndrome.

Active immunity. The form of adaptive immunity that is induced by exposure to a foreign antigen and activation of lymphocytes, in which the immunized individual plays an active role in responding to the antigen. Compare with **passive immunity.**

Acute phase response. The increase in plasma concentrations of several proteins, called acute phase reactants, that occurs as part of the innate immune response to infections. These proteins, including C-reactive protein, fibrinogen, and serum amyloid A protein, are synthesized by the liver in response to inflammatory cytokines, especially interleukin-6 and tumor necrosis factor.

Acute rejection. A form of graft rejection involving vascular and parenchymal injury mediated by T cells, macrophages, and antibodies, which usually begins after the first week of transplantation. The differentiation of the effector T cells and the production of antibodies that mediate acute rejection occur in response to graft antigens.

Adapter protein. Proteins involved in lymphocyte signal transduction pathways, which serve as bridge molecules or scaffolds for the recruitment of other signaling molecules. Adapter molecules involved in T cell activation include LAT, SLP-76, and Grb-2.

Adaptive immunity. The form of immunity that is mediated by lymphocytes and is stimulated by exposure to infectious agents. In contrast with innate immunity, adaptive immunity is characterized by exquisite specificity for distinct macromolecules, and by "memory," which is the ability to respond more vigorously to repeated exposures to the same microbe.

Adhesion molecule. A cell surface molecule whose function is to promote adhesive interactions with other cells or the extracellular matrix. Leukocytes express various types of adhesion molecules, such as selectins and integrins, and these molecules play important roles in cell migration and activation in innate and adaptive immune responses.

Adjuvant. A substance, distinct from antigen, that enhances T cell activation by promoting the accumulation of antigen-presenting cells at a site of antigen exposure and by enhancing the expression of costimulators and cytokines by the antigen-presenting cells.

Affinity. The strength of the binding between a single binding site of a molecule (e.g., an antibody) and a ligand (e.g., an antigen), represented by the dissociation constant (K_d). A smaller K_d indicates a stronger or higher-affinity interaction.

Affinity maturation. The process that leads to increased affinity of antibodies for a protein antigen as a humoral response progresses. Affinity maturation is the result of somatic mutation of immunoglobulin genes followed by selective survival of the B cells producing the highest-affinity antibodies.

AIRE. A transcription factor encoded by the *autoimmune regulator* (*AIRE*) gene, which promotes expression of peripheral tissue antigens in thymic epithelial cells and is essential for deletion (negative selection) of T cells specific for these antigens. Mutations in *AIRE* lead to the autoimmune polyendocrine syndrome type 1 (APS-1).

Allele. One of different forms of a gene present at a particular chromosomal locus. An individual who is heterozygous at a locus has two different alleles, each on a different chromosome, one inherited from the mother and one from the father. If there are many different alleles for a particular gene in a population, the gene or locus is said to be *polymorphic*. The major histocompatibility complex locus is extremely polymorphic.

Allelic exclusion. The expression of only one of two inherited alleles encoding immunoglobulin heavy and light chains and T cell receptor β chains. Allelic exclusion occurs when the protein product of one productively recombined antigen receptor locus on one chromosome blocks the rearrangement of the corresponding locus on the other chromosome.

Allergen. An antigen that elicits an immediate hypersensitivity (allergic) reaction. Allergens are proteins, or chemicals bound to proteins, that induce IgE antibody production in atopic individuals.

Allergy. A form of atopy or immediate hypersensitivity disease, often referring to the type of antigen that elicits the disease, such as food allergy, bee sting allergy, and penicillin allergy. All of these conditions are related to antigen-induced mast cell or basophil activation.

Alloantigen. A cell or tissue antigen that is present in some members of a species and not others and that is recognized as foreign on an allograft. Alloantigens are the products of polymorphic genes.

Allogeneic graft. An organ or tissue graft from a donor of the same species as, but genetically not identical to, the recipient (also called an allograft).

Alloreactive. Reactive to alloantigens; describes T cells or antibodies from one individual that will recognize antigens on cells or tissues of another, genetically nonidentical individual.

Altered peptide ligands (APLs). Peptides with altered T cell receptor contact residues that elicit responses different from the responses to the native peptide. APLs may be important in the regulation of T cell activation in physiologic, pathologic, or therapeutic situations.

Alternative pathway of complement activation. An antibody-independent pathway of activation of the complement system that occurs when the C3b protein binds to microbial cell surfaces. The alternative pathway is a component of the innate immune system and mediates inflammatory responses to infection, as well as direct lysis of microbes.

Anaphylatoxins. The C5a, C4a, and C3a complement fragments that are generated during complement activation. The anaphylatoxins bind specific cell surface receptors and promote acute inflammation by stimulating neutrophil chemotaxis and by activating mast cells.

Anaphylaxis. An extreme systemic form of immediate hypersensitivity reaction, also called anaphylactic shock, in which mast cell or basophil mediators cause bronchial constriction, massive tissue edema, and cardiovascular collapse.

Anergy. A state of unresponsiveness to antigenic stimulation. Lymphocyte anergy (also called clonal anergy) is the failure of clones of T or B cells to react to antigen, and this may be a mechanism of maintaining immunologic tolerance to self antigens. In clinical practice, anergy refers to a generalized defect in T cell–dependent cutaneous delayed-type hypersensitivity reactions to common antigens.

Antibody. A type of glycoprotein molecule, also called immunoglobulin (Ig), produced by B lymphocytes, that binds antigens, often with a high degree of specificity and high affinity. The basic structural unit of an antibody is composed of two identical heavy chains and two identical light chains. Amino-terminal variable regions of the heavy and light chains form the antigen binding sites, whereas the carboxy-terminal constant regions of the heavy chains functionally interact with other molecules in the immune system. In any individual, there are millions of different antibodies, each with a unique antigen-binding site. Secreted antibodies perform various effector functions, including neutralizing antigens, activating complement, and promoting phagocytosis and destruction of microbes.

Antibody-dependent cell-mediated cytotoxicity (ADCC). A process by which natural killer (NK) cells are targeted to IgG-coated cells, resulting in the lysis of the antibody-coated cells. A specific receptor for the constant region of IgG, called FcγRIII (CD16), is expressed on the NK cell membrane and mediates the binding to the IgG.

Antibody feedback. The down-regulation of antibody production by secreted IgG antibodies that occurs when antigen-antibody complexes simultaneously engage B cell membrane immunoglobulin (Ig) and Fcγ receptors. Under these conditions, the cytoplasmic tails of the Fcγ receptors deliver inhibitory signals to the B cell.

Antibody repertoire. The collection of different antibody specificities expressed in an individual.

Antibody-secreting cell. A B lymphocyte that has undergone differentiation and produces the secretory form of immunoglobulin (Ig). Antibody-secreting cells are produced in response to antigen and reside in lymphoid follicles in spleen and lymph node, as well as in the bone marrow. Plasma cells are typical antibody-secreting cells.

Antigen. A molecule that binds to an antibody or a T cell antigen receptor (TCR). Antigens that bind to antibodies include all classes of molecules. Most TCRs bind only peptide fragments of proteins complexed with major histocompatibility molecules; both the peptide ligand and the native protein from which it is derived are called T cell antigens.

Antigen presentation. The display of peptides bound by major histocompatibility molecules on the surface of an antigen-presenting cell, permitting specific recognition by T cell receptors and activation of T cells.

Antigen-presenting cell (APC). A cell that displays peptide fragments of protein antigens, in association with major histocompatibility (MHC) molecules on its surface, and activates antigen-specific T cells. In addition to displaying peptide-MHC complexes, APCs also must express costimulatory molecules to optimally activate T lymphocytes.

Antigen processing. The intracellular conversion of protein antigens derived from the extracellular space or the cytosol into peptides and loading of these peptides onto major histocompatibility complex molecules for display to T lymphocytes.

Antiserum. Serum from an individual previously immunized against an antigen that contains antibody specific for that antigen.

Apoptosis. A process of cell death that is characterized by DNA cleavage, nuclear condensation and fragmentation, and plasma membrane blebbing, leading to phagocytosis of the cell, without inducing an inflammatory response. This type of cell death is important in lymphocyte development, regulation of lymphocyte responses to foreign antigens, and maintenance of tolerance to self antigens.

Arthus reaction. A localized form of experimental immune complex–mediated vasculitis induced by injecting an antigen subcutaneously into a previously immunized animal or an animal that has been given intravenous antibody specific for the antigen. Circulating antibodies bind to the injected antigen, forming immune complexes that deposit in the walls of small arteries at the injection site, giving rise to a local cutaneous vasculitis with necrosis.

Atopy. The propensity of an individual to produce IgE antibodies in response to various environmental antigens and to develop strong immediate hypersensitivity (allergic) responses. People who have allergies to environmental antigens, such as pollen or house dust, are said to be atopic.

Autoantibody. An antibody specific for a self antigen. Autoantibodies can cause damage to cells and tissues and are produced in excess in many autoimmune diseases such as systemic lupus erythematosus.

Autoimmune disease. A disease caused by a breakdown of self-tolerance such that the adaptive immune system responds to self antigens and mediates cell and tissue damage. Autoimmune diseases can be organ-specific (e.g., thyroiditis or diabetes) or systemic (e.g., systemic lupus erythematosus).

Autoimmunity. The response of the adaptive immune system to self antigens that occurs when mechanisms of self-tolerance fail.

Autologous graft. A tissue or organ graft in which the donor and the recipient are the same individual. Autologous bone marrow and skin grafts commonly are performed in clinical medicine.

Avidity. The overall strength of interaction between two molecules, such as an antibody and an antigen. The avidity depends on both the affinity and the valency of interactions. Therefore, the avidity of a pentameric IgM antibody, with 10 antigen-binding sites, for a multivalent antigen may be much greater than the avidity of a dimeric IgG molecule for the same antigen. *Avidity* also can be used to describe the strength of cell–cell interactions, which are mediated by many binding interactions between cell surface molecules.

B lymphocyte. The only cell type capable of producing antibody molecules and therefore the central cellular component of humoral immune responses. B lymphocytes, or B cells, develop in the bone marrow, and mature B cells are found mainly in lymphoid follicles in secondary lymphoid tissues, in bone marrow, and in low numbers in the circulation.

B lymphocyte antigen receptor complex, or B cell receptor (BCR) complex. A multiprotein complex expressed on the surface of B lymphocytes that recognizes antigen and transduces activating signals. The BCR complex includes membrane immunoglobulin (Ig), which is responsible for binding antigen, and the associated Igα and Igβ proteins, which initiate signaling events.

B-1 B lymphocytes. A subset of B lymphocytes that develop earlier during ontogeny than do conventional B cells and that express a limited repertoire of V genes with little junctional diversity and secrete IgM antibodies that bind T-independent antigens. Many B-1 cells express the CD5 (Ly-1) molecule.

Bare lymphocyte syndrome. An immunodeficiency disease characterized by the lack of class II major histocompatibility complex (MHC) molecule expression, leading to defects in antigen presentation and cell-mediated immunity. The disease is caused by mutations in genes encoding factors that regulate class II MHC gene transcription.

Basophil. A type of bone marrow–derived circulating granulocyte with structural and functional similarities to mast cells, including granules containing many of the same inflammatory mediators as mast cells, and expression of a high-affinity Fc receptor for IgE. Basophils that are recruited into tissue sites where antigen is present may contribute to immediate hypersensitivity reactions.

Bone marrow. The central cavity of bone that is the site of generation of all circulating blood cells in the adult, including immature lymphocytes, and the site of B cell maturation.

Bone marrow transplantation. The transplantation of bone marrow stem cells that give rise to all mature blood cells and lymphocytes, performed clinically to treat hematopoietic or lymphopoietic disorders and malignancies; also used in various immunologic experiments in animals.

Bronchial asthma. An inflammatory disease usually caused by repeated immediate hypersensitivity reactions in the lung, leading to intermittent and reversible airway obstruction, chronic bronchial inflammation with eosinophils, and bronchial smooth muscle cell hypertrophy and hyperreactivity.

C3 convertase. A multiprotein enzyme complex generated by the early steps of complement activation, which cleaves C3, giving rise to two proteolytic products called C3a and C3b.

C5 convertase. A multiprotein enzyme complex generated by C3b binding to C3 convertase, which cleaves C5 and initiates the late steps of complement activation.

Caspases. Intracellular cysteine proteases that cleave substrates at the carboxy-terminal sides of aspartic acid residues and are components of enzymatic cascades that cause apoptotic death of cells. Lymphocyte caspases may be activated by two distinct pathways, one of which is associated with mitochondrial permeability changes in growth factor–deprived cells and the other with signals from death receptors in the plasma membrane.

CD molecules. Cell surface molecules expressed on various cell types in the immune system that are designated by the *cluster of differentiation* (CD) nomenclature. See Appendix II for a list of CD molecules.

Cell-mediated immunity. The form of adaptive immunity that is mediated by T lymphocytes and serves as the defense mechanism against microbes that survive within phagocytes or infect nonphagocytic cells. Cell-mediated immune responses include CD4+ T cell–mediated activation of macrophages that have phagocytosed microbes and CD8+ cytotoxic T lymphocyte killing of infected cells.

Central tolerance. A form of self-tolerance that is induced in generative ("central") lymphoid organs as a consequence of immature self-reactive lymphocytes recognizing self antigens, leading to their death or inactivation. Central tolerance prevents the emergence of lymphocytes with high-affinity receptors for ubiquitous self antigens that are present in the bone marrow or thymus and are likely to be present throughout the body. Central T cell tolerance to some peripheral tissue proteins may also occur due to AIRE-dependent expression of those proteins in the thymus.

Chédiak-Higashi syndrome. A rare autosomal recessive immunodeficiency disease due to a defect in cytoplasmic granules of various cell types that affects the lysosomes of neutrophils and macrophages, as well as the granules of cytotoxic T lymphocytes and natural killer cells. Patients show reduced resistance to infections with pyogenic bacteria.

Chemokine receptors. Cell surface receptors for chemokines that transduce signals, which stimulate migration of leukocytes. These receptors are members of the seven-transmembrane α-helical, G protein–linked family of receptors.

Chemokines. A large family of structurally homologous, low-molecular-weight cytokines that stimulate leukocyte movement and regulate the migration of leukocytes from the blood to tissues.

Chemotaxis. Movement of a cell directed by a chemical concentration gradient. The movement of lymphocytes, polymorphonuclear leukocytes, monocytes, and other leukocytes into various tissues often is directed by gradients of chemokines.

Chronic granulomatous disease (CGD). A rare inherited immunodeficiency disease due to a defect in the gene encoding a component of the phagocyte oxidase enzyme, which is needed for microbial killing by polymorphonuclear leukocytes and macrophages. The disease is characterized by recurrent intracellular bacterial and fungal infections, often accompanied by chronic cell-mediated immune responses and the formation of granulomas.

Chronic rejection. A form of allograft rejection characterized by fibrosis with loss of normal organ structures occurring over a prolonged period. In many cases, the major pathologic event in chronic rejection is graft arterial occlusion that occurs as a result of proliferation of intimal smooth muscle cells and is called graft arteriosclerosis.

Class I major histocompatibility complex (MHC) molecule. One of two forms of polymorphic, heterodimeric membrane proteins that bind and display peptide fragments of protein antigens on the surface of antigen-presenting cells for recognition by T lymphocytes. Class I MHC molecules display peptides derived from the cytoplasm of the cell.

Class II major histocompatibility complex (MHC) molecule. One of two forms of polymorphic, heterodimeric membrane proteins that bind and display peptide fragments of protein antigens on the surface of antigen-presenting cells for recognition by T lymphocytes. Class II MHC molecules display peptides derived from proteins that are internalized into phagocytic/endocytic vesicles.

Class II–associated invariant chain peptide (CLIP). A peptide remnant of the invariant chain that sits in the class II major histocompatibility complex (MHC) peptide-binding cleft and is removed by the action of the HLA-DM molecule before the cleft becomes accessible to peptides produced from endocytosed protein antigens.

Classical pathway of complement activation. The pathway of complement system activation that is initiated by binding of antigen-antibody complexes to the C1 molecule, inducing a proteolytic cascade involving multiple other complement proteins. The classical pathway is an effector arm of the humoral immune system that generates inflammatory mediators, opsonins for phagocytosis of antigens, and lytic complexes that destroy cells.

Clonal ignorance. A form of lymphocyte unresponsiveness in which self antigens are ignored by the immune system, even though lymphocytes specific for those antigens remain viable and functional.

Clonal selection. A fundamental feature of the immune system based on the fact that every individual possesses numerous clonally derived lymphocytes, each clone having arisen from a single precursor and being capable of recognizing and responding to a distinct antigenic determinant. When an antigen enters, it selects a specific preexisting clone and activates it.

Collectins. A family of proteins, including mannose-binding lectins, that are characterized by the presence of a collagen-like domain and a lectin (i.e., carbohydrate-binding) domain. Collectins play a role in the innate immune system by acting as microbial pattern recognition receptors, and they may activate the complement system by binding to C1q.

Colony-stimulating factors (CSFs). Cytokines that promote the expansion and differentiation of bone marrow progenitor cells. CSFs are essential for maturation of red blood cells, granulocytes, monocytes, and lymphocytes. Examples of CSFs are granulocyte-monocyte colony-stimulating factor, c-*kit* ligand, and interleukin-3.

Combinatorial diversity. A term describing lymphocyte antigen receptor diversity due to the many different combinations of variable, diversity, and joining segments (V, D, and J) that are possible as a result of somatic recombination of DNA in the immunoglobulin and T cell receptor loci during B cell or T cell development. This is one mechanism for the generation of large numbers of different antigen receptor genes from a limited number of gene segments.

Complement. A system of serum and cell surface proteins that interact with one another and with other molecules of the immune system to generate important effectors of innate and adaptive immune responses. There are three pathways of complement activation that differ in how they are initiated: the classical pathway, activated by antigen-antibody complexes; the alternative pathway, by microbial surfaces; and the lectin pathway, by plasma lectins that bind to microbes. Each complement pathway consists of a cascade of proteolytic enzymes that generate inflammatory mediators and opsonins and leads to the formation of a lytic complex that inserts in cell membranes.

Complement receptor, type 2 (CR2). A receptor expressed on B cells and follicular dendritic cells that binds proteolytic fragments of the C3 complement protein, including C3d, C3dg, and iC3b. CR2 functions to stimulate humoral immune responses by enhancing B cell activation by antigen and by promoting the trapping of antigen-antibody complexes in germinal centers. CR2 also is the receptor for Epstein-Barr virus.

Complementarity-determining region (CDR). Short segments of the immunoglobulin (Ig) and T cell receptor (TCR) proteins in which most of the sequence differences among different antibodies or TCRs are confined and which make contact with antigen. There are three CDRs in the variable domain of each antigen receptor polypeptide chain and six CDRs in an intact Ig or TCR molecule. These so-called hypervariable segments assume loop structures that together form a surface that is complementary to the three-dimensional structure of the bound antigen.

Constant (C) region. The portion of immunoglobulin (Ig) or T cell receptor (TCR) polypeptide chains that does not vary in sequence among different clones of B and T cells and is not involved in antigen binding. The C regions are encoded by DNA sequences in the Ig and TCR gene loci that are spatially separate from the sequences that encode the variable (V) regions.

Contact sensitivity. The propensity to develop a T cell–mediated, delayed-type hypersensitivity reaction in the skin on contact with a particular chemical agent. Chemicals that elicit contact sensitivity bind to and modify self proteins or molecules on the surfaces of antigen-presenting cells, which are then recognized by CD4+ or CD8+ T cells.

Co-receptor. A lymphocyte surface receptor that binds to a part of an antigen at the same time as when membrane immunoglobulin (Ig) or T cell receptor (TCR) binds the antigen and that delivers signals required for optimal lymphocyte activation. CD4 and CD8 are T cell co-receptors that bind nonpolymorphic regions of a major histocompatibility complex molecule concurrently with the TCR binding to polymorphic residues and the displayed peptide. The type 2 complement receptor (CR2) is a co-receptor on B cells that binds to complement-coated antigens, at the same time as when membrane Ig binds an epitope of the antigen.

Costimulator. A molecule on the surface of an antigen-presenting cell that provides a stimulus ("second signal") required for activation of naive T cells, in addition to antigen (the "first signal"). The best-defined costimulators are the CD80 and CD86 molecules on professional antigen-presenting cells that bind to the CD28 molecule on T cells.

Cross-matching. A screening test performed to minimize the chance of graft rejection, in which the patient in need of an allograft is tested for the presence of preformed antibodies against donor cell surface antigens (usually major histocompatibility antigens). The test involves mixing the recipient serum with leukocytes from potential donors, adding complement, and examining it to see if cell lysis occurs.

Cross presentation. A mechanism by which a professional antigen-presenting cell (APC) displays the antigens of another cell (e.g., a virus-infected or tumor cell) and activates (or primes) a naive CD8+ cytotoxic T lymphocyte. This occurs, for example, when an infected (often damaged) cell is ingested by a professional APC and the microbial antigens are processed and presented in association with major histocompatibility complex molecules, just like any other phagocytosed antigen. The professional APC also provides costimulation for the T cells. Also called *cross-priming.*

Cutaneous immune system. The components of the innate and adaptive immune systems found in the skin that function together in a specialized way to detect and respond to antigens that enter through the skin. Components of the cutaneous immune system include keratinocytes, Langerhans cells, intraepithelial lymphocytes, and dermal lymphocytes.

Cyclosporine. An immunosuppressive drug used to prevent allograft rejection, which functions by blocking T cell cytokine gene transcription. Cyclosporine binds to a cytosolic protein called cyclophilin, and cyclosporine-cyclophilin complexes bind to and inhibit the phosphatase calcineurin, thereby inhibiting activation and nuclear translocation of the transcription factor NFAT.

Cytokines. Secreted proteins that function as mediators of immune and inflammatory reactions. In innate immune responses, cytokines are produced by macrophages and natural killer cells and, in adaptive immune responses, mainly by T lymphocytes.

Cytotoxic (or cytolytic) T lymphocyte (CTL). A type of T lymphocyte whose major effector function is to recognize and kill host cells infected with viruses or other intracellular microbes. CTLs usually express CD8 and recognize microbial peptides displayed by class I major histocompatibility complex molecules. CTL killing of infected cells involves release of cytoplasmic granules whose contents include membrane pore-forming proteins and proteolytic enzymes.

Defensins. Cysteine-rich peptides, produced in epithelia and neutrophil granules, that act as broad-spectrum antibiotics that kill a wide variety of bacteria and fungi.

Delayed-type hypersensitivity (DTH). An immune reaction in which T cell–dependent macrophage activation and inflammation cause tissue injury. A DTH reaction to subcutaneous injection of antigen often is used as an assay for cell-mediated immunity (e.g., the purified protein derivative [PPD] skin test for immunity to *Mycobacterium tuberculosis*).

Dendritic cells. Bone marrow–derived cells, found in epithelia and most organs, characterized morphologically by thin membranous projections. Dendritic cells function as antigen-presenting cells for naive T lymphocytes and are important for initiation of adaptive immune responses to protein antigens.

Desensitization. A method for treating immediate hypersensitivity disease (e.g., allergies) that involves repetitive administration of low doses of an antigen to which the patient is allergic. This process often prevents severe allergic reactions on subsequent environmental exposure to the antigen, but the mechanisms are not well understood.

Determinant. The portion of a macromolecular antigen to which an antibody or T cell receptor binds. For a T cell, a determinant is the peptide portion of a protein antigen that binds to a major histocompatibility complex molecule and is recognized by the T cell receptor. It is synonymous with **epitope.**

DiGeorge syndrome. A T cell deficiency due to a congenital malformation that results in defective development of the thymus, parathyroid glands, and other structures that arise from the third and fourth pharyngeal pouches.

Direct antigen presentation. Presentation of cell surface allogeneic major histocompatibility complex (MHC) molecules by graft antigen-presenting cells to the recipient's T cells, leading to T cell activation, with no requirement for processing. Direct recognition of foreign MHC molecules is a cross-reaction of a normal T cell receptor that was selected to recognize a self MHC molecule plus foreign peptide, with an allogeneic MHC molecule plus peptide. (Contrasts with **indirect presentation of alloantigens.**)

Diversity. The existence of a large number of lymphocytes with different antigenic specificities in any individual (i.e., the lymphocyte repertoire is large and diverse). Diversity is a fundamental property of the adaptive immune system and is the result of variability in the structures of the antigen-binding sites of lymphocyte receptors for antigens (antibodies and T cell receptors).

Diversity (D) segments. Short coding sequences between the variable (V) and constant (C) gene segments in the immunoglobulin heavy chain and TCR γ and β loci, which, together with J segments, are somatically recombined with V segments during lymphocyte development. The resulting recombined V-D-J DNA codes for the antigen receptor V region.

DM. See **HLA-DM.**

DNA vaccine. A method for vaccination in which an individual is inoculated with a bacterial plasmid containing a complementary DNA encoding a protein antigen. DNA vaccines presumably work because professional antigen-presenting cells are transfected in vivo by the plasmid and express immunogenic peptides that elicit specific responses. Furthermore, the plasmid DNA includes unmethylated CpG nucleotides (typical of bacterial DNA) that act as adjuvants.

Double-negative thymocyte. A subset of developing T cells in the thymus that express neither CD4 nor CD8. Most double-negative thymocytes are at an early developmental stage and do not express antigen receptors. They will later express both CD4 and CD8 during the intermediate "double-positive" stage before further maturation to single-positive T cells expressing only CD4 or only CD8.

Double-positive thymocyte. A subset of developing T cells in the thymus, at an intermediate developmental stage, that express both CD4 and CD8. Double-positive thymocytes also express T cell receptors and are subject to selection processes, the survivors of which mature to single-positive T cells expressing only CD4 or only CD8.

Effector cells. The cells that perform effector functions during an immune response, such as secreting cytokines (e.g., helper T cells), killing microbes (e.g., macrophages, neutrophils, eosinophils), killing microbe-infected host cells (e.g., cytotoxic T lymphocytes), or secreting antibodies (e.g., differentiated B cells).

Endosome. An intracellular membrane-bound vesicle into which extracellular proteins are internalized during antigen processing. Endosomes have an acidic pH and contain proteolytic enzymes that degrade proteins into peptides that bind to class II major histocompatibility complex (MHC) molecules. A subset of class II MHC–rich endosomes, called MIIC, play a special role in antigen processing and presentation by the class II pathway.

Endotoxin. A component of the cell wall of Gram negative bacteria, also called lipopolysaccharide, that is released from dying bacteria and that stimulates many innate immune responses, including the secretion of cytokines and induction of microbicidal activities of macrophages and the expression of adhesion molecules for leukocytes on endothelium. Endotoxin contains both lipid components and carbohydrate (polysaccharide) moieties.

Endotoxin shock. See **Septic shock.**

Envelope glycoprotein (Env). A membrane glycoprotein encoded by a retrovirus that is expressed on the plasma membrane of infected cells and on the host cell–derived membrane coat of viral particles. Env proteins often are required for viral infectivity. The Env proteins of human immunodeficiency virus include gp41 and gp120, which bind to CD4 and chemokine receptors on human T cells and mediate fusion of the viral and T cell membranes.

Enzyme-linked immunosorbent assay (ELISA). A method for quantifying an antigen immobilized on a solid surface using a specific antibody with a covalently coupled enzyme. The amount of antibody that binds the antigen is proportional to the amount of antigen present and is determined by spectrophotometrically measuring the conversion of a clear substrate to a colored product by the coupled enzyme.

Eosinophil. A bone marrow–derived granulocyte that is abundant in the inflammatory infiltrates of immediate hypersensitivity late phase reactions and that contributes to many of the pathologic processes in allergic diseases. Eosinophils are important in defense against extracellular parasites, such as helminths.

Epitope. The specific portion of a macromolecular antigen to which an antibody binds. In the case of a protein antigen recognized by a T cell, an epitope is the peptide portion that is recognized by a TCR when it is displayed bound to a major histocompatibility complex molecule. It is synonymous with **determinant.**

Epstein-Barr virus (EBV). A double-stranded DNA virus of the herpesvirus family that is the etiologic agent of infectious mononucleosis and is associated with some B cell malignancies and nasopharyngeal carcinoma. EBV infects B lymphocytes and some epithelial cells by specifically binding to the complement receptor type 2 (CR2 or CD21).

F(ab′)₂ fragment. A proteolytic fragment of an IgG molecule that includes two complete light chains but only the variable domain, first constant domain, and hinge region of the two heavy chains. F(ab′)₂ fragments retain the entire bivalent antigen-binding region of an intact IgG but cannot bind complement or IgG Fc receptors. They are used in research and therapeutic applications when antigen binding is desired without antibody effector functions.

Fab fragment. A proteolytic fragment of an IgG antibody molecule that includes one complete light chain paired with one heavy chain fragment containing the variable domain and only the first constant domain. An Fab fragment retains the ability to bind an antigen but cannot interact with IgG Fc receptors on cells, or with complement. Therefore, Fab preparations are used in research and therapeutic applications when antigen binding is desired without activation of effector functions. (An Fab′ fragment retains the hinge region of the heavy chain.)

Fas. A member of the tumor necrosis factor receptor family that is expressed on the surface of T cells and many other cell types and that initiates a signaling cascade leading to the apoptotic death of the cell. The death pathway is initiated when Fas binds to Fas ligand expressed on activated T cells. Fas-mediated killing of self-reactive B cells and/or T cells, called activation-induced cell death, is postulated to be important for the maintenance of self-tolerance. Mutations in the *Fas* gene cause systemic autoimmune disease in mice and humans, called the autoimmune lymphoproliferative syndrome (ALPS). Also called CD95.

Fas ligand. A membrane protein that is a member of the tumor necrosis factor family of proteins that is expressed on activated T cells. Fas ligand binds to Fas, thereby stimulating a signaling pathway leading to apoptotic death of the Fas-expressing cell. Mutations in the Fas ligand gene, like mutations in Fas, cause systemic autoimmune disease in mice.

Fc (fragment crystalline). A proteolytic fragment of antibody that contains only the disulfide-linked carboxy-terminal regions of the two heavy chains. The Fc region mediates effector functions by binding to cell surface receptors of phagocytes and natural killer cells or the C1 complement protein. (Fc fragments are so named because they tend to crystallize out of solution.)

Fc receptor (FcR). A cell surface receptor specific for the carboxy-terminal constant region of an immunoglobulin (Ig) molecule. Fc receptors typically are multichain protein complexes that include Ig-binding components and signaling components. There are several types of Fc receptors, including those specific for different IgG isotypes, IgE, and IgA. Fc receptors mediate many of the effector functions of antibodies, including phagocytosis of antibody-coated (opsonized) microbes, antigen-induced activation of mast cells, and activation of natural killer cells.

FcεRI. A high-affinity receptor for the carboxy-terminal constant region of IgE molecules that is expressed on mast cells and basophils. FcεRI molecules on mast cells usually are occupied by IgE, and antigen-induced cross-linking of these IgE-FcεRI complexes activates the mast cell and initiates immediate hypersensitivity reactions.

Fcγ receptor (FcγR). A specific cell surface receptor for the carboxy-terminal constant region of IgG molecules. There are several different types of Fcγ receptors, including the high-affinity FcγRI, which mediates phagocytosis by macrophages and neutrophils; the low-affinity FcγRIIb, which transduces inhibitory signals in B cells; and the low-affinity FcγRIIIB, which mediates targeting and activation of natural killer cells.

Flow cytometry. A method of analysis of the phenotype of cell populations requiring a specialized instrument (flow cytometer) that can detect fluorescence on individual cells in a suspension and thereby determine the number of cells expressing the molecule to which a fluorescent probe binds. Suspensions of cells are incubated with fluorescently labeled antibodies or other probes, and the amount of probe bound by each cell in the population is measured by passing the cells one at a time through a fluorimeter with a laser-generated incident beam.

Fluorescence-activated cell sorter (FACS). An adaptation of the flow cytometer that is used for the purification of cells from a mixed population, depending on which and how much fluorescent probe the cells bind. Cells are first stained with fluorescently labeled probe, such as an antibody specific for a surface antigen of a cell population. The cells are then passed one at a time through a fluorimeter with a laser-generated incident beam and are differentially deflected by electromagnetic fields whose strength and direction are varied according to the measured intensity of the fluorescence signal.

Follicle. See **Lymphoid follicle.**

Follicular dendritic cells. Cells found in lymphoid follicles that express complement receptors, Fc receptors, and CD40 ligand and have long cytoplasmic processes that form a meshwork that is integral to the architecture of the lymphoid follicles. Follicular dendritic cells display antigens on their surface for recognition by B cells and are involved in the activation and selection of B cells expressing high-affinity membrane immunoglobulin during the process of affinity maturation.

Foxp3. A forkhead family transcription factor that is expressed in, and required for, the development of natural regulatory T cells. Genetic deficiencies in FoxP3 result in severe autoimmune disease.

G proteins. Proteins that bind guanyl nucleotides and act as exchange molecules, catalyzing the replacement of bound GDP by GTP. G proteins with bound GTP can activate a variety of cellular enzymes in different signaling cascades. Trimeric GTP-binding proteins are associated with the cytoplasmic portions of many cell surface receptors, such as chemokine receptors. Other small soluble G proteins, such as Ras and Raf, are recruited into signaling pathways by adapter proteins.

GATA3. A transcription factor that promotes the differentiation of T_H2 cells from naive T cells.

Generative lymphoid organs. Organs in which lymphocytes develop from immature precursors. The bone marrow and thymus are the major generative lymphoid organs in which B cells and T cells develop, respectively.

Germinal center. A central, light-staining region within a lymphoid follicle in spleen, lymph node, or mucosal lymphoid tissue that forms during T cell–dependent humoral immune responses and is the site of B cell affinity maturation.

Glomerulonephritis. Inflammation of the renal glomeruli, often initiated by immunopathologic mechanisms, such as deposition of circulating antigen-antibody complexes in the glomerular basement membrane or binding of antibodies to antigens expressed in the glomerulus. The antibodies can activate complement and phagocytes, and the resulting inflammatory response can lead to renal failure.

Graft. A tissue or organ that is removed from one site and is placed in another site, usually in a different individual.

Graft arteriosclerosis. Occlusion of graft arteries due to proliferation of intimal smooth muscle cells. This process is evident within 6 months to 1 year after transplantation and is responsible for chronic rejection of vascularized organ grafts. The mechanism is likely to be a result of a chronic immune response to vessel wall alloantigens. It also is called accelerated arteriosclerosis.

Graft rejection. A specific immune response to an organ or tissue graft that leads to inflammation, damage, and possibly graft failure.

Graft-versus-host disease. A disease occurring in bone marrow transplant recipients that is caused by the reaction of mature T cells in the marrow graft against alloantigens on host cells. The disease most often affects skin, liver, and intestines.

Granulocyte colony-stimulating factor (G-CSF). A cytokine made by activated T cells, macrophages, and endothelial cells at sites of infection that acts on bone marrow to increase production of and mobilize neutrophils to replace those consumed in inflammatory reactions.

Granulocyte-monocyte colony-stimulating factor (GM-CSF). A cytokine made by activated T cells, macrophages, endothelial cells, and bone marrow stromal fibroblasts that acts on progenitors in the bone marrow to increase production of neutrophils and monocytes.

Granuloma. A nodule of inflammatory tissue composed of clusters of activated macrophages and T lymphocytes, often with associated necrosis and fibrosis. Granulomatous inflammation is a form of chronic delayed-type hypersensitivity, often occurring in response to persistent microbes, such as *Mycobacterium tuberculosis* and some fungi, or in response to particulate antigens that are not readily phagocytosed.

Granzyme. A serine protease enzyme found in the granules of cytotoxic T lymphocytes and natural killer cells that is released by exocytosis, enters target cells, mainly through perforin-created "holes," and proteolytically cleaves and activates caspases, which in turn cleave several substrates and induce target cell apoptosis.

H-2 molecule. A major histocompatibility complex (MHC) molecule in the mouse. The mouse MHC originally was called the H-2 locus.

Haplotype. The set of major histocompatibility complex alleles inherited from one parent and therefore located on one chromosome.

Hapten. A small chemical that can bind to an antibody but must be attached to a macromolecule (carrier) to stimulate an adaptive immune response specific for that chemical. For example, immunization with dinitrophenol

(DNP) alone does not stimulate an anti-DNP antibody response, but immunization with the DNP hapten attached to a protein does stimulate anti-DNP antibody production.

Heavy chain. See **Immunoglobulin (Ig) heavy chain.**

Heavy chain class (isotype) switching. The process by which a B lymphocyte changes the isotype of the antibodies it produces, from IgM to IgG, IgE, or IgA, without changing the specificity of the antibody. Heavy chain class switching is regulated by helper T cell cytokines and CD40 ligand and involves recombination of heavy chain VDJ segments with downstream constant region gene segments.

Helminth. A parasitic worm. Helminthic infections often elicit T$_H$2 responses with eosinophil-rich inflammatory infiltrates and IgE production.

Helper T lymphocytes. The functional subset of T lymphocytes whose main effector functions are to activate macrophages in cell-mediated immune responses and promote B cell antibody production in humoral immune responses. These effector functions are mediated by secreted cytokines and by T cell CD40 ligand binding to macrophage or B cell CD40. Most helper T cells express the CD4 molecule.

Hematopoiesis. The development of mature blood cells, including erythrocytes, leukocytes, and platelets, from pluripotential stem cells in the bone marrow and fetal liver. Hematopoiesis is regulated by several different cytokines produced by bone marrow stromal cells, T cells, and other cell types.

High endothelial venule (HEV). Specialized venules that are the sites of lymphocyte extravasation from the blood into the stroma of a peripheral lymph node or mucosal lymphoid tissues. HEVs are lined by plump endothelial cells that protrude into the vessel lumen and express unique adhesion molecules involved in binding naive T cells.

Hinge region. A region of immunoglobulin heavy chains between the first two constant domains that can assume multiple conformations, thereby imparting a flexibility in the orientation of the two antigen-binding sites. Because of the hinge region, an antibody molecule can simultaneously bind two epitopes that are anywhere within reach of one another.

Histamine. A vasoactive amine, stored in the granules of mast cells, that is one of the important mediators of immediate hypersensitivity. Histamine binds to specific receptors in various tissues and causes increased vascular permeability and contraction of bronchial and intestinal smooth muscle.

HLA. See **Human leukocyte antigens (HLA).**

HLA-DM (also called DM). A peptide exchange molecule that plays a critical role in the class II major histocompatibility complex (MHC) pathway of antigen presentation. HLA-DM is found in the specialized MIIC endosomal compartment and facilitates the removal of the class II–associated invariant chain peptide (CLIP) and the binding of other peptides to class II MHC molecules. HLA-DM is encoded by a gene in the MHC and is structurally similar to class II MHC molecules, but it is not polymorphic. Called H-2M in the mouse.

Homeostasis. In the adaptive immune system, the maintenance of a constant number and diverse repertoire of lymphocytes, despite the emergence of new lymphocytes and tremendous expansions of individual clones that may occur during responses to microbial antigens. Homeostasis is achieved by regulated pathways of lymphocyte production, death and inactivation.

Homing of lymphocytes. The directed migration of subsets of circulating lymphocytes into particular tissue sites. Lymphocyte homing is regulated by the selective expression of adhesion molecules, called homing receptors, on the lymphocytes and the tissue-specific expression of endothelial ligands for these homing receptors, called addressins, in different vascular beds. For example, some T lymphocytes preferentially home to intestinal lymphoid tissue (e.g., Peyer's patches), and this is regulated by binding of the $\alpha_4\beta_1$ integrin on the T cells to the MAdCAM (mucosal addressin cell adhesion molecule) on Peyer's patch endothelium.

Homing receptor. Adhesion molecules expressed on the surface of lymphocytes that are responsible for the different pathways of lymphocyte recirculation and tissue homing. Homing receptors bind to ligands (called addressins) expressed on endothelial cells in particular vascular beds.

Human immunodeficiency virus (HIV). The etiologic agent of acquired immunodeficiency syndrome (AIDS). HIV is a retrovirus that infects a variety of cell types, including CD4-expressing helper T cells, macrophages, and dendritic cells, and causes a chronic progressive destruction of the immune system.

Human leukocyte antigen (HLA). Major histocompatibility complex (MHC) molecule expressed on the surface of human cells. Human MHC molecules were first identified as alloantigens on the surface of white blood cells (leukocytes) that bound serum antibodies from people previously exposed to cells from another person (e.g., mother, transfusion recipient).

Humanized antibody. A monoclonal antibody encoded by a recombinant hybrid gene and composed of the antigen-binding sites from a murine monoclonal antibody and the constant region of a human antibody. Humanized antibodies are less likely than mouse monoclonal antibodies to induce an anti-antibody response in humans; they are used clinically in the treatment of tumors and various inflammatory diseases.

Humoral immunity. The type of adaptive immune response mediated by antibodies that are produced by plasma cells. Humoral immunity is the principal defense mechanism against extracellular microbes and their toxins.

Hybridoma. A cell line derived by cell fusion, or somatic cell hybridization, between a normal lymphocyte and an immortalized lymphocyte tumor line. B cell hybridomas, created by fusion of normal B cells of defined antigen specificity with a myeloma cell line, are used to produce monoclonal antibodies. T cell hybridomas, created by fusion of a normal T cell of defined specificity with a T cell tumor line, commonly are used in research.

Hyperacute rejection. A form of allograft or xenograft rejection that begins within minutes to hours after transplantation and is characterized by thrombotic occlusion of the graft vessels. Hyperacute rejection is mediated by preexisting antibodies in the host circulation that bind to donor endothelial antigens such as blood group antigens or major histocompatibility complex (MHC) molecules.

Hypersensitivity diseases. Disorders caused by immune responses. Hypersensitivity diseases include autoimmune diseases, in which immune responses are directed against self antigens, and diseases that result from uncontrolled or excessive responses against foreign antigens, such as microbes and allergens. The tissue damage that occurs in hypersensitivity diseases is the result of the same effector mechanisms used by the immune system to protect against microbes.

Hypervariable region. Short segments of about 10 amino acid residues within the variable regions of antibody or T cell receptor (TCR) proteins, which form loop structures that contact antigen. There are three hypervariable regions, also called **complementarity-determining regions**, in each antibody heavy chain and light chain and in each TCR α and β chain. Most of the variability between different antibodies or TCRs is located within these regions.

Idiotope. A unique determinant on an antibody or T cell receptor molecule, usually formed by one or more of the hypervariable regions. Idiotopes may be recognized as "foreign" in an individual because they usually are present in quantities too low to induce self-tolerance.

Idiotype. The unique structures present in the antigen-binding regions of the antibodies or T cell receptors produced by a single clone of lymphocytes. A theory called

the *network hypothesis* postulates that a network of complementary interactions involving idiotypes and anti-idiotypes reach a steady state at which the immune system is at homeostasis, and that antigen perturbs this steady state. The importance of such a network has not been established.

Igα and Igβ. Proteins that are required for surface expression and signaling functions of membrane immunoglobulin (Ig) on B cells. Igα and Igβ pairs are disulfide-linked to one another and noncovalently associated with the cytoplasmic tail of membrane Ig, forming the B cell receptor complex. The cytoplasmic domains of Igα and Igβ contain immunoreceptor tyrosine-based activation motifs (ITAMs) that are involved in early signaling events during antigen-induced B cell activation.

Immature B lymphocyte. A membrane IgM+, IgD+ B cell, recently derived from marrow precursors, that does not proliferate or differentiate in response to antigens but rather may undergo apoptotic death or become functionally unresponsive. Immature B cells that are specific for self antigens present in the bone marrow are negatively selected by encounter with these antigens and do not complete their maturation.

Immediate hypersensitivity. The type of immune reaction responsible for allergic diseases and dependent on IgE plus antigen-mediated stimulation of tissue mast cells and basophils. The mast cells and basophils release mediators that cause increased vascular permeability, vasodilation, bronchial and visceral smooth muscle contraction, and inflammation.

Immune complex. A complex of one or more antibody molecules with bound antigen. Because each antibody molecule has a minimum of two antigen-binding sites and many antigens contain multiple epitopes, immune complexes can vary greatly in size. Immune complexes activate effector mechanisms of humoral immunity, such as the classical complement pathway and Fc receptor–mediated phagocyte activation. Deposition of circulating immune complexes in blood vessel walls, renal glomeruli, and joint synovia can lead to inflammation and disease.

Immune complex disease. An inflammatory disease caused by deposition of antigen-antibody complexes in blood vessel walls, resulting in local complement activation and phagocyte recruitment. Immune complexes may form because of overproduction of antibodies to microbial antigens or because of autoantibody production in the setting of an autoimmune disease such as systemic lupus erythematosus. Immune complex deposition in arteries, kidney glomeruli, and joint synovia may cause vasculitis, glomerulonephritis, and arthritis, respectively.

Immune-privileged site. A site in the body that is inaccessible to, or actively suppresses, immune responses. The anterior chamber of the eye, the testes, and the brain are examples of immune-privileged sites.

Immune response. A collective and coordinated response to the introduction of foreign substances in an individual mediated by the cells and molecules of the immune system.

Immune surveillance. The concept that a physiologic function of the immune system is to recognize and destroy clones of transformed cells before they grow into tumors and to kill tumors after they are formed. This term sometimes is used in a general sense to describe the function of T lymphocytes in detecting and destroying any cell, not necessarily a tumor cell, that is expressing a foreign antigen (e.g., if it is infected with an intracellular microbe).

Immune system. The molecules, cells, tissues, and organs that collectively function to provide immunity, or protection, against infectious pathogens.

Immunodominant epitope. The portion of an antigen that is recognized by a majority of the lymphocytes specific for that antigen. For T cells, immunodominant epitopes correspond to the peptides generated within antigen-presenting cells that bind most avidly to major histocompatibility complex (MHC) molecules and are most likely to stimulate T cells.

Immunofluorescence. A technique in which a molecule is detected using an antibody labeled with a fluorescent probe. For example, in immunofluorescence microscopy, cells that express a particular surface antigen can be stained with a fluorescein-conjugated antibody specific for the antigen and then visualized under a fluorescent microscope.

Immunogen. An antigen that induces an immune response. Not all antigens are immunogens. For example, small-molecular-weight compounds (haptens) may not stimulate an immune response unless they are linked to macromolecules.

Immunoglobulin. Synonymous with **antibody**.

Immunoglobulin (Ig) domain. A three-dimensional globular structural motif found in many proteins in the immune system, including immunoglobulins, T cell receptors, and major histocompatibility complex molecules. Ig domains are about 110 amino acid residues in length, include an internal disulfide bond, and contain two layers of β-pleated sheet, each layer composed of three to five strands of antiparallel polypeptide chain.

Immunoglobulin (Ig) heavy chain. One of two types of polypeptide chains that compose an antibody molecule. The basic structural unit of an antibody includes two identical, disulfide-linked heavy chains and two identical light chains. Each heavy chain is composed of a variable (V) Ig domain and three or four constant (C) Ig domains. The different antibody isotypes, including IgM, IgD, IgG, IgA, and IgE, are distinguished by structural differences in their heavy chain constant regions. The heavy chain constant regions also mediate effector functions, such as complement activation and engagement of phagocytes.

Immunoglobulin (Ig) light chain. One of two types of polypeptide chains that compose an antibody molecule. The basic structural unit of an antibody includes two identical light chains, each disulfide-linked to one of two identical heavy chains. Each light chain is composed of one variable (V) Ig domain and one constant (C) Ig domain. There are two light chain isotypes, called κ and λ, both functionally identical. About 60% of human antibodies have κ light chains and 40% have λ light chains.

Immunoglobulin (Ig) superfamily. A large family of proteins that contain a globular structural motif called an immunoglobulin (Ig) domain, or Ig fold, originally described in antibodies. Many proteins of importance in the immune system are members of this superfamily, including antibodies, T cell receptors, major histocompatibility complex molecules, CD4, and CD8.

Immunohistochemistry. A technique used to detect the presence of an antigen in histologic tissue sections using an enzyme-coupled antibody that is specific for the antigen. The enzyme converts a colorless substrate to a colored insoluble substance that precipitates at the site where the antibody, and thus the antigen, are localized. The position of the colored precipitate, and therefore the antigen, in the tissue section is observed by conventional light microscopy. Immunohistochemistry is a routine technique in diagnostic pathology and in various fields of research.

Immunoperoxidase. A common immunohistochemical technique in which a horseradish peroxidase–coupled antibody is used to identify the presence of an antigen in a tissue section. The peroxidase enzyme converts a colorless substrate to an insoluble brown product that is observable by light microscopy.

Immunoprecipitation. A technique for the isolation of a molecule from a solution by binding it to an antibody and then rendering the antigen-antibody complex insoluble, either by precipitation with a second anti-antibody or by coupling the first antibody to an insoluble particle or bead.

Immunoreceptor tyrosine-based activation motif (ITAM). A conserved motif composed of two copies of the sequence tyrosine-X-X-leucine (where X is an unspecified amino acid) found in the cytoplasmic tails of various membrane proteins in the immune system that are involved in signal transduction. ITAMs are present in the ζ and CD3 proteins of the T cell receptor complex, in the Igα and Igβ proteins in the B cell receptor complex, and in signaling subunits of several Ig Fc receptors. When these receptors bind their ligands, the tyrosine residues of the ITAMs become phosphorylated, forming docking sites for other molecules involved in propagating cell-activating signal transduction pathways.

Immunoreceptor tyrosine-based inhibition motif (ITIM). A 6-amino-acid (isoleucine-X-tyrosine-X-X-leucine, where X is an unspecified amino acid) motif found in the cytoplasmic tails of various inhibitory receptors in the immune system, including FcγRIIB on B cells, and the killer inhibitory receptor on natural killer cells. When these receptors bind their ligands, the ITIMs become phosphorylated on their tyrosine residues, forming a docking site for protein tyrosine phosphatases, which in turn function to inhibit other signal transduction pathways.

Immunosuppression. Inhibition of one or more components of the adaptive or the innate immune system, resulting from an underlying disease or intentionally induced by drugs for the purpose of preventing or treating graft rejection or autoimmune disease. A commonly used immunosuppressive drug is cyclosporine, which blocks T cell cytokine production.

Immunotherapy. The treatment of a disease using therapeutic agents that promote immune responses. Cancer immunotherapy, for example, involves promoting active immune responses to tumor antigens or administering antitumor antibodies or T cells to establish passive immunity.

Immunotoxins. Reagents that may be used in the treatment of cancer that consist of covalent conjugates of a potent cellular toxin, such as ricin or diphtheria toxin, with antibodies specific for antigens expressed on the surface of tumor cells. It is hoped that such reagents can specifically target and kill tumor cells without damaging normal cells, but safe and effective immunotoxins have yet to be developed.

Inbred mouse strain. A strain of mice created by repetitive mating of siblings, characterized by homozygosity at every genetic locus. Every mouse of an inbred strain is genetically identical (syngeneic) to every other mouse of the same strain.

Indirect antigen presentation. In transplantation immunology, a pathway of presentation of donor (allogeneic) major histocompatibility complex (MHC) molecules by recipient antigen-presenting cells (APCs) involving the same mechanisms used to present microbial proteins. The allogeneic MHC proteins are processed by recipient pro-

fessional APCs, and peptides derived from the allogeneic MHC molecules are presented, in association with recipient (self) MHC molecules, to host T cells. This is in contrast with direct antigen presentation, which involves recipient T cell recognition of unprocessed allogeneic MHC molecules on the surface of graft cells.

Inflammation. A complex reaction of the innate immune system in vascularized tissues that involves accumulation and activation of leukocytes and plasma proteins at a site of infection, toxin exposure, or cell injury. Inflammation is initiated by changes in blood vessels that promote leukocyte recruitment and movement of fluid and plasma proteins into tissue. Local adaptive immune responses can promote inflammation. Although inflammation serves a protective function in controlling infections and promoting tissue repair, it also can cause tissue damage and disease.

Inflammatory bowel disease (IBD). A group of disorders, including ulcerative colitis and Crohn's disease, characterized by chronic inflammation in the gastrointestinal tract. The etiology of IBD is not known, but there is evidence that immune mechanisms may be involved: IBD develops in gene knockout mice lacking the interleukins IL-2 or IL-10 or the T cell receptor α chain.

Innate immunity. Protection against infections that relies on mechanisms that exist before infection, are capable of rapid responses to microbes, and react in essentially the same way to repeat infections. The innate immune system includes epithelial barriers; phagocytic cells (neutrophils, macrophages); natural killer cells; the complement system; and cytokines, largely made by mononuclear phagocytes, that regulate and coordinate many of the activities of the cells of innate immunity.

Insulin-dependent diabetes mellitus (IDDM). A disease, also called type 1 diabetes, characterized by a lack of insulin, which leads to various metabolic and vascular abnormalities. The insulin deficiency results from destruction of the insulin-producing β cells of the islets of Langerhans in the pancreas, usually a result of T cell–mediated autoimmunity.

Integrins. Heterodimeric cell surface proteins whose major functions are to mediate adhesion of leukocytes to other leukocytes, endothelial cells, and extracellular matrix proteins. Integrins are important for T cell interactions with antigen-presenting cells and for migration of leukocytes from blood into tissues. The ligand-binding affinity of the integrins can be regulated by various stimuli, and the cytoplasmic domains of integrins bind to the cytoskeleton. There are two subfamilies of integrins, and the members of each family express a conserved β chain (β_1, or CD18, and β_2, or CD29) associated with different α

chains. VLA-4 is a β_1 integrin expressed on T cells, and LFA-1 is a β_2 integrin expressed on T cells and phagocytes.

Interferon-γ (IFN-γ). A cytokine produced by T lymphocytes and natural killer cells whose principal function is to activate macrophages in both innate immune responses and adaptive cell-mediated immune responses. (In the past, IFN-γ also was called immune or type II interferon.)

Interleukin. Another name for a cytokine that acts on leukocytes, originally used to describe a cytokine made by leukocytes. It is now generally used with a numerical suffix to designate a structurally defined cytokine regardless of source or target.

Interleukin-1 (IL-1). A cytokine produced mainly by activated mononuclear phagocytes whose principal function is to mediate host inflammatory responses in innate immunity. There are two forms of IL-1 (α and β) that bind to the same receptors and have identical biologic effects, including induction of endothelial cell adhesion molecules, stimulation of chemokine production by endothelial cells and macrophages, stimulation of synthesis of acute-phase reactants by the liver, and fever.

Interleukin-10 (IL-10). A cytokine produced by activated macrophages and some helper T cells whose major function is to inhibit activated macrophages and therefore maintain homeostatic control of innate and cell-mediated immune reactions.

Interleukin-12 (IL-12). A cytokine produced by mononuclear phagocytes and dendritic cells that serves as a mediator of the innate immune response to intracellular microbes and is a key inducer of cell-mediated immune responses to these microbes. IL-12 activates natural killer (NK) cells, promotes interferon-γ production by NK cells and T cells, enhances cytolytic activity of NK cells and cytotoxic T lymphocytes, and promotes the development of T_H1 cells.

Interleukin-15 (IL-15). A cytokine produced by mononuclear phagocytes and other cells in response to viral infections whose principal function is to stimulate the proliferation of natural killer cells. It is structurally similar to IL-2.

Interleukin-17 (IL-17). A cytokine produced mainly by the T_H17 subset of CD4+ helper T cells, which promotes inflammatory responses that are protective against certain bacterial infections and are implicated in the pathogenesis of several autoimmune diseases.

Interleukin-18 (IL-18). A cytokine produced by macrophages in response to lipopolysaccharide (LPS) and other microbial products, which functions together with IL-12 as an inducer of cell-mediated immunity. IL-18 synergizes with IL-12 in stimulating the production of interferon-γ by natural killer cells and T cells. IL-18 is structurally homologous to, but is functionally very different from, IL-1.

Interleukin-2 (IL-2). A cytokine produced by antigen-activated T cells that acts in an autocrine manner to stimulate effector T cell proliferation and also promotes regulatory T cell growth and survival. Thus, IL-2 is required for both induction and regulation of T cell–mediated immune responses. IL-2 also stimulates proliferation and differentiation of natural killer cells and B cells.

Interleukin-3 (IL-3). A cytokine produced by CD4+ T cells that promotes the expansion of immature marrow progenitors of all blood cells. IL-3 also is known as multilineage colony-stimulating factor (multi-CSF).

Interleukin-4 (IL-4). A cytokine produced mainly by the T_H2 subset of CD4+ helper T cells whose functions include inducing differentiation of T_H2 cells from naive CD4+ precursors, stimulation of IgE production by B cells, and suppression of interferon-γ–dependent macrophage functions.

Interleukin-5 (IL-5). A cytokine produced by CD4+ T_H2 cells and activated mast cells that stimulates the growth and differentiation of eosinophils and activates mature eosinophils.

Interleukin-6 (IL-6). A cytokine produced by many cell types, including activated mononuclear phagocytes, endothelial cells, and fibroblasts, that functions in both innate and adaptive immunity. IL-6 stimulates the synthesis of acute phase proteins by hepatocytes and stimulates the growth of antibody-producing B lymphocytes.

Interleukin-7 (IL-7). A cytokine secreted by bone marrow stromal cells that stimulates survival and expansion of immature precursors of B and T lymphocytes.

Intracellular bacterium. A bacterium that survives and replicates within cells, usually in phagolysosomes. The principal defense against intracellular bacteria, such as *Mycobacterium tuberculosis*, is cell-mediated immunity.

Intraepidermal lymphocyte. T lymphocytes found within the epidermal layer of the skin. In the mouse, most of the intraepidermal T cells express the γδ form of T cell receptor. (See **Intraepithelial T lymphocytes.**)

Intraepithelial T lymphocytes. T lymphocytes that are present in the epidermis of the skin and in mucosal epithelia that typically express a very limited diversity of antigen receptors. Some of these lymphocytes may recognize microbial products, such as glycolipids, associated with nonpolymorphic class I major histocompatibility complex–like molecules. Intraepithelial T lymphocytes may be considered effector cells of innate immunity and function in host defense by secreting cytokines and activating phagocytes and by killing infected cells.

Invariant chain (I$_i$). A nonpolymorphic protein that binds to newly synthesized class II major histocompatibility complex (MHC) molecules in the endoplasmic reticulum (ER). The invariant chain prevents loading of the class II MHC peptide-binding cleft with peptides present in the ER, leaving such peptides to bind to class I molecules. The invariant chain also promotes folding and assembly of class II molecules and directs newly formed class II molecules to the specialized endosomal MIIC compartment in which peptide loading takes place.

Isotype. A type of antibody determined by which of five different forms of heavy chain is present. Antibody isotypes include IgM, IgD, IgG, IgA, and IgE, and each isotype performs a different set of effector functions. Additional structural variations characterize distinct subtypes of IgG and IgA.

J chain. A protein produced in mature B cells that binds to secreted forms of IgM and IgA molecules and brings together five and two of these molecules, respectively. (Not to be confused with the J segment of antigen receptor genes.)

Joining (J) segments. Short coding sequences, between the variable (V) and constant (C) gene segments in all immunoglobulin and T cell receptor loci, that together with D segments are somatically recombined with V segments during lymphocyte development. The resulting recombined V(D)J DNA codes for antigen receptor V regions.

Junctional diversity. The diversity in the antibody and T cell receptor repertoires that is attributed to the random addition or the removal of nucleotide sequences at junctions between V, D, and J gene segments.

Killer cell immunoglobulin-like receptors (KIRs). Receptors on natural killer cells that recognize self class I major histocompatibility complex (MHC) molecules and deliver inhibitory signals that prevent activation of natural killer (NK) cell cytolytic mechanisms. These receptors ensure that NK cells do not kill normal host cells, which express class I MHC molecules, while permitting lysis of virus-infected cells in which class I MHC expression is suppressed.

Kinase (protein kinase). An enzyme that adds phosphate groups to the side chains of certain amino acid residues of proteins. Protein kinases in lymphocytes, such as Lck, are involved in signal transduction and the activation of transcription factors. Most protein kinases are specific for tyrosine residues.

Knockout mice. Mice with a targeted disruption of one or more genes, created by homologous recombination techniques. Knockout mice lacking functional genes encoding cytokines, cell surface receptors, signaling molecules, and transcription factors have provided extensive information about the roles of these molecules in the immune system.

Langerhans cells. Immature dendritic cells found as a continuous meshwork in the epidermal layer of the skin, whose major function is to trap and transport protein antigens to draining lymph nodes. During their migration to the lymph nodes, Langerhans cells mature into lymph node dendritic cells that can efficiently process and present antigen to naive T cells.

Large granular lymphocyte (LGL). Another name for a natural killer (NK) cell based on the morphologic appearance of this cell type in the blood.

Late phase reaction. A component of the immediate hypersensitivity reaction that ensues several hours after mast cell and basophil degranulation and is characterized by an inflammatory infiltrate of eosinophils, basophils, neutrophils, and lymphocytes. Repeated bouts of late phase reactions can cause tissue damage.

Lck. An Src family nonreceptor tyrosine kinase that noncovalently associates with the cytoplasmic tails of CD4 and CD8 molecules in T cells and is involved in the early signaling events of antigen-induced T cell activation. Lck mediates tyrosine phosphorylation of the cytoplasmic tails of CD3 and ζ proteins of the T cell receptor complex.

Lectin pathway of complement activation. A pathway of complement activation triggered, in the absence of antibody, by the binding of microbial polysaccharides to circulating lectins like plasma mannose-binding lectin (MBL). MBL is structurally similar to C1q and activates the C1r-C1s enzyme complex (like C1q) or activates another serine esterase, called mannose-binding protein–associated serine esterase. The remaining steps of the lectin pathway, beginning with cleavage of C4, are the same as the classical pathway.

Leishmania. An obligate intracellular protozoal parasite that infects macrophages and can cause a chronic inflammatory disease involving many tissues. *Leishmania* infection in mice has served as a model system for the study of the effector functions of several cytokines and the helper T cell subsets that produce them. T$_H$1 responses to *Leishmania major* and associated interferon-γ production control infection, whereas T$_H$2 responses with IL-4 production lead to disseminated lethal disease.

Leukemia. A malignancy of bone marrow precursors of blood cells. Large numbers of leukemic cells usually occupy the bone marrow and often circulate in the blood stream. Lymphocytic leukemias are derived from B or T cell precursors, myelogenous leukemias are derived from granulocyte or monocyte precursors, and erythroid leukemias are derived from red blood cell precursors.

Leukocyte adhesion deficiency (LAD). A rare group of immunodeficiency diseases caused by defective expression of leukocyte adhesion molecules required for tissue recruitment of phagocytes and lymphocytes. LAD I is due to mutations in the gene encoding the CD18 protein, which is part of β_2 integrins. LAD II is caused by mutations in a gene that encodes an enzyme involved in the synthesis of leukocyte ligands for endothelial selectins.

Leukotrienes. A class of arachidonic acid–derived lipid inflammatory mediators produced by the lipoxygenase pathway in many cell types. Mast cells make abundant leukotriene C_4 (LTC$_4$) and its degradation products LTD$_4$ and LTE$_4$, which bind to specific receptors on smooth muscle cells and cause prolonged bronchoconstriction. Leukotrienes contribute to the pathology of bronchial asthma. Collectively, LTC$_4$, LTD$_4$, and LTE$_4$ constitute what was once called "slow-reacting substance of anaphylaxis."

Lipopolysaccharide (LPS). Synonymous with **endotoxin.**

Lymph node. Small nodular, encapsulated aggregates of lymphocyte-rich tissue situated along lymphatic channels throughout the body, where adaptive immune responses to lymph-borne antigens are initiated.

Lymphatic system. A system of vessels throughout the body that collects tissue fluid called lymph, originally derived from the blood, and returns it, via the thoracic duct, to the circulation. Lymph nodes are interspersed along these vessels and trap and retain antigens present in the lymph.

Lymphocyte. A cell type found in the blood, lymphoid tissues, and virtually all organs, that expresses receptors for antigens and mediates immune responses. Lymphocytes include B and T cells (the cells of adaptive immunity and natural killer (NK) cells (mediators of some innate immune responses).

Lymphoid follicle. A B cell–rich region of a peripheral lymphoid organ, such as a lymph node or the spleen, that is the site of antigen-induced B cell proliferation and differentiation. In T cell–dependent B cell responses to protein antigens, a germinal center forms within the follicles.

Lymphokine. An old name for cytokines produced by T lymphocytes. It is now known that the same cytokines may be produced by other cell types.

Lymphokine activated killer (LAK) cell. Natural killer cells with enhanced cytotoxic activity for tumor cells as a result of exposure to high doses of interleukin-2. LAK cells generated in vitro have been adoptively transferred back into cancer patients to treat their tumors.

Lymphoma. A malignant tumor of B or T lymphocytes, arising in and spreading between lymphoid tissues. Lymphomas often express phenotypic characteristics of the normal lymphocytes from which they were derived.

Lymphotoxin (LT, TNF-β). A cytokine produced by T cells, which is homologous to, and binds to the same receptors as those for, tumor necrosis factor (TNF). Like TNF, LT has proinflammatory effects, including endothelial and neutrophil activation. LT also is critical for the normal development of lymphoid organs.

Lysosome. A membrane-bound, acidic organelle, abundant in phagocytic cells, that contains proteolytic enzymes that degrade proteins derived mainly from the extracellular environment. Lysosomes are involved in the class II major histocompatibility complex (MHC) pathway of antigen processing.

Macrophage. A tissue-based phagocytic cell, derived from blood monocytes, that plays important roles in innate and adaptive immune responses. Macrophages are activated by microbial products, such as endotoxin, by molecules such as CD40 ligand, and by T cell cytokines such as interferon-γ. Activated macrophages phagocytose and kill microorganisms, secrete proinflammatory cytokines, and present antigens to helper T cells. Macrophages may assume different morphologic forms in different tissues, including the microglial cells of the central nervous system, Kupffer cells in the liver, alveolar macrophages in the lung, and osteoclasts in bone.

Major histocompatibility complex (MHC). A large genetic locus (on human chromosome 6 and mouse chromosome 17) that includes the highly polymorphic genes encoding the peptide-binding molecules recognized by T lymphocytes. The MHC locus also includes genes encoding cytokines, molecules involved in antigen processing, and complement proteins.

Major histocompatibility complex (MHC) molecule. A heterodimeric membrane protein encoded in the major histocompatibility complex (MHC) locus that serves as a peptide display molecule for recognition by T lymphocytes. Two structurally distinct types of MHC molecules exist: Class I MHC molecules are present on nucleated cells, bind peptides derived from cytosolic proteins, and are recognized by CD8+ T cells. Class II MHC molecules are restricted largely to professional antigen-presenting cells, macrophages, and B lymphocytes; bind peptides derived from endocytosed proteins; and are recognized by CD4+ T cells.

Mannose receptor. A carbohydrate-binding receptor (lectin) expressed by macrophages that binds mannose and fucose residues on microbial cell walls and mediates phagocytosis of the organisms.

Marginal zone. A peripheral region of splenic lymphoid follicles that contains macrophages that are particularly efficient at trapping polysaccharide antigens. Such antigens may either persist for prolonged periods on the surfaces of marginal zone macrophages, where they are recognized by specific B cells, or they may be transported into follicles.

Marginal zone B lymphocytes. A subset of B lymphocytes, found exclusively in the marginal zone of the spleen, that respond rapidly to blood-borne microbial antigens by producing IgM antibodies with limited diversity.

Mast cell. The major effector cell of immediate hypersensitivity (allergic) reactions. Mast cells are derived from bone marrow precursors, reside in tissues adjacent to blood vessels, express a high-affinity Fc receptor for IgE, and contain numerous mediator-filled granules. Antigen-induced cross-linking of IgE bound to the mast cell Fc receptors causes release of their granule contents as well as synthesis and secretion of other mediators, and this leads to the immediate hypersensitivity reaction.

Maturation of lymphocytes. The process by which pluripotent bone marrow precursor cells develop into mature antigen receptor–expressing naive B or T lymphocytes that populate peripheral lymphoid tissues. This process takes place in the specialized environments of the bone marrow (for B cells) and the thymus (for T cells).

Mature B cell. IgM- and IgD-expressing functionally competent naive B cells that represent the final stage of B cell maturation that takes place outside the bone marrow and that populate peripheral lymphoid organs.

Membrane attack complex (MAC). A lytic complex of the terminal components of the complement cascade, including multiple copies of C9, that forms in the membranes of target cells on which complement is activated. The MAC causes lethal ionic and osmotic changes of cells.

Memory. The ability of the adaptive immune system to mount more rapid, larger, and more effective responses to repeat encounters with the same antigen.

Memory lymphocytes. B or T lymphocytes that mediate rapid and enhanced (i.e., memory) responses to second and subsequent exposures to antigens. Memory B and T cells are produced by antigen stimulation of naive lymphocytes and survive in a functionally quiescent state for many years after the antigen is eliminated.

MHC restriction. The characteristic of T lymphocytes that they recognize a foreign peptide antigen only when it is bound to a particular allelic form of a major histocompatibility complex (MHC) molecule.

β_2-Microglobulin. The light chain of a class I major histocompatibility (MHC) molecule. β_2-Microglobulin is an extracellular protein encoded by a nonpolymorphic gene outside the MHC complex and is structurally homologous to an Ig domain and is invariant among all class I molecules.

Migration of lymphocyte. The movement of lymphocytes from the bloodstream into tissues.

Mitogen-activated protein (MAP) kinase cascade. A signal transduction cascade initiated by the active form of the Ras protein and involving the sequential activation of three serine-threonine kinases, the last one being the MAP kinase. MAP kinase, in turn, phosphorylates and activates other enzymes or transcription factors. The MAP kinase pathway is one of several signal pathways activated by antigen binding to the T cell receptor.

Mixed leukocyte reaction (MLR). An in vitro reaction of alloreactive T cells from one individual against major histocompatibility complex antigens on blood cells from another individual. The MLR involves proliferation of and cytokine secretion by both CD4+ and CD8+ T cells and is used as a screening test to assess the compatibility of a potential graft recipient with a potential donor.

Molecular mimicry. A postulated mechanism of autoimmunity, which is triggered by infection with a microbe that contains antigens that cross-react with self antigens, so that immune responses to the microbe result in reactions against self tissues.

Monoclonal antibody. An antibody that is specific for one antigen and is produced by a B cell hybridoma (a cell line derived by the fusion of a single normal B cell and an immortal B cell tumor line). Monoclonal antibodies are widely employed in research and clinical diagnosis and therapy.

Monocyte. A type of bone marrow–derived circulating blood cell that is the precursor of tissue macrophages. Monocytes are actively recruited into inflammatory sites, where they differentiate into macrophages.

Monocyte colony-stimulating factor (M-CSF). A cytokine made by activated T cells, macrophages, endothelial cells, and bone marrow stromal fibroblasts that stimulates the production of monocytes from bone marrow precursor cells.

Monokines. An old name for cytokines produced by mononuclear phagocytes. It is now known that the same cytokines are produced by many cell types.

Mononuclear phagocytes. Cells with a common bone marrow lineage whose primary function is phagocytosis. These cells function as antigen-presenting cells in the recognition and activation phases of adaptive immune responses and as effector cells in innate and adaptive immunity. Mononuclear phagocytes circulate in the blood in an incompletely differentiated form called monocytes, and once they settle in tissues they mature into cells called macrophages.

Mucosal immune system. A part of the immune system that responds to and protects against microbes that enter the body through mucosal surfaces, such as the gastrointestinal and respiratory tracts. The mucosal immune system is composed of collections of lymphocytes and antigen-presenting cells in the epithelia and lamina propria of mucosal surfaces. The mucosal immune system includes intraepithelial lymphocytes, mainly T cells, and organized collections of lymphocytes, often rich in B cells, below mucosal epithelia, such as Peyer's patches in the gut or tonsils in the pharynx.

Mucosal immunity. The form of protective immunity that acts at mucosal surfaces of the gastrointestinal and respiratory tracts to prevent colonization by ingested and inhaled microbes. The secretion of IgA antibody is an important component of mucosal immunity.

Multiple myeloma. A malignant tumor of antibody-producing B cells that often secretes an immunoglobulin or part of an immunoglobulin molecule. The monoclonal antibodies produced by multiple myelomas were critical for the early biochemical analyses of antibody structure.

Multivalency. The presence of multiple identical copies of an epitope on a single antigen molecule, cell surface, or particle. Multivalent antigens, such as bacterial capsular polysaccharides, often are capable of activating B lymphocytes independent of helper T cells.

Mycobacterium. A genus of bacteria, many species of which can survive within phagocytes and cause disease. The principal host defense against mycobacteria such as *Mycobacterium tuberculosis* is cell-mediated immunity.

Naive lymphocyte. A mature B or T lymphocyte that has not previously encountered antigen or is not the progeny of an antigen-stimulated mature lymphocyte. When naive lymphocytes are stimulated by antigen, they differentiate into effector lymphocytes, such as antibody-secreting B cells or helper T lymphocytes. Naive lymphocytes have surface markers and recirculation patterns that are distinct from those of previously activated lymphocytes.

Natural antibodies. IgM antibodies, largely produced by B-1 or marginal zone B cells, specific for bacteria that are common in the environment. Normal individuals contain natural antibodies without any evidence of infection, and these antibodies serve as a preformed defense mechanism against microbes that succeed in penetrating epithelial barriers. Some of these antibodies cross-react with ABO blood group antigens and are responsible for transfusion reactions.

Natural killer (NK) cells. A subset of bone marrow–derived lymphocytes, distinct from B and T cells, that function in innate immune responses to kill microbe-infected cells and to activate phagocytes by secreting interferon-γ. NK cells do not express clonally distributed antigen receptors like immunoglobulin or T cell receptors, and their activation is regulated by a combination of cell surface stimulatory and inhibitory receptors, the latter recognizing self major histocompatibility complex molecules.

Negative selection. The process by which developing lymphocytes that express antigen receptors specific for self antigens are eliminated, thereby contributing to the maintenance of self-tolerance. Negative selection of developing T lymphocytes (thymocytes) is best understood and involves high-avidity binding of an immature T cell to self major histocompatibility complex molecules with bound self peptides on thymic antigen-presenting cells, leading to apoptotic death of the T cell.

Neonatal immunity. Passive humoral immunity to infections in mammals in the first months of life, before full development of the immune system. Neonatal immunity is mediated by maternally produced antibodies, which are transported across the placenta into the fetal circulation before birth or are derived from ingested milk and transported across the gut epithelium.

Neutrophil. The most abundant circulating white blood cell, also called a **polymorphonuclear leukocyte (PMN),** which is recruited to inflammatory sites and is capable of phagocytosing and enzymatically digesting microbes.

Nitric oxide. A biologic effector molecule with a broad range of activities that, in macrophages, functions as a potent microbicidal agent that kills ingested organisms. Production of nitric oxide (NO) is dependent on an enzyme called NO synthase, which converts L-arginine into NO. Macrophages express an inducible form of NO synthase on activation by various microbial or cytokine stimuli.

N-nucleotides. The name given to nucleotides randomly added to the junctions between V, D, and J gene segments in immunoglobulin or T cell receptor (TCR) genes during lymphocyte development. The addition of up to 20 of these nucleotides, which is mediated by the enzyme terminal deoxyribonucleotidyl transferase, contributes to the diversity of the antibody and TCR repertoires.

Nuclear factor of activated T cells (NFAT). A transcription factor required for the expression of the interleukins IL-2 and IL-4, tumor necrosis factor, and other cytokine genes. There are four different NFATs, each encoded by a separate gene; NFAT1 and NFAT4 are found in T cells. Cytoplasmic NFAT is activated by Ca^{2+}-calmodulin–dependent, calcineurin-mediated dephosphorylation that permits NFAT to translocate into the nucleus and bind to consensus-binding sequences in the regulatory regions of IL-2, IL-4, and other cytokine genes, usually in association with other transcription factors, such as AP-1.

Nuclear factor-κB (NF-κB). A family of transcription factors composed of homodimers or heterodimers of proteins homologous to the c-Rel protein. NF-κκB proteins are important in the transcription of many genes in both innate and adaptive immune responses.

Oncofetal antigens. Proteins that are expressed at high levels on some types of cancer cells and in normal developing (fetal) but not adult tissues. Antibodies specific for these proteins often are used in histopathologic identification of tumors or to follow the progression of tumor growth in patients. Carcinoembryonic antigen (CEA) (i.e., CD66) and α-fetoprotein (AFP) are two oncofetal antigens that commonly are expressed by certain carcinomas.

Opsonin. A macromolecule that becomes attached to the surface of a microbe that can be recognized by surface receptors of neutrophils and macrophages and that increases the efficiency of phagocytosis of the microbe. Opsonins include IgG antibodies, which are recognized by Fcγ receptors on phagocytes, and fragments of complement proteins, which are recognized by the type 1 complement receptor (CR1) (i.e., CD35) and by the leukocyte integrin Mac-1.

Opsonization. The process of attaching opsonins, such as IgG or complement fragments, to microbial surfaces to target the microbes for phagocytosis.

Oral tolerance. The suppression of systemic humoral and cell-mediated immune responses to an antigen after the oral administration of that antigen, due to anergy of antigen-specific T cells or the production of immunosuppressive cytokines such as transforming growth factor-β. Oral tolerance is a possible mechanism for preventing immune responses to food antigens and to bacteria that normally reside as commensal organisms in the intestinal lumen.

Passive immunity. The form of immunity to an antigen that is established in one individual by transfer of antibodies or lymphocytes from another individual known to be immune to that antigen. The recipient of such a transfer can become immune to the antigen without ever having been exposed to or having responded to the antigen. An example of passive immunity is the transfer of human sera containing antibodies specific for certain microbial toxins or snake venoms to a previously unimmunized individual.

Pathogenicity. The ability of a microorganism to cause disease. Multiple mechanisms may contribute to pathogenicity, including production of toxins, the stimulation of host inflammatory responses, and the perturbation of host cell metabolism.

Pattern recognition receptors. Receptors of the innate immune system that recognize frequently encountered structures called *molecular patterns* produced by microorganisms and that facilitate innate immune responses against the microorganisms. Examples of pattern recognition receptors of phagocytes are Toll-like receptors, which bind bacterial endotoxin, and the mannose receptor, which binds microbial glycoproteins or glycolipids with terminal mannose residues.

Pentraxins. A family of plasma proteins that contain five identical globular subunits; includes the acute phase reactant C-reactive protein.

Peptide-binding cleft. The portion of a major histocompatibility complex (MHC) molecule that binds peptides for display to T cells. The cleft is composed of paired α-helices resting upon a floor made up of an eight-stranded β-pleated sheet. The polymorphic residues, which are the amino acids that vary among different MHC alleles, are located in and around this cleft.

Perforin. A pore-forming protein, homologous to the C9 complement protein, that is present as a monomer in the granules of cytotoxic T lymphocytes (CTLs) and natural killer (NK) cells. When perforin monomers are released from granules of activated CTLs or NK cells, they undergo polymerization in the lipid bilayer of the target cell plasma membrane, forming a large aqueous channel. This pore may serve as a channel for influx of enzymes derived from the CTL granules.

Periarteriolar lymphoid sheath (PALS). A cuff of lymphocytes surrounding small arterioles in the spleen, which contains mainly T lymphocytes, about two thirds of which are CD4+ and one third of which are CD8+.

Peripheral lymphoid organs/tissues. Organized collections of lymphocytes and accessory cells, including the spleen, lymph node, and mucosa-associated lymphoid tissues, in which adaptive immune responses are initiated.

Peripheral tolerance. Physiologic unresponsiveness to self antigens that are present in peripheral tissues and usually not in the generative lymphoid organs. Peripheral tolerance is induced by the recognition of the antigens without adequate levels of the costimulators that are required for lymphocyte activation or by persistent and repeated stimulation by these self antigens.

Peyer's patches. Organized lymphoid tissues in the lamina propria of the small intestine in which immune responses to ingested antigens may be initiated. Peyer's patches are composed mostly of B cells, with smaller numbers of T cells and antigen-presenting cells, all arranged in follicles similar to those found in lymph nodes, often with germinal centers.

Phagocytosis. The process by which certain cells of the innate immune system, including macrophages and neutrophils, engulf large particles (greater than 0.5 μm in diameter) such as intact microbes. The cell surrounds the particle with extensions of its plasma membrane by an energy- and cytoskeleton-dependent process, leading to formation of an intracellular vesicle called a phagosome, which contains the ingested particle.

Phagosome. A membrane-bound intracellular vesicle that contains microbes or particulate material from the extracellular environment. Phagosomes are formed during the process of phagocytosis and fuse with other vesicular structures such as lysosomes, leading to the enzymatic degradation of the ingested material.

Phosphatase (protein phosphatase). An enzyme that removes phosphate groups from the side chains of certain amino acid residues of proteins. Protein phosphatases in lymphocytes, such as CD45 or calcineurin, regulate the activity of various signal transduction molecules and transcription factors. Some protein phosphatases may be specific for phosphotyrosine residues and others for phosphoserine and phosphothreonine residues.

Phospholipase C (PLCγl). An enzyme that catalyzes the hydrolysis of the plasma membrane phospholipid phosphatidylinositol 4,5-bisphosphate (PIP_2), generating two signaling molecules, inositol 1,4,5-trisphosphate (IP_3) and diacylglycerol (DAG). PLCγl becomes activated in lymphocytes by antigen binding to the antigen receptor.

Phytohemagglutinin (PHA). A polymeric carbohydrate-binding protein, or lectin, produced by plants, that crosslinks human T cell surface molecules, including the T cell receptor, thereby inducing activation and agglutination of T cells. Because PHA activates all T cells, regardless of antigen specificity, it is called a **polyclonal activator.** In clinical medicine, PHA is used to assess whether a patient's

T cells are functional or to induce T cell mitosis for the purpose of producing chromosomal spreads for karyotyping.

Plasma cell. A terminally differentiated antibody-secreting B lymphocyte with a characteristic histologic appearance, including oval shape, eccentric nucleus, and a perinuclear halo.

Pluripotent stem cell. An undifferentiated bone marrow cell that divides continuously and gives rise to additional stem cells and to cells of multiple different lineages. A hematopoietic stem cell in the bone marrow will give rise to cells of lymphoid, myeloid, and erythrocytic lineages.

Polyclonal activators. Agents that are capable of activating many clones of lymphocytes, regardless of their antigen specificities. Examples of polyclonal activators are anti-IgM antibodies for B cells and anti-CD3 antibodies and phytohemagglutinin for T cells.

Poly-Ig receptor. An Fc receptor expressed by mucosal epithelial cells that mediates the transport of IgA and IgM through the epithelial cells into the intestinal lumen. (Also called secretory component.)

Polymorphism. The existence of two or more alternative forms, or variants, of a particular gene that are present at stable frequencies in a population. Each common variant of a polymorphic gene is called an **allele,** and one individual may carry two different alleles of a gene, each inherited from a different parent. The major histocompatibility complex genes are the most polymorphic genes in the mammalian genome.

Polymorphonuclear leukocyte (PMN). A phagocytic cell, also called a **neutrophil,** characterized by a segmented multilobed nucleus and cytoplasmic granules filled with degradative enzymes. PMNs are the most abundant type of circulating white blood cells and are the major cell type mediating acute inflammatory responses to bacterial infections.

Polyvalency. See **Multivalency.**

Positive selection. The process by which developing T cells in the thymus (thymocytes) whose antigen receptors bind to self major histocompatibility complex (MHC) molecules are rescued from programmed cell death, while thymocytes whose receptors do not recognize self MHC molecules die by default. Positive selection ensures that mature T cells are self MHC restricted, and that CD8+ T cells are specific for complexes of peptides with class I MHC molecules and CD4+ T cells for complexes of peptides with class II MHC molecules.

Pre-B cell. A developing B cell present only in hematopoietic tissues at a maturational stage characterized by expression of cytoplasmic immunoglobulin (Ig) μ heavy chains but not Ig light chains. Pre-B cell receptors composed of μ chains and surrogate light chains deliver signals that stimulate further maturation of the pre-B cell into an immature B cell.

Pre-B cell receptor. A receptor expressed on maturing B lymphocytes at the pre-B cell stage composed of an immunoglobulin (Ig) μ heavy chain and an invariant surrogate light chain. The surrogate light chain is composed of two proteins, including the λ5 protein that is homologous to λ light chain C domain and the V pre-B protein that is homologous to a V domain. The pre-B cell receptor associates with the Igα and Igβ signal transduction proteins to form the pre-B cell receptor complex. Pre-B cell receptors are required for stimulating the proliferation and continued maturation of the developing B cell. It is not known if the pre-B cell receptor binds a specific ligand.

Pre-T cell. A developing T lymphocyte in the thymus at a maturational stage characterized by expression of the T cell receptor (TCR) β chain, but not the α chain, and not CD4 or CD8. In pre-T cells, the TCR β chain is found on the cell surface as part of the pre-T cell receptor.

Pre-T cell receptor (Pre-TCR). A receptor expressed on the surface of pre-T cells, composed of the T cell receptor (TCR) β chain and an invariant pre-Tα protein. This receptor associates with the CD3 and ζ molecules, forming the pre-TCR complex. The function of this complex is similar to that of the pre-B cell receptor in B cell development, namely, the delivery of signals that stimulate further proliferation, antigen receptor gene rearrangements, and maturation. It is not known if the pre-TCR binds a specific ligand.

Primary immune response. An adaptive immune response that occurs after the first exposure of an individual to a foreign antigen. Primary responses are characterized by relatively slow kinetics and small magnitude, compared with responses after a second or subsequent exposure.

Primary immunodeficiency. A genetic defect that results in a deficiency in some component of the innate or adaptive immune systems, leading to an increased susceptibility to infections that frequently is manifested early in infancy and childhood but sometimes is clinically detected later in life.

Pro-B cell. A developing B cell in the bone marrow that is the earliest cell committed to the B lymphocyte lineage. Pro-B cells do not produce immunoglobulin, but they can be distinguished from other immature cells by the expression of B-lineage–restricted surface molecules such as CD19 and CD10.

Professional antigen-presenting cells. Antigen-presenting cells (APCs) for T lymphocytes that are capable of displaying peptides bound to major histocompatibility complex molecules and expressing costimulators. The most important professional APCs for initiating primary T cell responses are dendritic cells.

Programmed cell death. A pathway of cell death by apoptosis, which occurs in lymphocytes deprived of necessary survival stimuli, such as growth factors or costimulators. Programmed cell death, also called "death by neglect," is characterized by release of mitochondrial cytochrome *c* into the cytoplasm, activation of caspase-9, and initiation of the apoptotic pathway.

Prostaglandins. A class of lipid inflammatory mediators derived from arachidonic acid in many cell types via the cyclooxygenase pathway. Activated mast cells make prostaglandin D_2 (PGD_2), which binds to receptors on smooth muscle cells and acts as a vasodilator and as a bronchoconstrictor. PGD_2 also promotes neutrophil chemotaxis and accumulation at inflammatory sites.

Pro-T cell. A developing T cell in the thymic cortex that is a recent arrival from the bone marrow and does not express T cell receptors, CD3, or ζ chains, or CD4 or CD8 molecules. Pro-T cells also are called double-negative thymocytes.

Proteasome. A large multiprotein enzyme complex with a broad range of proteolytic activity, which is found in the cytoplasm of most cells and which generates from cytosolic proteins the peptides that bind to class I major histocompatibility complex molecules. Proteins are targeted for proteasomal degradation by covalent linkage of ubiquitin molecules.

Protein kinase C (PKC). Any of several isoforms of an enzyme that mediates the phosphorylation of serine and threonine residues in many different protein substrates and thereby serves to propagate various signal transduction pathways leading to transcription factor activation. In T and B lymphocytes, PKC is activated by diacylglycerol, which is generated in response to antigen receptor ligation.

Protein tyrosine kinase (PTK). See Kinase.

Protozoa. Complex single-celled eukaryotic organisms, many of which are human parasites and cause diseases. Examples of pathogenic protozoa are *Entamoeba histolytica,* causing amebic dysentery; *Plasmodium,* causing malaria; and *Leishmania,* causing leishmaniasis. Protozoa stimulate both innate and adaptive immune responses.

Provirus. A DNA copy of the genome of a retrovirus, which is integrated into the host cell genome, and from which viral genes are transcribed and the viral genome is reproduced. Human immunodeficiency virus (HIV) proviruses can remain inactive for long periods of time, so the presence of such proviruses represents a latent form of HIV infection that is not accessible to immune defense.

Purified antigen (subunit) vaccine. Vaccines composed of purified antigens or subunits of microbes. Examples of this type of vaccine are diphtheria and tetanus toxoids, *Pneumococcus* and *Haemophilus influenzae* polysaccharide vaccines, and purified polypeptide vaccines against hepatitis B virus and influenza virus. Purified antigen vaccines may stimulate antibody and helper T cell responses, but they do not generate cytolytic T lymphocyte responses.

Pyogenic bacteria. Bacteria, such as the gram-positive staphylococci and streptococci, that induce inflammatory responses rich in polymorphonuclear leukocytes (giving rise to pus). Antibody responses to these bacteria greatly enhance the efficacy of innate immune effector mechanisms to clear infections.

Radioimmunoassay (RIA). A highly sensitive and specific immunologic method for quantifying the concentration of an antigen in a solution, which relies on a radioactively labeled antibody specific for the antigen. Usually, two antibodies specific for the antigen are employed. The first antibody is unlabeled but attached to a solid support, where it binds and immobilizes the antigen whose concentration is being determined. The amount of the second, labeled antibody that binds to the immobilized antigen, determined by radioactive decay detectors, is proportional to the concentration of antigen in the test solution.

Reactive oxygen species (ROS). Highly reactive metabolites of oxygen, including superoxide anion, hydroxyl radical, and hydrogen peroxide, which are produced by activated phagocytes. ROS are used by the phagocytes to form oxyhalides, which damage ingested bacteria. ROS also may be released from the cells and promote inflammatory responses or cause tissue damage.

Receptor editing. A process by which some immature B cells that recognize self antigens in the bone marrow may be induced to change their immunoglobulin (Ig) specificities. Receptor editing involves reactivation of the RAG genes, additional light chain V-J recombinations, and production of a new Ig light chain, allowing the cell to express a different antigen receptor that is not self-reactive.

Recirculation of lymphocytes. The continuous movement of naive lymphocytes via the bloodstream and lymphatics, between lymph nodes or spleen, and, if activated, to peripheral inflammatory sites.

Recombination activating gene 1 and 2 (RAG-1 and RAG-2). The genes encoding RAG-1 and RAG-2 proteins, which are the lymphocyte-specific components of the V(D)J recombinase and are critical for DNA recombi-

nation events that form functional immunoglobulin and T cell receptor genes. The RAG proteins are expressed in developing B and T cells and bind to recombination recognition sequences, which consist of a highly conserved stretch of 7 nucleotides, called the hepatamer, located adjacent to the V, D, or J coding sequence, followed by a spacer of exactly 12 or 23 nonconserved nucleotides, followed by a highly conserved stretch of 9 nucleotides, called the nonamer. Therefore, RAG proteins are required for expression of the antigen receptors and for the maturation of B and T lymphocytes.

Red pulp. An anatomic and functional compartment of the spleen composed of vascular sinusoids, scattered among which are large numbers of macrophages, dendritic cells, sparse lymphocytes, and plasma cells. Red pulp macrophages clear the blood of microbes, other foreign particles, and damaged red blood cells.

Regulatory T cells. A population of T cells that regulate the activation or effector functions of other T cells and may be necessary to maintain tolerance to self antigens. Most regulatory T cells express CD4, CD25 and FoxP3. Regulatory T cells that develop in the thymus as a consequence of self antigen recognition sometimes are called "natural" regulatory T cells.

Repertoire. The complete collection of antigen receptors, and therefore antigen specificities, expressed by all of the B and T lymphocytes of an individual.

Reverse transcriptase. An enzyme encoded by retroviruses, such as human immunodeficiency virus (HIV), which synthesizes a DNA copy of the viral genome from the RNA template of the virus. Purified reverse transcriptase is used widely in molecular biology research for purposes of cloning complementary DNAs encoding a gene of interest from messenger RNA. Reverse transcriptase inhibitors are used as drugs to treat HIV-1 infection.

Rheumatoid arthritis. An autoimmune disease characterized primarily by inflammatory damage to joints and sometimes inflammation of blood vessels, lungs, and other tissues. CD4+ T cells, activated B lymphocytes, and plasma cells are found in the inflamed joint lining (synovium), and numerous proinflammatory cytokines, including interleukin-1 and tumor necrosis factor, are present in the synovial (joint) fluid.

Scavenger receptors. A family of cell surface receptors expressed on macrophages, originally defined as receptors that mediate endocytosis of oxidized or acetylated low-density lipoprotein particles but that also bind and mediate phagocytosis of a variety of microbes.

SCID mouse. A mouse strain in which B and T cells are absent because of an early block in maturation from bone marrow precursors. SCID mice carry a mutation in a component of the enzyme DNA-dependent protein kinase, which is required for double-stranded DNA break repair. Deficiency of this enzyme results in abnormal joining of immunoglobulin and T cell receptor gene segments during recombination, and therefore a failure to express antigen receptors.

Secondary immune response. An adaptive immune response that occurs on second exposure to an antigen. A secondary response is characterized by more rapid kinetics and greater magnitude relative to the primary immune response that occurs on first exposure.

Secretory component. The proteolytically cleaved portion of the extracellular domain of the poly-Ig receptor, which remains bound to IgA molecules secreted into the intestinal lumen.

Selectin. Any one of three separate but closely related carbohydrate-binding proteins that mediate adhesion of leukocytes to endothelial cells. Each of the selectin molecules is a single-chain transmembrane glycoprotein with a similar modular structure, including an extracellular calcium-dependent lectin domain. The selectins include L-selectin (CD62L) expressed on leukocytes, P-selectin (CD62P) expressed on platelets and activated endothelium, and E-selectin (CD62E) expressed on activated endothelium.

Self major histocompatibility complex (MHC) restriction. The limitation (or restriction) of antigens that can be recognized by an individual's T cells to complexes of peptides bound to MHC molecules that were present in the thymus during T cell maturation (i.e., self MHC molecules). The T cell repertoire is self MHC restricted as a result of the process of positive selection.

Self-tolerance. Unresponsiveness of the adaptive immune system to self antigens, largely as a result of inactivation or death of self-reactive lymphocytes induced by exposure to those self antigens. Self-tolerance is a cardinal feature of the normal immune system, and failure of self-tolerance leads to autoimmune diseases.

Septic shock. An often lethal complication of severe gram-negative bacterial infection with spread to the bloodstream (sepsis), which is characterized by vascular collapse, disseminated intravascular coagulation, and metabolic disturbances. This syndrome is due to effects of bacterial lipopolysaccharide (LPS) and cytokines, including tumor necrosis factor, interleukin-12 (IL-12), and IL-1. Septic shock also is called **endotoxin shock.**

Seroconversion. The production of detectable antibodies in the serum specific for a microorganism, during the course of an infection or in response to an immunization.

Serology. The study of blood (serum) antibodies and their reactions with antigens. The term *serology* often is used to refer to the diagnosis of infectious diseases by detection of microbe-specific antibodies in the serum.

Serotype. An antigenically distinct subset of a species of an infectious organism that is distinguished from other subsets by serologic (i.e., serum antibody) tests. Humoral immune responses to one serotype of microbes (e.g., influenza virus) may not be protective against another serotype.

Serum. The cell-free fluid that remains when blood or plasma forms a clot. Blood antibodies are found in the serum fraction.

Serum sickness. A disease caused by injection of large doses of a protein antigen into the blood, characterized by the deposition of antigen-antibody (immune) complexes in blood vessel walls, especially in kidneys and joints. The immune complex deposition leads to complement activation and leukocyte recruitment, causing glomerulonephritis and arthritis. Serum sickness originally was described as a disorder that occurred in patients receiving injections of horse serum containing antitoxin antibodies to prevent diphtheria; these patients made antibodies against horse proteins followed by formation of immune complexes composed of these antibodies and the injected antigens.

Severe combined immunodeficiency (SCID). Immunodeficiency disease in which both B and T lymphocytes do not develop or do not function properly; therefore, both humoral immunity and cell-mediated immunity are impaired. Children with SCID usually present with infections during the first year of life and succumb to these infections unless the immunodeficiency is treated. There are several different genetic causes of SCID.

Signal transducer and activator of transcription (STAT). A member of a family of proteins that function as signaling molecules and transcription factors in response to cytokines binding to type I and type II cytokine receptors. The STATs are present as inactive monomers in the cytoplasm of cells and are recruited to the cytoplasmic tails of cross-linked cytokine receptors, where they are tyrosine-phosphorylated by Janus kinases. The phosphorylated STAT proteins dimerize and move to the nucleus, where they bind to specific sequences in the promoter regions of various genes and stimulate their transcription. Different STATs are activated by different cytokines.

Single-positive thymocyte. A maturing T cell precursor in the thymus that expresses CD4 or CD8 molecules but not both. Single-positive thymocytes are found mainly in the medulla and have matured from the double-positive stage, during which thymocytes express both CD4 and CD8 molecules.

Smallpox. A disease caused by variola virus. Smallpox was the first infectious disease shown to be preventable by vaccination, and the first disease to be completely eradicated by a worldwide vaccination program.

Somatic hypermutation. High-frequency point mutations in immunoglobulin heavy and light chains that occur in germinal center B cells. Mutations that lead to increased affinity of antibodies for antigen impart a selective survival advantage to the B cells producing those antibodies, leading to affinity maturation of a humoral immune response.

Somatic recombination. The process of DNA recombination by which the genes encoding the variable regions of antigen receptors are formed during lymphocyte development. A relatively limited set of inherited, or germline, DNA sequences that are initially separate from one another are brought together by enzymatic deletion of intervening sequences and religation. This process occurs only in developing B and T lymphocytes.

Specificity. A cardinal feature of the adaptive immune system, referring to the ability of immune responses to distinguish between distinct antigens or small parts of macromolecular antigens. This fine specificity is attributed to lymphocyte antigen receptors that may bind to one molecule but not to another with only minor structural differences from the first.

Spleen. A peripheral lymphoid organ located in the left upper quadrant of the abdomen. The spleen is the major site for adaptive immune responses to blood-borne antigens. The red pulp of the spleen is composed of blood-filled vascular sinusoids lined by phagocytes that ingest opsonized microbes and damaged red blood cells. The white pulp of the spleen contains lymphocytes and lymphoid follicles.

Stem cell. An undifferentiated cell that divides continuously and gives rise to additional stem cells and to cells of multiple different lineages. For example, all blood cells arise from a common hematopoietic stem cell in the bone marrow.

Superantigen. A protein that binds to and activates all of the T cells in an individual that express a particular set or family of Vβ T cell receptor (TCR) genes. Superantigens are presented to T cells by binding to nonpolymorphic regions of class II major histocompatibility complex molecules on antigen-presenting cells, and they interact with conserved regions of TCR Vβ domains. Several staphylococcal enterotoxins are superantigens. Their importance lies in their ability to activate many T cells, resulting in large amounts of cytokine production and a clinical syndrome called **toxic shock syndrome** that is similar to septic shock.

Suppressor T cell. T cells that block the activation and functions of other effector T lymphocytes. Some suppressor cells may function by producing cytokines that inhibit immune responses.

Surrogate light chain. A complex of two nonvariable proteins that associate with immunoglobulin μ heavy chains in pre-B cells to form the pre-B cell receptor. The two surrogate light chain proteins include V pre-B protein, which is homologous to a light chain V domain, and λ5, which is covalently attached to the μ heavy chain by a disulfide bond.

Switch recombination. The molecular mechanism underlying immunoglobulin heavy chain class, or isotype, switching, in which a rearranged VDJ gene segment in an antibody-producing B cell recombines with a downstream C gene and the intervening C genes are deleted. DNA recombination events in switch recombination are triggered by CD40 ligation and cytokines and involve nucleotide sequences called switch regions, located in the introns at the 5′ end of each C_H locus.

Syngeneic. Genetically identical. All animals of an inbred strain and monozygotic twins of any species are syngeneic.

Syngeneic graft. A graft from a donor who/that is genetically identical to the recipient. Syngeneic grafts are not rejected.

Systemic lupus erythematosus (SLE). A chronic systemic autoimmune disease that affects predominantly women and is characterized by rashes, arthritis, glomerulonephritis, hemolytic anemia, thrombocytopenia, and central nervous system involvement. Many different autoantibodies are found in patients with SLE, particularly anti-DNA antibodies. Many of the manifestations of SLE are due to formation of immune complexes composed of autoantibodies and their antigens and deposition of these complexes in small blood vessels in various tissues. The underlying mechanism for the breakdown of self-tolerance in SLE is not understood.

γδ T cell. A subset of T cells that express a form of antigen receptor (T cell receptor [TCR]) that is distinct from the more common αβ TCR found on CD4+ and CD8+ T cells. These T cells are abundant in epithelia. They recognize lipids and other nonprotein antigens of microbes.

T cell receptor (TCR). The clonally distributed antigen receptor on CD4+ and CD8+ T lymphocytes that recognizes complexes of foreign peptides bound to self major histocompatibility complex molecules on the surface of antigen-presenting cells. The most common form of TCR is composed of a heterodimer of two disulfide-linked transmembrane polypeptide chains, designated α and β, each containing one amino-terminal Ig-like variable (V) domain, one Ig-like constant (C) domain, a hydrophobic transmembrane region, and a short cytoplasmic region. (Another less common type of TCR, composed of γ and δ chains, is found on a small subset of T cells and recognizes different forms of antigen.)

T cell receptor (TCR) complex. A multiprotein plasma membrane complex on T lymphocytes composed of the highly variable, antigen-binding TCR heterodimer and the invariant signaling proteins CD3 γ, δ, and ε and the ζ chain.

T lymphocyte. The cell type that mediates cell-mediated immune responses in the adaptive immune system. T lymphocytes mature in the thymus, circulate in the blood, populate secondary lymphoid tissues, and are recruited to peripheral sites of antigen exposure. They express antigen receptors (T cell receptors) that recognize peptide fragments of foreign proteins bound to self major histocompatibility complex molecules. Functional subsets of T lymphocytes include CD4$^+$ helper T cells and CD8$^+$ cytolytic T lymphocytes.

T-bet. A T-box family transcription factor that promotes the differentiation of T_H1 cells from naive T cells.

T-dependent antigen. An antigen that requires both B cells and helper T cells to stimulate an antibody response. T-dependent antigens are all protein antigens that contain some epitopes recognized by T cells and other epitopes recognized by B cells. The helper T cells produce cytokines and cell surface molecules that stimulate B cell growth and differentiation into antibody-secreting cells. Humoral immune responses to T-dependent antigens are characterized by isotype switching, affinity maturation, and memory.

T_H1 cells. A functional subset of helper T cells that secretes a particular set of cytokines, including interferon-γ, and whose principal function is to stimulate phagocyte-mediated defense against infections, especially with intracellular microbes.

T_H2 cells. A functional subset of helper T cells that secretes a particular set of cytokines, including the interleukins IL-4 and IL-5, and whose principal functions are to stimulate immunoglobulin E (IgE) and eosinophil/mast cell–mediated immune reactions and to down-regulate T_H1 responses.

T_H17 cells. A functional subset of CD4$^+$ helper T cells that secrete a particular set of inflammatory cytokines, including interleukin-17, which are protective against certain bacterial infections and also mediate pathogenic responses in autoimmune diseases.

Thymocyte. A precursor of a mature T lymphocyte present in the thymus.

Thymus. A bilobed organ situated in the anterior mediastinum, which is the site of maturation of T lymphocytes from bone marrow–derived precursors. The thymus is divided into an outer cortex and an inner medulla and contains epithelial cells, macrophages, dendritic cells, and numerous T cell precursors (thymocytes) at various stages of maturation.

T-independent antigen. Nonprotein antigens, such as polysaccharides and lipids, that can stimulate antibody responses without a requirement for antigen-specific helper T lymphocytes. T-independent antigens usually contain multiple identical epitopes that can cross-link antigen receptors of B cells and thereby activate the cells. Humoral immune responses to T-independent antigens show relatively little heavy chain isotype switching or affinity maturation, two processes that require signals from helper T cells.

Tissue typing. The determination of the particular major histocompatibility complex (MHC) alleles expressed by an individual for the purposes of matching allograft donors and recipients. Tissue typing, also called human leukocyte antigen (HLA) typing, usually is done by testing whether sera known to be reactive with certain MHC gene products mediate complement-dependent lysis of an individual's lymphocytes. Polymerase chain reaction (PCR) techniques now also are used to determine if an individual carries a particular MHC allele.

Tolerogen. An antigen that induces immunologic tolerance, in contrast with an immunogen, which induces an immune response. Many antigens can be either tolerogens or immunogens, depending on how they are administered. Tolerogenic forms of antigens include large doses of the proteins administered without adjuvants, altered peptide ligands, and orally administered antigens.

Toll-like receptors (TLRs). Cell surface and endosomal receptors expressed by many cell types, which are pattern recognition receptors for many different pathogen-associated molecular patterns, such as lipopolysaccharides and microbial nucleic acids. TLRs are linked to signal transduction pathways, which activate genes that promote inflammation and resistance to viral infection.

Toxic shock syndrome. An acute illness characterized by shock, skin exfoliation, conjunctivitis, and diarrhea, associated with tampon use and caused by a *Staphylococcus aureus* superantigen.

Transforming growth factor-β (TGF-β). A cytokine produced by activated T cells, mononuclear phagocytes, and other cells, whose principal actions are to inhibit the proliferation and differentiation of T cells, to inhibit the activation of macrophages, and to counteract the effects of proinflammatory cytokines.

Transfusion. Transplantation of circulating blood cells, platelets, or plasma from one individual to another. Transfusions are performed to treat blood loss due to hemorrhage or to treat a deficiency in one or more blood cell types due to inadequate production or excess destruction.

Transfusion reaction. An immunologic reaction against transfused blood products, usually mediated by preformed antibodies in the recipient that bind to donor blood cell antigens, such as ABO blood group antigens or histocompatibility antigens. Transfusion reactions can lead to intravascular lysis of red blood cells and, in severe cases, kidney damage, fever, shock, and disseminated intravascular coagulation.

Transgenic mouse. A mouse that expresses an exogenous gene that has been introduced into the genome by injection of a DNA sequence into the pronuclei of fertilized mouse eggs. Transgenes insert randomly at chromosomal breakpoints and subsequently are inherited as simple mendelian traits. By designing transgenes with tissue-specific regulatory sequences, mice can be produced that express a particular gene only in certain tissues. Transgenic mice are used extensively in immunology research to study the functions of various cytokines, cell surface molecules, and intracellular signaling molecules.

Transporter associated with antigen processing (TAP). An ATP-dependent peptide transporter that mediates the active transport of peptides from the cytosol to the site of assembly of class I major histocompatibility complex (MHC) molecules inside the endoplasmic reticulum. TAP is a heterodimeric molecule composed of TAP-1 and TAP-2 polypeptides, both encoded by genes in the MHC. Because peptides are required for stable assembly of class I MHC molecules, TAP-deficient animals express very few cell surface class I MHC molecules, resulting in diminished development and activation of CD8+ T cells.

Tumor immunity. Protection against the development of tumors mediated by the immune system. Strong immune responses are induced by tumors that express immunogenetic antigens (e.g., tumors that are caused by oncogenic viruses and therefore express viral antigens).

Tumor necrosis factor (TNF). A cytokine produced mainly by activated mononuclear phagocytes that functions to stimulate the recruitment of neutrophils and monocytes to sites of infection and to activate these cells to eradicate microbes. TNF stimulates vascular endothelial cells to express adhesion molecules and induces macrophages and endothelial cells to secrete chemokines. In severe infections, TNF is produced in large amounts and has systemic effects, including induction of fever, synthesis of acute phase proteins by the liver, and cachexia. Production of very large amounts of TNF can lead to intravascular thrombosis and shock (the clinical syndrome of septic shock).

Tumor-infiltrating lymphocytes (TILs). Lymphocytes isolated from the inflammatory infiltrates present in and around surgical resection samples of solid tumors, which are enriched for tumor-specific cytolytic T lymphocytes and natural killer cells. In an experimental model of cancer treatment, TILs isolated from a patient with a tumor are expanded in vitro by culture with high concentrations of interleukin-2 and are then transferred back into the patient.

Tumor-specific transplantation antigen (TSTA). An antigen expressed on experimental animal tumor cells that can be detected by induction of immunologic rejection of tumor transplants. TSTAs originally were defined on chemically induced rodent sarcomas and were shown to stimulate cytolytic T lymphocyte–mediated tumor transplant rejection of transplanted tumors.

Two-signal hypothesis. A proven hypothesis stating that the activation of lymphocytes requires two distinct signals, the first being antigen and the second either microbial products or components of innate immune responses to microbes. The requirement for antigen (so-called signal 1) ensures that the ensuing immune response is specific. The requirement for additional stimuli triggered by microbes or innate immune reactions (signal 2) ensures that immune responses are induced when they are needed (i.e., against microbes and other noxious substances) and not against harmless substances, including self antigens. Signal 2 often is referred to as costimulation.

Type I interferons (IFN-α, IFN-β). A family of cytokines, including several structurally related interferon-α (IFN-α) proteins and a single IFN-β protein, all of which have potent antiviral actions. The major source of IFN-α is mononuclear phagocytes, and IFN-β is produced by many cells, including fibroblasts. Both IFN-α and IFN-β bind to the same cell surface receptor and induce similar biologic responses. Type I IFNs inhibit viral replication, increase the lytic potential of natural killer cells, increase expression of class I major histocompatibility complex molecules on virus-infected cells, and stimulate the development of T_H1 cells, especially in humans.

Urticaria. Localized transient swelling and redness of the skin due to leakage of fluid and plasma proteins from small vessels into the dermis during an immediate hypersensitivity reaction.

V gene segment. A DNA sequence that encodes the variable domain of an immunoglobulin heavy chain or light chain or a T cell receptor α, β, γ, or δ chain. Each antigen receptor locus contains many different V gene segments, any one of which may recombine with downstream D or J segments during lymphocyte maturation to form functional antigen receptor genes.

Vaccine. A preparation of microbial antigen, often combined with adjuvants, that is administered to individuals to induce protective immunity against microbial infections. The antigen may be in the form of live but avirulent microorganisms, killed microorganisms, or purified macromolecular components of microorganisms.

Variable region. The extracellular amino-terminal region of an immunoglobulin heavy or light chain or a T cell receptor α, β, γ, or δ chain that contains variable amino acid sequences that differ between every clone of lymphocytes and that are responsible for specificity for antigen. The antigen-binding variable sequences are localized to hypervariable segments.

V(D)J recombinase. A collection of enzymes that together mediate the somatic recombination events that result in formation of functional antigen receptor genes in developing B and T lymphocytes. Some of the enzymes, such as RAG-1 and RAG-2, are found only in developing lymphocytes, and others are DNA repair enzymes found in most cell types.

Virus. A primitive obligate intracellular parasitic organism or infectious particle that consists of a simple nucleic acid genome packaged in a protein capsid, sometimes surrounded by a lipid envelope. There are many pathogenic animal viruses that cause a wide range of diseases. Humoral immune responses to viruses can be effective in blocking infection of cells, and natural killer cells and cytolytic T lymphocytes are necessary to kill already infected cells.

Western blot. An immunologic technique to determine the presence of a protein in a biologic sample. The method involves separation of proteins in the sample by electrophoresis, transfer of the protein array from the electrophoresis gel to a support membrane by capillary action (blotting), and finally detection of the protein by binding of an enzymatically or radioactively labeled antibody specific for that protein.

Wheal and flare reaction. Local swelling and redness in the skin at a site of an immediate hypersensitivity reaction. The wheal reflects increased vascular permeability, and the flare results from increased local blood flow, both changes resulting from mediators, such as histamine, released from activated dermal mast cells.

White pulp. The part of the spleen that is composed predominantly of lymphocytes, arranged in periarteriolar lymphoid sheaths (PALS) and follicles. The remainder of the spleen contains vascular sinusoids lined with phagocytic cells and filled with blood, called the **red pulp.**

Wiskott-Aldrich syndrome. An X-linked disease characterized by eczema, thrombocytopenia (reduced blood platelets), and immunodeficiency manifested as susceptibility to bacterial infections. The defective gene encodes a cytosolic protein involved in signaling cascades and regulation of the actin cytoskeleton.

Xenoantigen. An antigen on a graft from another species.

Xenogeneic graft. An organ or tissue graft derived from a different species from that of the recipient. Transplantation of xenogeneic grafts (e.g., pig) to humans is not yet practical because of special problems related to immunologic rejection.

X-linked agammaglobulinemia. An immunodeficiency disease, also called Bruton's agammaglobulinemia, characterized by a block in early B cell maturation and an absence of serum immunoglobulin. Patients suffer from pyogenic bacterial infections. The disease is caused by mutations or deletions in the gene encoding B cell tyrosine kinase (Btk), an enzyme involved in signal transduction in developing B cells.

X-linked hyper-IgM syndrome. A rare immunodeficiency disease caused by mutations in the CD40 ligand gene and characterized by a failure of B cell heavy chain isotype switching and cell-mediated immunity. Patients suffer from both pyogenic bacterial and intracellular microbial infections.

Zeta-associated protein of 70 kD (ZAP-70). An Src family cytoplasmic protein tyrosine kinase that is critical for early signaling steps in antigen-induced T cell activation. ZAP-70 binds to phosphorylated tyrosines in the cytoplasmic tails of the ζ chain of the T cell antigen-receptor complex and, in turn, phosphorylates adapter proteins that recruit other components of the signaling cascade.

ζ chain. A transmembrane protein, expressed in T cells as part of the T cell receptor complex, that contains immunoreceptor tyrosine-based activation motifs in its cytoplasmic portion and that binds the ZAP-70 protein tyrosine kinase during T cell activation.

PRINCIPAL FEATURES OF CD MOLECULES

The following table lists selected CD molecules, many of which are referred to in the text. We have not included cytokine receptors and Toll-like receptors, many of which have been assigned CD numbers, because we refer to these molecules by the more descriptive names throughout the book. Many other molecules that have CD number designations are not described in the text, so they are not included in the table. A complete and up-to-date listing of CD molecules may be found online at http://www.hcdm.org (Human Cell Differentiation Molecules workshop).

CD Designation*	Common Synonym(s)	Molecular Structure, Family	Main Cellular Expression	Known or Proposed Function(s)
CD1a-d	T6	43-49 kD; class I MHC family; β_2-microglobulin–associated	Thymocytes, dendritic cells (including Langerhans cells)	Presentation of nonpeptide (lipid and glycolipid) antigens to NK-T cells
CD2	T11; LFA-2	50 kD; Ig superfamily; CD2/CD48/CD58 family	T cells, thymocytes, NK cells	Binds CD58; T cell activation; CTL- and NK cell–mediated killing
CD3γ	T3; Leu-4	25-28 kD; associated with CD3δ and CD3ϵ in TCR complex; Ig superfamily; ITAM in cytoplasmic tail	T cells, thymocytes	Cell surface expression of and signal transduction by the T cell antigen receptor
CD3δ	T3; Leu-4	20 kD; associated with CD3δ and CD3ϵ in TCR complex; Ig superfamily; ITAM in cytoplasmic tail	T cells, thymocytes	Cell surface expression of and signal transduction by the T cell antigen receptor

Continued

273

CD Designation*	Common Synonym(s)	Molecular Structure, Family	Main Cellular Expression	Known or Proposed Function(s)
CD3ε	T3; Leu-4	20 kD; associated with CD3δ and CD3ε in TCR complex; Ig superfamily; ITAM in cytoplasmic tail	T cells, thymocytes	Required for cell surface expression of and signal transduction by the T cell antigen receptor
CD4	T4; Leu-3; L3T4	55 kD; Ig superfamily; CD2/CD48/CD58 family	Class II MHC–restricted T cells; thymocyte subsets; monocytes/macrophages, dendritic cells	Signaling co-receptor in class II MHC–restricted antigen-induced T cell activation (binds to class II MHC molecules) and thymocyte development; receptor for HIV
CD5	T1; Ly-1;	67 kD; scavenger receptor family	T cells; thymocytes; B cell subset	Signaling molecule; binds CD72
CD8α	T8; Leu2; Lyt2	34 kD; expressed as homodimer or heterodimer with CD8β	Class I MHC–restricted T cells; thymocyte subsets	Signaling co-receptor in class I MHC–restricted antigen-induced T cell activation (binds to class I MHC molecules) and thymocyte development
CD8β	T8; Leu2; Lyt2	34 kD; expressed as heterodimer with CD8α; Ig superfamily	Same as for CD8α	Same as for CD8α
CD10	Common acute lymphoblastic leukemia antigen (CALLA); neutral endopeptidase; metalloendopeptidase; enkephalinase	100 kD; type II membrane protein	Immature and some mature B cells; lymphoid progenitors, granulocytes	?Role in B cell development
CD11a	LFA-1 α chain; αL integrin subunit	180 kD; noncovalently linked to CD18 to form LFA-1 integrin	Leukocytes	Cell–cell adhesion; binds to ICAM-1 (CD54), ICAM-2 (CD102), and ICAM-3 (CD50)

CD Designation*	Common Synonym(s)	Molecular Structure, Family	Main Cellular Expression	Known or Proposed Function(s)
CD11b	Mac-1; Mo1;CR3 (iC3b receptor) αM integrin chain	165 kD; noncovalently linked to CD18 to form Mac-1 integrin	Granulocytes, monocytes/ macrophages, dendritic cells, NK cells	Phagocytosis of iC3b-coated particles; neutrophil and monocyte adhesion to endothelium (binds CD54) and extracellular matrix proteins
CD11c	p150/95; CR4 α chain; αX integrin chain	145 kD; noncovalently linked to CD18 to form p150,95 integrin	Monocytes/ macrophages, granulocytes, NK cells	Similar functions to those for CD11b; major CD11CD18 integrin on macrophages
CD14	Mo2; LPS receptor	53 kD; GPI-linked	Monocytes, macrophages, granulocytes	Binds complex of LPS and LPS-binding protein; required for LPS-induced macrophage activation
CD16a	FcγRIIIA	50-70 kD; transmembrane protein; Ig superfamily	NK cells, macrophages	Binds Fc region of IgG; phagocytosis and ADCC
CD16b	FcγRIIIB	50-70 kD; GPI-linked; Ig superfamily	Neutrophils	Binds Fc region of IgG; synergy with FcγRII in immune complex–mediated neutrophil activation
CD18	β chain of LFA-1 family; β2 integrin subunit	95 kD; noncovalently linked to CD11a, CD11b, or CD11c to form β2 integrins	Leukocytes	See **CD11a, CD11b, CD11c**

Continued

CD Designation*	Common Synonym(s)	Molecular Structure, Family	Main Cellular Expression	Known or Proposed Function(s)
CD19	B4	95 kD; Ig superfamily	Most B cells	B cell activation; forms a co-receptor complex with CD21 and CD81 that delivers signals that synergize with signals from B cell antigen receptor complex
CD20	B1	35-37 kD; tetraspan (TM4SF) family	Most or all B cells	?Role in B cell activation or regulation; calcium ion channel
CD21	CR2; C3d receptor; B2	145 kD; regulators of complement activation	Mature B cells, follicular dendritic cells	Receptor for complement fragment C3d; forms a co-receptor complex with CD21 and CD81 that delivers activating signals in B cells; Epstein-Barr virus receptor
CD23	FcεRIIb; low-affinity IgE receptor	45 kD; C-type lectin	Activated B cells, monocytes/ macrophages	Low-affinity Fcε receptor; ?regulation of IgE synthesis
CD25	IL-2 receptor α chain; TAC; p55	55 kD; regulators of complement activation family; noncovalently associates with IL-2Rβ (CD122) and IL-2Rγ (CD132) chains to form high-affinity IL-2 receptor	Activated T and B cells, regulatory T cells, activated macrophages	Binds IL-2; subunit of IL-2R
CD28	Tp44	Homodimer of 44 kD chains; Ig superfamily	T cells (all CD4+, most CD8+ cells)	T cell receptor for costimulator molecules CD80 (B7-1) and CD86 (B7-2)

CD Designation*	Common Synonym(s)	Molecular Structure, Family	Main Cellular Expression	Known or Proposed Function(s)
CD29	β chain of VLA antigens; β1 integrin subunit; platelet gpIIa	130 kD; noncovalently linked with CD49a-d chains to form VLA (β1) integrins	T cells, B cells, monocytes, granulocytes	Leukocyte adhesion to extracellular matrix proteins and endothelium (see **CD49**)
CD30	Ki-1	120 kD; TNF-R family	Activated T and B cells; NK cells, monocytes, Reed-Sternberg cells in Hodgkin's disease	Binds to CD153 (CD30L) on neutrophils, activated T cells, and macrophages
CD31	PECAM-1; platelet gpIIa	130-140 kD; Ig superfamily	Platelets; monocytes, granulocytes, B cells, endothelial cells	Adhesion molecule involved in leukocyte migration through endothelium
CD32	FcγRIIA; FcγRIIB; FcγRIIC	40 kD; Ig superfamily; ITIM in cytoplasmic tail; A, B, and C forms are products of different but homologous genes	B cells, macrophages, granulocytes, dendritic cells, eosinophils, platelets	Fc receptor for aggregated IgG; inhibitory receptor that terminates activation signals initiated by the B cell antigen receptor, ?inhibits dendritic cells
CD34	gp105-gp120	105-120 kD; sialomucin	Precursors of hemopoietic cells; endothelial cells in high endothelial venules	Cell–cell adhesion; binds CD62L (L-selectin)
CD35	CR1; C3b receptor	190-285 kD (four products of polymorphic alleles); regulator of complement activation family	Granulocytes, monocytes, erythrocytes, B cells, T cell subsets, follicular dendritic cells	Binds C3b and C4b; promotes phagocytosis of C3b- or C4b-coated particles and immune complexes; regulates complement activation

Continued

CD Designation*	Common Synonym(s)	Molecular Structure, Family	Main Cellular Expression	Known or Proposed Function(s)
CD36	Platelet gpIIIb; gpIV	85-90 kD	Platelets, monocytes and macrophages, microvascular endothelial cells	Scavenger receptor for oxidized low-density lipoprotein; platelet adhesion; phagocytosis of apoptotic cells
CD40		Homodimer of 44- to 48-kD chains; TNF-R family	B cells, macrophages, dendritic cells, endothelial cells	Binds CD154 (CD40 ligand); role in T cell–dependent B cell activation, and macrophage, dendritic cell, and endothelial cell activation
CD44	Pgp-1; Hermes	80-100 kD, highly glycosylated; cartilage link protein family	Leukocytes, erythrocytes	Binds hyaluronan; involved in leukocyte adhesion to endothelial cells and extracellular matrix
CD45	Leukocyte common antigen (LCA); T200; B220	Multiple isoforms, 180-220 kD (see CD45R); protein tyrosine phosphatase receptor family; fibronectin type III family	Hematopoietic cells	Tyrosine phosphatase; role in T and B cell antigen receptor–mediated signaling
CD45R	Forms of CD45 with restricted cellular expression	CD45RO:180 kD CD45RA: 220 kD CD45RB: 190-, 205-, and 220-kD isoforms	CD45RO: memory T cells; subset of B cells, monocytes, macrophages CD45RA: naive T cells, B cells, monocytes CD45RB: B cells, subset of T cells	See **CD45**
CD46	Membrane cofactor protein (MCP)	52-58 kD; regulators of complement activation family	Leukocytes, epithelial cells, fibroblasts	Regulation of complement activation

CD Designation*	Common Synonym(s)	Molecular Structure, Family	Main Cellular Expression	Known or Proposed Function(s)
CD49d	α_4 integrin subunit	150 kD; noncovalently linked to CD29 to form VLA-4 ($\alpha_4\beta_1$) integrin	T cells, monocytes, B cells, NK cells, eosinophils, dendritic cells, thymocytes	Leukocyte adhesion to endothelium and extracellular matrix; binds to VCAM-1 and MAdCAM-1; binds fibronectin and collagens
CD54	ICAM-1	75-114 kD; Ig superfamily	Endothelial cells, T cells, B cells, monocytes, endothelial cells (cytokine-inducible)	Cell-cell adhesion; ligand for CD11aCD18 (LFA-1) and CD11bCD18 (Mac-1); receptor for rhinovirus
CD55	Decay-accelerating factor (DAF)	55-70 kD; GPI-linked; regulators of complement activation family	Broad	Regulation of complement activation; binds C3b, C4b
CD58	LFA-3	55-70 kD; GPI-linked or integral membrane protein; CD2/CD48/CD58 family	Broad	Leukocyte adhesion; binds CD2
CD59	Membrane inhibitor of reactive lysis (MIRL)	18-20 kD; GPI-linked; Ly-6 superfamily	Broad	Binds C9; inhibits formation of membrane attack complex of complement
CD62E	E-selectin; ELAM-1	115 kD; selectin family	Endothelial cells	Leukocyte-endothelial adhesion
CD62L	L-selectin; LAM-1; MEL-14	74-95 kD; selectin family	B cells, T cells, monocytes, granulocytes, some NK cells	Leukocyte-endothelial adhesion; homing of naive T cells to peripheral lymph nodes

Continued

CD Designation*	Common Synonym(s)	Molecular Structure, Family	Main Cellular Expression	Known or Proposed Function(s)
CD62P	P-selectin; gmp140; PADGEM	140 kD; selectin family	Platelets, endothelial cells (present in granules, translocated to cell surface on activation)	Leukocyte adhesion to endothelium, platelets; binds CD162 (PSGL-1)
CD64	FcγRI	72 kD; Ig superfamily; noncovalently associated with the common FcR γ chain	Monocytes, macrophages, activated neutrophils	High-affinity Fcγ receptor; role in phagocytosis, ADCC, macrophage activation
CD66e	Carcinoembryonic antigen (CEA)	180-220 kD; Ig superfamily; CEA family	Colonic and other epithelial cells	?Adhesion; clinical marker of carcinoma burden
CD74	Class II MHC invariant (γ) chain; Ii	33-, 35-, and 41-kD isoforms	B cells, monocytes, macrophages; other class II MHC–expressing cells	Binds to and directs intracellular sorting of newly synthesized class II MHC molecules
CD79a	Igα, MB1	33, 45 kD; forms dimer with CD79β; Ig superfamily; ITAM in cytoplasmic tail	Mature B cells	Required for cell surface expression of and signal transduction by the B cell antigen receptor complex
CD79b	Igβ, B29	37-39 kD; forms dimer with CD79α; Ig superfamily; ITAM in cytoplasmic tail	Mature B cells	See **CD79a**
CD80	B7-1; BB1	60 kD; Ig superfamily	Dendritic cells, activated B cells and macrophages	Costimulator for T lymphocyte activation; ligand for CD28 and CD152 (CTLA-4)

CD Designation*	Common Synonym(s)	Molecular Structure, Family	Main Cellular Expression	Known or Proposed Function(s)
CD81	Target for antiproliferative antigen-1 (TAPA-1)	26 kD; tetraspan (TM4SF)	T cells, B cells, NK cells, dendritic cells, thymocytes, endothelium	B cell activation; forms a co-receptor complex with CD19 and CD21 that delivers signals that synergize with signals from B cell antigen receptor complex
CD86	B7-2	80 kD; Ig superfamily	B cells, monocytes; dendritic cells; some T cells	Costimulator for T lymphocyte activation; ligand for CD28 and CD152 (CTLA-4)
CD88	C5a receptor	43 kD; G-protein–coupled, seven-membrane spanning receptor family	Granulocytes, monocytes, dendritic cells, mast cells	Receptor for C5a complement fragment; role in complement-induced inflammation
CD94	Kp43; KIR	43 kD; C-type lectin; on NK cells, covalently assembles with other C-type lectin molecules (NKG2)	NK cells; subset of CD8+ T cells	CD94/NKG2 complex functions as an NK cell inhibitory receptor; binds HLA-E class I MHC molecule
CD95	Fas antigen, APO-1	Homotrimer of 45 kD chains; TNF receptor family	Multiple cell types	Binds Fas ligand; mediates signals leading to activation-induced cell death
CD106	VCAM-1; INCAM-110	100-110 kD; Ig superfamily	Endothelial cells, macrophages, follicular dendritic cells, marrow stromal cells	Adhesion; receptor for CD49dCD29 (VLA-4) integrin; role in lymphocyte trafficking, activation; role in hematopoiesis

Continued

CD Designation*	Common Synonym(s)	Molecular Structure, Family	Main Cellular Expression	Known or Proposed Function(s)
CD152	CTLA-4	33, 50 kD; Ig superfamily	Activated T lymphocytes	Inhibitory signaling in T cells; binds CD80 (B7-1) and CD86 (B7-2) on antigen presenting cells
CD154	CD40 ligand (CD40L); TNF-related activation protein (TRAP); gp39	Homotrimer of 32- to 39-kD chains; TNF receptor family	Activated CD4+ T cells	Activates B cells, macrophages and endothelial cells; ligand for CD40
CD273	B7DC, PD-L2	25 kD; Ig superfamily; B7 costimulator family	Dendritic cells, monocytes, macrophages	Binds PD-1; inhibition of T cell activation
CD274	B7-H1, PD-L1	33 kD; Ig superfamily; B7 costimulator family	Leukocytes	Binds PD-1; inhibition of T cell activation
CD275	B7-H2, ICOS ligand, B7-RP1	60 kD; Ig superfamily; B7 costimulator family	B cells, dendritic cells, monocytes	Binds ICOS (CD278); T cell costimulation
CD278	ICOS	55-60 kD; Ig superfamily; CD28 costimulator family	Activated T cells	Binds ICOS-L (CD275); T costimulation
CD279	PD1	55 kD; Ig superfamily; CD28 costimulator family	Activated T cells activated B cells	Binds B7-H1 (CD274(and B7-DC (CD273); regulation of T cell activation

ADCC, antibody-dependent cell-mediated cytotoxicity; CTL, cytotoxic T lymphocyte; CTLA-4, cytotoxic T lymphocyte-associated protein-4; ELAM-1, endothelial-leukocyte adhesion molecule-1; gp, glycoprotein; GPI, glycophosphatidylinositol; HIV, human immunodeficiency virus; HLA, human leukocyte antigen; ICAM, intercellular adhesion molecule; ICOS, inducible costimulatory molecule; Ig, immunoglobulin; IL, interleukin; ITAM, immunoreceptor tyrosine-based activation motif; ITIM, immunoreceptor tyrosine-based inhibition motif; kD, kilodalton; LAM-1, leukocyte adhesion molecule-1; LFA, lymphocyte function–associated antigen; LPS, lipopolysaccharide; MHC, major histocompatibility complex; NK, natural killer; TCR, T cell receptor; TNF, tumor necrosis factor; VCAM, vascular cell adhesion molecule; VLA, very late antigen.

*The lowercase letters affixed to some CD numbers refer to complex CD molecules that are encoded by multiple genes or that belong to families of structurally related proteins. For instance, CD11a, CD11b, and CD11c are structurally related but distinct forms of an integrin family α chain.

CLINICAL CASES

This appendix presents five clinical cases illustrating various diseases involving the immune system. These cases are not meant to teach clinical skills but rather show how the basic science of immunology contributes to our understanding of human diseases. Each case illustrates typical ways in which a disease manifests, what tests are used in diagnosis, and common modes of treatment. The appendix was compiled with the assistance of Dr. Richard Mitchell, Department of Pathology, Brigham and Women's Hospital, Boston, Massachusetts, and Dr. James Faix, Department of Pathology, Stanford University School of Medicine, Palo Alto, California.

CASE 1: LYMPHOMA

E.B. was a 38-year-old chemical engineer who had been well all of his life. One morning, he noticed a lump in his left groin while showering. It was not tender, and the overlying skin appeared normal. After a few weeks, he began to worry about it because it did not "go away," and he finally made an appointment with a doctor after 2 months. On physical examination, the physician noted a subcutaneous firm, movable nodule, about 3 cm in diameter, in the left inguinal region. The doctor asked E.B. if he had recently noticed any infections of his left foot or leg (which E.B. hadn't). The doctor also found some slightly enlarged lymph nodes in E.B.'s right neck. Otherwise, the physical examination findings were normal. The doctor explained that the nodule probably was a lymph node that was enlarged as a result of a reaction to some infection. However, he advised E.B. to see a surgeon, who would remove the lymph node so that a pathologist could examine it to be sure that it was not malignant.

The lymph node was removed, and histologic examination revealed an expansion of the node by follicular structures composed of monotonous collections of enlarged, activated ("lymphoblastoid") cells (Fig. A-1). Immunohistochemical studies revealed that these cells expressed B cell surface molecules. Also, polymerase chain reaction (PCR) analysis of DNA from the lymph node showed a clonal rearrangement of the immunoglobulin (Ig) heavy chain gene.

On this basis, the diagnosis of follicular lymphoma was made.

1. Why does the presence of a clonal rearrangement of Ig heavy chain genes in the lymph node indicate a neoplasm rather than a response to an infection?

E.B.'s lymphoma was treated with chemotherapy. The lymphadenopathy in his neck (which was due to his lymphoma) regressed, but unfortunately, a new enlarged lymph node appeared in his left cervical area about a year later. This lymph node was removed, and it showed follicular lymphoma, with the same histologic features as those of the original.

2. If an anti-idiotypic antibody was developed against the surface Ig present on E.B.'s original lymphoma cells, it might not recognize the cells responsible for his recurrence. Why not?

The oncologist caring for E.B. is now planning to administer chemotherapy and radiation therapy to kill all the tumor cells, followed by bone marrow transplantation.

3. Why would it be necessary to perform the bone marrow transplantation, and what will be the status of the patient's immune system after the recommended treatment?

ANSWERS TO QUESTIONS FOR CASE 1

1. In an infection, many different clones of lymphocytes are activated. More than one clone may be specific for the same microbial antigen, and different clones may be responding to different antigens produced by the microbe. Furthermore, even in a lymph node draining a site of infection, there are many clones of normal B cells not specific for the microbe. Because each clone of B cells has a unique rearrangement of its Ig heavy and light chain genes (see Chapter 4), the analysis of heavy chain genes in the polyclonal mixture of B cells in a lymph node draining a site of infection reveals many different (polyclonal) rearrangements. By contrast, B cell lymphomas arise from a single cell with a unique Ig heavy chain rearrangement, and after the tumor has grown for some time, it represents a majority of cells in the lymph node.

283

FIGURE A-1   Lymph node biopsy with follicular lymphoma. The microscopic appearance of the patient's inguinal lymph node is shown. The follicular structures are abnormal, composed of a monotonous collection of neoplastic cells. By contrast, a lymph node with reactive hyperplasia would have follicles with germinal center formation, containing a heterogeneous mixture of cells.

Therefore, analysis of heavy chain genes in a lymph node with a B cell lymphoma reveals a single dominant heavy chain rearrangement. PCR assay often is used for analysis of clonality of B cell tumors. In this method, specific sequences of the tumor DNA are amplified by the use of complementary DNA primers and a DNA polymerase. The size of the amplified products is analyzed by gel electrophoresis. Two primers typically are used, one corresponding to a consensus sequence common to most V segments and the other to a sequence common to most J segments. The length of the amplified PCR product is determined by the unique sequences generated during VDJ joining in each clone of B cells. With a normal population of B cells, many PCR products of different sizes are generated, and these appear as a smear on the gel. In the case of lymphoma, all of the B cells have the same VDJ rearrangement, and the PCR product is of one size, appearing as a single band on the gel.

2. An anti-idiotypic antibody would recognize the portions of the Ig that are unique to the original tumor—that is, the hypervariable portions of the antigen receptors of this clone of B cells. During their lives, the Ig genes of B cells often undergo extensive somatic mutations; in humoral immune responses to protein antigens, this process accounts for affinity maturation (see Chapter 7). Somatic mutations of the Ig genes may occur in the tumor cells also, resulting in the appearance of B cells that express a new Ig that is not recognized by the anti-idiotypic antibody.

3. The chemotherapy and radiation treatment, which kills the tumor cells, also destroys the normal hematopoietic cells in the bone marrow. This would be lethal because the patient would not be able to produce red blood cells for oxygen transport, leukocytes for immunity, and platelets to control bleeding. By injecting hematopoietic stem cells from another donor, hematopoiesis can be restored. The stem cells may be administered in the form of whole bone marrow or stem cells purified from the peripheral blood of a donor. Sometimes, the patient's own marrow is harvested before the chemotherapy and irradiation, treated in vitro to destroy tumor cells specifically, and then transplanted back into the patient after the antitumor treatments. Early after bone marrow transplantation, patients often show considerable immune deficiencies. Because B and T lymphocyte progenitors arise from bone marrow stem cells, bone marrow transplantation can lead to reconstitution of the patient's adaptive immune system over time.

CASE 2: HEART TRANSPLANTATION COMPLICATED BY ALLOGRAFT REJECTION

C.M., a computer software salesman, was 48 years old when he came to his primary care physician because of fatigue and shortness of breath. He had not seen a doctor on a regular basis before this visit and felt well up until 1 year ago, when he began experiencing difficulty climbing stairs or playing basketball with his children. Over the past 6 months he had had trouble breathing when he lay down in bed. He did not remember ever experiencing significant chest pain and had no family history of heart disease. He did recall that about 18 months ago he had to take 2 days off from work because of a severe flulike illness.

On examination, he had a pulse of 105 beats per minute, a respiratory rate of 32 breaths per minute, and a blood pressure of 100/60 mm Hg and was afebrile. His doctor heard rales (evidence of abnormal fluid accumulation) in the bases of both lungs. His feet and ankles were swollen. A chest x-ray film showed pulmonary edema and pleural effusions and a significantly enlarged left ventricle. C.M. was admitted to the cardiology service of the University Hospital. On the basis of further tests, including coronary angiography and echocardiography, a diagnosis of dilated cardiomyopathy was made. The doctors explained to the patient that his heart muscle had been damaged. The cause may have been an episode of inflammation as a complication of a viral infection some time ago, but they could not be sure. The only lifesaving treatment for his condition would be to receive a heart transplant.

A panel-reactive antibody (PRA) test was performed on C.M.'s serum to determine whether he had been previously sensitized to alloantigens. This test showed the patient had no circulating antibodies against human leukocyte antigens (HLA), and no further immunologic testing was performed. Two weeks later in a nearby city, a donor heart was removed from a victim of a construction-site accident. The donor had the same ABO blood group type as C.M.'s. The transplant surgery, performed 4 hours after the donor heart was removed, went well, and the allograft was functioning properly postoperatively.

1. What problems might arise if the transplant recipient and the donor have different blood types, or if the recipient has high levels of anti-HLA antibodies?

C.M. was placed on immunosuppressive therapy the day after transplantation, which included daily doses of cyclosporine, mycophenolic acid, and prednisone. Endomyocardial biopsy was performed 1 week after surgery and showed no evidence of myocardial injury or inflammatory cells. He was sent home 10 days after surgery, and within a month he was able to do light exercise without problems. On routinely scheduled endomyocardial biopsy performed within the first 3 months after transplantation, findings were normal, but a biopsy performed 14 weeks after surgery showed the presence of numerous lymphocytes within the myocardium and a few apoptotic muscle fibers (Fig. A-2). The findings were interpreted as evidence of acute allograft rejection.

2. What was the patient's immune system responding to, and what were the effector mechanisms in the acute rejection episode?

C.M.'s serum creatinine level, an indicator of renal function, was high (2.2 mg/dL; normal, less than 1.5 mg/dL). His doctors therefore did not want to increase his cyclosporine

FIGURE A-2 Endomyocardial biopsy showing acute cellular rejection. The heart muscle is infiltrated by lymphocytes, and necrotic muscle fibers are present. (Courtesy of Dr. Richard Mitchell, Department of Pathology, Brigham and Women's Hospital, Boston.)

FIGURE A-3 Coronary artery with transplant-associated arteriosclerosis. This histologic section was taken from a coronary artery of a cardiac allograft that was removed from a patient 5 years after transplantation because of graft failure. The lumen is markedly narrowed by the presence of intimal smooth muscle cells. (Courtesy of Dr. Richard Mitchell, Department of Pathology, Brigham and Women's Hospital, Boston.)

dose because this drug can be toxic to the kidneys. He was given three additional doses of a steroid drug over 18 hours, and a repeat endomyocardial biopsy 1 week later showed only a few scattered macrophages and a small focus of healing tissue. C.M. went home feeling well, and he was able to live a relatively normal life, taking cyclosporine, mycophenolic acid, and prednisone daily.

3. What is the goal of the immunosuppressive drug therapy?

Coronary angiograms performed yearly since the transplant showed a gradual narrowing of the lumens of the coronary arteries. In the sixth year after transplantation, C.M. began experiencing some shortness of breath after mild exercise and showed some left ventricular dilatation on radiographic examination. An intravascular ultrasound examination demonstrated significant thickening of the walls and narrowing of the lumen of the coronary arteries (Fig. A-3). An endomyocardial biopsy showed areas of ischemic necrosis. C.M. and his physicians are now considering the possibility of a second cardiac transplant.

4. What process has led to failure of the graft after 6 years?

ANSWERS TO QUESTIONS FOR CASE 2

1. If the recipient and the heart donor had different blood types, or if the recipient had high levels of anti-HLA antibodies, a form of rejection called hyperacute rejection might occur after transplantation (see Chapter 10).

People with type A, B, or O blood have circulating IgM antibodies against the antigens they do not possess (B, A, or both, respectively). People who have received previous blood transfusions or transplants, or were previously pregnant, may have circulating anti-HLA antibodies. Blood group antigens and HLA antigens are present on endothelial cells. Preformed antibodies, already present in the recipient at the time of transplantation, can bind to these antigens on graft endothelial cells, causing complement activation, leukocyte recruitment, and thrombosis. As a result, the graft blood supply becomes impaired and the organ can rapidly undergo ischemic necrosis. The PRA test typically is performed to determine whether a patient needing a transplant has preexisting antibodies specific for HLA antigens from a random collection of subjects. The test is performed by mixing the patient's serum with a panel of lymphocytes from a random set of various donors, adding anti-immunoglobulin antibody (to amplify the reaction) and complement, and examining to see if the lymphocytes are lysed. The results are expressed as the percentage of donor cells from a panel of donors with which a potential graft recipient's serum reacts. The higher the PRA value obtained, the greater the chance that the recipient will reject a graft.

2. In the acute rejection episode, the patient's immune system is responding to alloantigens in the graft (see Chapter 10). These antigens are likely to include donor major histocompatibility complex (MHC) molecules encoded by alleles not shared by the recipient, as well as unshared allelic variants of other proteins (minor histocompatibility antigens). These alloantigens may be expressed on the graft endothelial cells, leukocytes, and parenchymal cells within the donor heart. The effector mechanisms in the acute rejection episode include both cell-mediated and humoral immune responses. Recipient CD4+ T cells secrete cytokines that promote macrophage activation and inflammation, which causes myocyte or endothelial cell injury and dysfunction, and CD8+ cytotoxic T lymphocytes directly kill graft cells. Recipient antibodies, produced in response to the graft antigens, bind to graft cells, leading to complement activation and leukocyte recruitment.

3. The goal of the immunosuppressive drug therapy is to impair the recipient's immune response to alloantigens present in the graft, thereby preventing rejection. The drugs work by blocking T cell activation (cyclosporine), lymphocyte proliferation (mycophenolic acid), and inflammatory cytokine production (prednisone). An attempt is made to preserve some immune function to combat infections.

4. The graft has failed as a result of chronic rejection manifested as a thickening of the walls and narrowing of the lumens of the graft arteries (see Chapter 10). This vascular change, called graft arteriosclerosis, or transplant-associated arteriosclerosis, leads to ischemic damage to the heart and is the most frequent reason for chronic graft failure. It may be caused by a chronic delayed-type hypersensitivity reaction against vessel wall alloantigens, resulting in cytokine-stimulated smooth muscle cell migration into the intima and proliferation of the smooth muscle cells.

CASE 3: ALLERGIC ASTHMA

I.E. was a 10-year-old girl who was brought to her pediatrician's office in November because of frequent coughing for the past 2 days, wheezing, and a feeling of tightness in her chest. Her symptoms had been especially severe at night. In addition to her routine checkups, she had visited the doctor in the past for occasional ear and upper respiratory tract infections but had not previously experienced wheezing or chest tightness. She had eczema, but otherwise, she was in good health and was developmentally normal. Her immunizations were up to date. She lived at home with her mother, father, and two sisters, ages 12 and 4, and a pet cat. Both of her parents smoked cigarettes, her father suffered from hay fever, and her older sister had a history of sinus infections.

At the time of her examination, I.E. had a temperature of 37° C (98.6° F), blood pressure of 105/65 mm Hg, and a respiratory rate of 28 breaths per minute. She did not appear short of breath. There were no signs of ear infection or pharyngitis. Auscultation of the chest revealed diffuse wheezing in both lungs without signs of congestive heart failure (rales). There was no evidence of pneumonia. The doctor made a presumptive diagnosis of bronchospasm and referred I.E. to a pediatric allergist-immunologist who was associated with his physicians' group. In the meantime, the patient was given a prescription for a short-acting β_2-adrenergic agonist bronchodilator inhaler, and the child was instructed to administer the drug every 6 hours to relieve symptoms. This drug binds to β_2-adrenergic receptors on bronchial smooth muscle cells and causes them to relax, resulting in dilatation of the bronchioles.

1. Asthma is an example of *atopy*. What are the different ways in which atopy may manifest clinically?

One week later, I.E. was seen by the allergist. He auscultated her lungs and confirmed the presence of wheezing. I.E. was instructed to blow into a flowmeter, and the doctor determined that her peak expiratory flow rate was 65% of normal, indicating airway obstruction. The doctor then administered a nebulized bronchodilator, and 10 minutes

FIGURE A-4   A positive result on skin testing for environmental antigens. Small doses of the antigens are injected intradermally. If mast cells are present with bound IgE specific for the test antigen, the antigen will cross-link the Fc receptors to which the IgE is bound. This induces degranulation of the mast cells and the release of mediators that cause the wheal-and-flare reaction.

later performed the test again. The repeat flow rate was 85% of normal, indicating reversibility of the airway obstruction. Blood was drawn and sent for total and differential blood cell count and determination of IgE levels. In addition, a skin test was performed to determine hypersensitivity to various antigens and showed a positive result for cat dander and house dust (Fig. A-4). The patient was instructed to begin using an inhaled corticosteroid and to use her bronchodilator only as needed for respiratory symptoms. Her parents were instructed to make a return appointment 2 weeks later for reevaluation of I.E. and discussion of blood test results.

2. What is the immunologic basis for a "positive" skin test?

At I.E.'s return appointment 2 weeks later, laboratory tests revealed that she had a serum IgE level of 1200 IU/mL (normal range, 0–180) and a total white blood cell count of 7000/mm^3 with 3% eosinophils (normal, less than 0.5%). When she returned to the allergist's office another week later, her respiratory status on physical examination was significantly improved, with no audible wheezing. I.E.'s peak expiratory airflow had improved to 90% of predicted. The family was told that I.E. had reversible airway obstruction, possibly triggered by a viral illness and possibly related to cat and dust allergies. The doctor advised that the cat should either be given to a friend or at least kept out of I.E.'s bedroom. The mother was told that smoking in the house probably was contributing to I.E.'s symptoms. The doctor recommended that I.E. continue to use the short-acting inhaler for acute episodes of wheezing or shortness of breath. I.E. was asked to return in 3 months,

and sooner if she used the inhaler more than twice per month.

3. What is the mechanism for the increased IgE levels seen in patients who suffer from allergic symptoms?

The family cat was given to a neighbor, and I.E. did well on the therapy for about 6 months, experiencing only mild wheezing a few times. The next spring, she began to have more frequent episodes of coughing and wheezing. During a soccer game one Saturday, she became very short of breath, and her parents brought her to the emergency department of the local hospital. After confirming that she was experiencing marked upper airway constriction, the emergency department physician treated her with a nebulized β$_2$-agonist bronchodilator and an oral corticosteroid. After 6 hours, her symptoms resolved, and she was sent home. I.E. was brought to her allergist the next week, who changed her maintenance medication to a different inhaled corticosteroid. She has subsequently been well, with occasional mild "attacks" that are cleared by the bronchodilator inhaler.

4. What are the therapeutic approaches to allergic asthma?

ANSWERS TO QUESTIONS FOR CASE 3

1. *Atopic* reactions to essentially harmless antigens are mediated by IgE on mast cells but may manifest in a variety of ways (see Chapter 11). The signs and symptoms usually reflect the site of entry of the allergen. Hay fever (allergic rhinitis) and asthma usually are responses to inhaled allergens, whereas urticaria and eczema more commonly occur with skin exposure. Although food allergies may cause gastrointestinal symptoms in small children, in adults they usually also provoke systemic urticaria. The most dramatic presentation of allergies to insect venom, foods, or drugs is anaphylaxis, an allergic reaction characterized by systemic vasodilatation, increased vascular permeability, and bronchoconstriction. These pathologic changes may progress to asphyxia and cardiovascular collapse.

2. Immediate release of histamine from triggered mast cells produces a central *wheal* of edema (due to leakage of plasma) and the surrounding *flare* of vascular congestion (due to vessel dilation). However, it is the subsequent *late phase reaction*, characterized by cellular inflammation, that is more characteristic of the damage to tissue affected by allergic diseases. (See Chapter 11.) The allergy skin test should not be confused with the skin test used to assess prior sensitization to certain infectious agents such as *Mycobacterium tuberculosis*. A positive tuberculosis skin test is an example of a delayed-type hypersensitivity (DTH) reaction, mediated by antigen-stimulated helper T cells, which release cytokines such

as interferon-γ, leading to macrophage activation and inflammation. (See Chapter 6.)

3. For unknown reasons, patients with atopy mount helper T cell responses of the T_H2 type to a variety of essentially harmless protein antigens, and the T_H2 cells produce the interleukins IL-4 and IL-5. IL-4 induces IgE synthesis by B cells, and IL-5 promotes eosinophil production and activation (see Chapter 5 and Chapter 11). Because atopy appears to run in families, genetic susceptibility is clearly involved. Attention has been focused especially on genes on the long arm of chromosome 5 (5q) (that encode several T_H2 cytokines) and on 11q (where the gene for a chain of the IgE receptor is located).

4. A major therapeutic approach for allergies is prevention by avoidance of precipitating allergens, if known. Although pharmacologic therapy previously has been focused on treating the symptoms of bronchoconstriction by elevating intracellular cyclic adenosine monophosphate (cAMP) levels (using β_2-adrenergic agents and inhibitors of cAMP degradation), the balance of therapy has shifted to use of anti-inflammatory agents in recent years. These include corticosteroids (which block cytokine release) and cromolyn (which may inhibit release of mast cell mediators). Newer approaches include use of receptor antagonists for lipid mediators and inhibitors of leukocyte adhesion.

CASE 4: SYSTEMIC LUPUS ERYTHEMATOSUS

N.Z. was a 25-year-old unmarried woman who presented to her primary care physician with complaints of joint pain involving her wrists, fingers, and ankles. When seen in the physician's office, N.Z. had normal body temperature, heart rate, blood pressure, and respiratory rate. There was a noticeable red rash on her cheeks, most marked around her nose, and on questioning she said the redness got worse after being out in the sun for 1 or 2 hours. The joints of her fingers and her wrists were swollen and tender. The remainder of the findings on the physical examination were unremarkable.

Her doctor took a blood sample for various tests. Her hematocrit was 35% (normal, 37% to 48%). The total white blood cell count was 9800/mm³ (within normal range) with a normal differential count. The erythrocyte sedimentation rate was 40 mm per hour (normal, 1-20). Her serum antinuclear antibody (ANA) test was positive at 1:256 dilution (normally, negative at 1:8 dilution). Other laboratory findings were unremarkable. On the basis of these findings, a diagnosis of systemic lupus erythematosus

(SLE) was made. N.Z.'s physician prescribed oral prednisone, a corticosteroid, and with this treatment, her joint pain subsided.

1. What is the significance of the positive result for the ANA test?

Three months later, N.Z. began feeling unusually tired and thought that she had the "flu." For about a week she had noticed that her ankles were swollen, and she had difficulty putting on her shoes. She returned to her primary care physician. Her ankles and feet showed severe edema (swollen as a result of extra fluid in the tissue). Her abdomen appeared slightly distended, with a mild shifting dullness to percussion (a sign of an abnormally high amount of fluid in the peritoneal cavity). Her physician ordered several laboratory tests. Her ANA test result was still positive, with a titer of 1:256, and her erythrocyte sedimentation rate was 120 mm per hour. Serum albumin was 0.8 g/dL (normal, 3.5-5.0). Measurement of serum complement proteins revealed a C3 of 42 mg/dL (normal, 80–180) and a C4 of 5 mg/dL (normal, 15–45). Urinalysis showed 4+ proteinuria, both red and white blood cells, and numerous hyaline and granular casts. A 24-hour urine sample contained 4 g of protein.

2. What is the likely reason for the decreased complement levels and the abnormalities in blood and urinary proteins?

Because of the abnormal urinalysis findings, the doctor recommended that a renal biopsy be taken. This was performed a week later in the outpatient surgery department of the community hospital next door to the doctor's office. The biopsy specimen was examined by routine histologic methods, immunofluorescence, and electron microscopy (Fig. A-5).

3. What is the explanation for the pathologic changes seen in the kidney?

The physician made the diagnosis of proliferative lupus glomerulonephritis and prescribed a higher dose of prednisone than what N.Z. was taking previously. The proteinuria and edema subsided over a 2-week period, and serum C3 levels returned to normal. Her corticosteroid dose was tapered down to a lower amount. Over the next few years, she has had intermittent flare-ups of her disease, with joint aches and tissue swelling and laboratory tests indicating depressed C3 levels and proteinuria. These have been effectively managed with corticosteroids, and she has been able to lead an active life.

4. Some autoimmune diseases are thought to be caused by lymphocytes specific for microbes that are activated by an infection and that cross-react with self antigens. Why is this not likely to be a valid explanation for how SLE develops?

Granular deposits of immunoglobulin
and complement in the basement membrane

FIGURE A-5   Glomerulonephritis with immune complex deposition in systemic lupus erythematosus. A, A light micrograph of a renal biopsy specimen in which neutrophilic infiltration in a glomerulus can be seen. **B,** An immunofluorescence micrograph showing granular deposits of immunoglobulin G (IgG) along the basement membrane. (In this technique, called immunofluorescence microscopy, a frozen section of the kidney is incubated with a fluorescein-conjugated antibody against IgG, and the site of deposition of the IgG is defined by determining where the fluorescence is located.) **C,** An electron micrograph of the same tissue revealing immune complex deposition. (Courtesy of Dr. Helmut Rennke, Department of Pathology, Brigham and Women's Hospital, Boston.)

ANSWERS TO QUESTIONS FOR CASE 4

1. A positive ANA test reveals the presence of serum antibodies that bind to components of cellular nuclei. The test is performed by placing different dilutions of the patient's serum on top of a monolayer of human cells on a glass slide. A second fluorescently labeled anti-immunoglobulin is then added, and the cells are examined with a fluorescent microscope to detect if any serum antibodies bound to the nuclei. The ANA titer is the maximum dilution of the serum that still produces detectable nuclear staining. Patients with SLE often have ANAs, which may be specific for histones, other nuclear proteins, or double-stranded DNA. These are autoantibodies, and their production is evidence of autoimmunity. Autoantibodies may be produced against red blood cell membrane proteins and many other self antigens.

2. Some of the autoantibodies form circulating immune complexes by binding to antigens in the blood. When these immune complexes deposit in the basement membranes of vessel walls, they may activate the classical pathway of complement, leading to depletion of complement proteins through consumption. Inflammation caused by the immune complexes in the kidney leads to leakage of protein and red blood cells into the urine. The loss of protein in the urine results in reduced plasma albumin, reduction of osmotic pressure of the plasma, and fluid loss into the tissues, leading to edema of the feet and abdominal distention.

3. The pathologic changes in the kidney are the result of the deposition of circulating immune complexes in the basement membranes of renal glomeruli. These deposits can be seen by immunofluorescence and electron microscopy. The immune complexes activate complement, and leukocytes are recruited by complement byproducts (C3a, C5a) and by binding of leukocyte Fc receptors to the antibodies in the complexes. These leukocytes are activated, and they produce reactive oxygen species and lysosomal enzymes that damage the glomerular basement membrane. These findings are characteristic of immune complex–mediated tissue injury, and complexes may deposit in joints and small blood vessels anywhere in the body, as well as in the kidney. SLE is a prototype of an immune complex disease (see Chapter 11).

4. The autoantibodies in patients with SLE are specific for a wide range of structurally unrelated self antigens. It is therefore unlikely that the presence of these antibodies represents a cross-reaction with one or a few microbial antigens (so-called molecular mimicry); rather, this wide-ranging specificity of autoantibodies implicates a fundamental dysregulation of the mechanisms of self-tolerance that affects many different clones of lymphocytes (see Chapter 9).

CASE 5: HUMAN IMMUNODEFICIENCY VIRUS INFECTION AND ACQUIRED IMMUNODEFICIENCY SYNDROME

J.C. was a 28-year-old assistant carpenter with a history of human immunodeficiency virus (HIV) infection who came to the emergency department of his local hospital complaining of difficulty breathing and chills. The patient had a history of intravenous heroin abuse, with an admission to the same hospital 7 years earlier because of a drug overdose. At that time he had tested positive for both anti-HIV and anti-hepatitis B virus antibodies by enzyme-linked immunosorbent assay (ELISA). On discharge from the hospital, he was referred to an HIV clinic, where Western blot testing confirmed the presence of anti-HIV antibodies. A reverse transcriptase PCR test for viral RNA in the blood revealed 15,000 copies/mL of viral genome. His CD4+ T cell count was 800/mm^3 (normal, 500 to 1500/mm^3). There was no evidence of opportunistic infections at that time.

1. What major risk factor did this patient have for acquiring HIV infection? What are other risk factors for HIV infection?

J.C. began taking anti-HIV medications including two nucleoside reverse transcriptase inhibitors and one viral protease inhibitor. He also attended a drug abuse rehabilitation program (and has not used illegal drugs since the time of his overdose). He became steadily employed and acquired health insurance benefits. After a year of his triple-drug therapy, J.C.'s CD4+ T cell count remained about 800/mm^3, and a viral load test indicated less than 100 copies/mL. Over the next 5 years, however, his CD4+ T cell count gradually declined to 300/mm^3. He assured his doctors that he rarely missed a dose of his medication, which was changed to different reverse transcriptase inhibitors three times, and a different protease inhibitor once, in an attempt to stop the

decline in his CD4+ count. He felt well and was able to work regularly, with the only sign of his HIV disease being multiple enlarged lymph nodes. He was started on antibiotic prophylaxis for *Pneumocystis jiroveci* pneumonia 3 years after his initial diagnosis.

2. What caused the gradual decline in the CD4+ T cell count?

After 6 years from the time of initial diagnosis, J.C. began to lose weight. At a clinic visit around this time, he complained of a sore throat and had white plaque lesions in his mouth. Flow cytometry indicated a CD4+ count of 64/mm^3 (Fig. A-6), and the viral load was more than 500,000 copies/mL. A diagnosis of acquired immunodeficiency syndrome (AIDS) was made.

3. What is the likely reason for why the anti-HIV drugs given to this patient became ineffective over time?

Six months later, the patient came to the emergency department with a temperature of 39°C (102.2°F), blood pressure of 160/55 mm Hg, and shallow respirations, with a respiratory rate of 40 breaths per minute. He had lost 10 kg of body weight since his last clinic visit. Several red skin nodules were present on the patient's chest and arms. A chest radiograph showed a diffuse pneumonia. Intravenous antibiotics were administered for presumed *Pneumocystis jiroveci* pneumonia, and the patient was admitted to the infectious disease service.

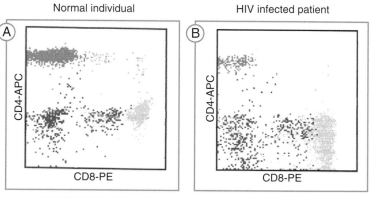

FIGURE A-6　**Flow cytometry analysis of a human immunodeficiency virus (HIV)-infected patient's CD4+ and CD8+ T cells.** A suspension of the patient's white blood cells was incubated with monoclonal antibodies specific for CD4 and CD8. The anti-CD4 antibody was labeled with the fluorochrome allophycocyanin (APC), and the anti-CD8 antibody was labeled with the fluorochrome phycoerythrin (PE). These two fluorochromes emit light of different colors when excited by the appropriate wavelengths. The cell suspensions were analyzed in a flow cytometer, which can enumerate the number of cells stained by each of the differently labeled antibodies. In this way, the number of CD4+ and CD8+ T cells can be determined. Shown here are two-color plots of a control blood sample (**A**) and that of the patient (**B**). The CD4+ T cells are shown in orange *(upper left quadrant)*, and the CD8+ T cells are shown in green *(lower right quadrant)*. (These are not the colors of light emitted by the APC and PE fluorochromes.)

That night, a sputum sample was collected, and the following day, skin biopsy specimens were taken from his chest. Staining of the sputum sample revealed numerous *Pneumocystis jiroveci* organisms. The skin biopsy specimens showed Kaposi's sarcoma. Despite intensive care, the patient's pneumonia progressed, and he died 3 days later.

4. Why are patients with AIDS at high risk for developing opportunistic infections such as *Pneumocystis jiroveci* and malignancies such as Kaposi's sarcoma?

ANSWERS TO QUESTIONS FOR CASE 5

1. Intravenous drug use is the major risk factor for HIV infection in this patient. Shared needles among drug addicts transmit blood-borne viral particles from one infected person to others. Other major risk factors for HIV infection include sexual intercourse with an infected person, transfusion of contaminated blood products, and birth from an infected mother. (See Chapter 12.)

2. After initial infection, the HIV rapidly enters various types of cells in the body, including CD4+ T lymphocytes, dendritic cells, mononuclear phagocytes, and others. Once in an intracellular location, the virus is safe from antibody neutralization. The gradual decline in CD4+ T cells in this patient was caused by repetitive cycles of HIV infection and death of CD4+ T cells in lymphoid organs. The symptoms of AIDS do not usually occur until the blood count of CD4+ T cells is below 200/mm^3, reflecting a severe depletion of T cells in the lymphoid organs. (See Chapter 12.)

3. HIV has a very high mutation rate. Mutations in the reverse transcriptase gene that render the enzyme resistant to nucleoside inhibitors occur frequently in patients receiving these drugs. Resistance to protease inhibitors may come about by similar mechanisms.

4. The deficiencies in T cell–mediated immunity in patients with AIDS lead to impaired immunity to viruses, fungi, and protozoa, which otherwise are easily controlled by normal immune system. *Pneumocystis jiroveci* is a fungal organism and usually is eradicated by the action of activated CD4+ T cells. Many of the malignancies that are frequent in patients with AIDS are associated with oncogenic viruses. For example, Kaposi's sarcoma is associated with human herpesvirus 8 infection. Many of the lymphomas that occur in patients with AIDS are associated with the Epstein-Barr virus, and many of the skin and cervical carcinomas that occur in these patients are associated with human papillomavirus.

INDEX

AP-1 (activating protein-1), 100f, 101, 136f
APC. *See* Antigen-presenting cells
Apoptosis, 21
  of B lymphocytes in central tolerance, 181, 181f
  and decline of immune response, 110
  definitions of, 247, 265
  of immature lymphocytes, 79, 85, 85f
  of T lymphocytes
    in central tolerance, 174–176, 175f, 176f
    in peripheral tolerance, 176, 179f, 179–181
Arachidonic acid in immediate hypersensitivity reactions, 209, 211f
Arteriosclerosis, graft, 200, 253, 286
Arthritis, rheumatoid, 96, 219f, 266
  as autoimmune disease, 184f
  definition of, 266
Arthus reaction, 217, 217f, 247
Asthma, 248
  clinical case on, 286–288, 287f
  in immediate hypersensitivity, 206, 212, 212f
    treatment of, 212, 213f
    triggering factors in, 212
Ataxia-telangiectasia, 230
Atopy, 247
  asthma in, 286, 287, 288
  and immediate hypersensitivity, 206–212
Autoantibody, 213, 247
  in lupus erythematosus, 289
Autocrine actions of cytokines, 38
Autoimmune diseases, 173, 182–187, 205, 216f, 247
  genetic factors in, 182–185, 183f, 184f, 185f, 187
  infections as triggering factor in, 182, 183f, 185–187
  lupus erythematosus in, 288–289
Autoimmune lymphoproliferative syndrome (ALPS), 180
Autoimmune polyendocrine syndrome, 175, 185f
Autoimmune regulator (AIRE), 175, 185f, 246
Autologous grafts, 247
Avidity, 72, 86, 247

B

B-1 B lymphocytes, 36, 84, 133, 133f
  definition of, 247–248
  as IgA source, 144, 167

B7 costimulators, 42f, 137
  B7-1 (CD80), 95, 280
  B7-2 (CD86), 95, 281
  in cancer immunotherapy, 195f, 196
  in T cell activation, 95, 96, 101, 137
    and anergy, 176–177
  as therapy target, 96
B lymphocyte(s), 8, 9, 10f, 21
  activation of, 20, 42f, 132–150
    and anergy, 182, 182f
    complement system in, 135–137, 137f, 162
    congenital disorders of, 229
    functional consequences of, 137–138, 138f
    helper T cells in, 133, 137–147
    mechanisms in, 140–141, 141f
    regulation of, 149f, 149–150
    signals in, 72–74, 135, 136f, 150
  anergy of, 182, 182f
  antibodies produced by, 4, 8, 17, 20–21, 64, 72, 86, 132
  and antibody isotypes, 72, 73f
    in heavy chain class switching, 141–144
  antigen presentation to, 13
    by follicular dendritic cells, 64
  in antigen presentation to helper T cells, 140, 140f
  antigen recognition, 13, 45, 46, 64, 65, 68, 76, 77f
    effector functions in, 10f
    phases of humoral immune response in, 132, 132f
    proliferation and differentiation in, 10f, 12f, 42f
    stimulation of humoral immune response in, 135–138
  apoptosis in central tolerance, 181, 181f
  clones of, 67, 132, 137
  compared to T cells, 4
  congenital disorders of, 224, 224f, 225f, 226f, 227
  definition of, 247
  effector functions, 10f, 12f, 13, 17, 21, 132
  follicular, 19, 36, 64, 84, 133, 133f, 150
    high-affinity, 144–145, 146f
  in humoral immunity, 4, 8, 20, 45, 50, 64, 131–150
    activation process, 42f, 72–74, 132–137
    functions of, 5f, 9f
    interaction with helper T cells, 137–147
  immature, 83f, 84, 255

B lymphocyte(s) *(Continued)*
  in innate immune response, 36
  interaction with helper T cells, 14, 16, 20, 62, 133, 137–147
    mechanisms of B cell activation in, 140–141, 141f
  in lymph nodes, 18, 64
    in lymphoma, 283–284
    segregation from T cells, 14f, 15, 16f
  marginal zone, 36, 84, 133, 133f, 148–149
    definition of, 261
  maturation of, 9, 11f, 76–79, 83–84
    congenital defects in, 224, 225, 225f, 227
    recombination and diversity in, 79–83
    steps in, 76–77, 78f, 83f
  mature, 83f, 84, 261
  memory cells, 12f, 134f, 147, 147f, 154
  migration of, 150
    toward T cells, 139, 139f
  naive, 12f, 131
    antigen receptors of, 135
  pre-B cells, 83, 83f, 264–265
  pro-B cells, 83, 83f, 265
  proliferation and differentiation of, 137, 146, 147f
    antigen recognition by, 10f, 12f, 42f
    and maturation, 77–78, 78f
  recirculation of, 11f
  repertoire of, 84
  specificity of, 68
  stimulation of, 135–138, 154
  subsets of, 133, 133f
  tolerance in, 181–182
    central, 181, 181f, 187
    peripheral, 181–182, 182f, 187
  in transplantation response, 200
B lymphocyte receptor, 8, 20, 45, 64, 67–70
  compared to T cell receptor, 76, 77f
  diversity of, 79–83
  and pre-B cell receptor, 83–84
  receptor editing process, 84
B lymphocyte receptor complex, 70, 135, 247
Bacteria
  encapsulated, 157
  evasion of humoral immunity, 168, 168f
  extracellular, 40
    antibody-mediated phagocytosis of, 156–157, 158f
  innate immune response to, 24, 26, 27f, 40
    toll-like receptors in, 26, 43

Cytotoxic T lymphocyte-associated protein
4 (CTLA-4, CD152), 93f, 97, 282
in cancer immunotherapy, 196
and immunosuppressive therapy, 202f
in T lymphocyte anergy, 176–177,
177f
Cytotoxic T lymphocytes (CTLs), 11, 21
activation of, 98, 125f, 125–126
in adaptive immune response, 9, 10f,
18, 46
antigen recognition, 10f, 50, 124–125
CD8+ cells as, 11, 20, 62, 63f
clonal expansion of, 104
definition of, 250
differentiation of, 109, 111, 125
effector functions, 9f, 10f, 12f, 109,
124–126, 125f
in HIV infection, 98, 236
in hypersensitivity reactions, 218, 218f
in intracellular antigen response, 9, 20,
46, 50, 113–114, 114f
mechanism of actions, 124–126, 125f
and natural killer cells, 34, 35–36
in transplant rejection, 199
in tumor response, 191f, 192f, 192–194,
203
and immunotherapy, 194

D

Death receptors in activation-induced cell
death, 179f, 179–180
Decay-accelerating factor, 164–165, 165t,
166f
Decline of immune response, 7, 21, 110,
149
Defensins, 250
Delayed-type hypersensitivity, 119, 121f,
123, 219
compared to other hypersensitivity
reactions, 207f
in contact sensitivity, 249–250
definition of, 250
mechanisms of tissue injury in, 218,
218f
in transplantation, 199
δ chains, of T cell receptor, 28, 72, 94
Dementia in HIV infection, 236
Dendritic cells, 9f, 13, 32
activation of, 48
as antigen-presenting cells, 9f, 13,
47–51
capture and display of microbial
antigens, 19, 47–51
and CD4+ T cells, 50
and CD8+ T cells, 50

Dendritic cells, follicular (*Continued*)
costimulator expression stimulating
adaptive immune response, 41, 42f
cytokine production, 32, 38, 39f, 41,
42f
definition of, 250
in epithelium, 13, 19, 47–48, 48f
follicular, 9f, 13, 15
in affinity maturation, 145
antigen display to B cells, 64
definition of, 253
in HIV infection, 235
immature, 48, 48f
in innate immunity, 32, 43
in lymph nodes, 14, 48–49
maturation of, 48, 49f
migration of, 48, 49f
in spleen, 15
subsets of, 50
in tumor therapy, 194
Desensitization, 212, 213f, 250
Determinant portion of antigen, 20
definitions of, 250, 252
immunodominant, 58, 75, 256
spreading phenomenon, 219
Diabetes mellitus, 184f, 219f, 257
DiGeorge syndrome, 225f, 226f, 227, 237,
250–251
Diphtheria, 2f, 156
Direct antigen presentation, 198–199,
199f, 251
Diversity
of antigen receptors, 76, 78, 79–83
combinatorial, 79–80, 82f, 249
junctional, 79–80, 82f, 83, 259
mechanisms in, 82f
definitions of, 251, 259
Diversity gene segments, 79–83, 82f, 87,
251
DM (HLA-DM), 57, 254
DNA recombinant technology, 74
DNA vaccine, 169f, 251
Donor of graft, 196
Double-negative T cells, 84, 85, 85f, 251
Double-positive T cells, 85, 85f, 86, 251
DP genes, 53
DQ genes, 53
DR genes, 53

E

Effector cells, 9f, 11, 12f, 13
B lymphocyte, 10f, 12f, 13, 17, 21, 132
definition of, 251
granulocyte, 9f, 13
macrophage, 9f, 13

Effector cells (*Continued*)
migration of, 16–17, 17f
to sites of infection, 95, 114–119,
117f, 128
T lymphocyte, 12f, 13, 17–18, 20, 21,
113–129
CD4+ helper cells, 119–124
CD8+ cytotoxic cells, 124–126
differentiation of naive cells into,
90–91, 91f, 92, 104–109, 116
in eradication of intracellular
microbes, 113–129
microbe resistance to, 126–128
migration to sites of infection, 95,
114–119, 117f, 128
time of response, 3f
types of, 9f, 10f
Endocytosis, 140, 140f
Endoplasmic reticulum (ER)
synthesis of MHC molecules in, 57, 58f,
59, 60f
transporter associated with antigen
processing in, 59, 61f
Endosomes, 57, 251
Endothelial cells
adhesion molecules on, 30, 31, 116
chemokines and, 30, 31, 39f, 116
cytokine effects on, 38, 39f, 116
delayed type hypersensitivity reaction
and, 121
leukocyte adhesion to, 30–31
T cell migration and, 115f, 116, 117f,
118f
Toll like receptor expression by, 26,
27f
Endotoxin, 156
definitions of, 251, 260
phagocyte receptors for, 24
second signal induced by, 64
Endotoxin shock, 38, 267
Envelope glycoprotein, 251
gp120, 168
in HIV infection, 231, 232f, 233f,
236, 237
Environmental factors in autoimmune
disorders, 182, 183, 183f, 185–187
Enzyme-linked immunosorbent assay, 251
Eosinophils
definition of, 251–252
in helminth infections, 104, 107, 108f,
123, 141, 158–159, 212
in immediate hypersensitivity, 210
Epithelium
antigen-presenting cells in, 13
barrier function in innate immunity, 3,
3f, 18, 28, 28f, 43